Calderwood's
Orthopedic nursing

SIXTH EDITION

Calderwood's Orthopedic nursing

CARROLL B. LARSON, M.D., F.A.C.S.

Professor of Orthopedic Surgery and Chairman of the Department of Orthopedic Surgery, State University of Iowa, Iowa City, Iowa

MARJORIE GOULD, R.N., B.S., M.S.

Supervisor of Orthopedic Nursing, State University of Iowa, Iowa City, Iowa; formerly Instructor, Advanced Orthopedic Nursing, Boston University, Boston, Mass.

With 359 figures

THE C. V. MOSBY COMPANY

Saint Louis 1965

Preface to sixth edition

Innovations in medical therapy, such as intensive care units, pneumatic mattresses, and devices for lifting patients; the gradual disappearance of poliomyelitis and bone tuberculosis; and an increased interest in rheumatoid arthritis and rehabilitation of amputees are only a few of the reasons why orthopedic nursing texts need revision to keep abreast of the times. Teachers of orthopedic nursing have responded to requests for suggestions of revision that would improve the scope, simplicity, and usefulness of this book in their teaching programs.

In the revision of this book, we have added what is new in orthopedic nursing and deleted the obsolete; expanded the important areas in depth; remained comprehensive in coverage of the art as well as in the science of orthopedic nursing; and rearranged the material for easy reference.

Numerous new illustrations have been included to clarify many discussions; preventive nursing is stressed throughout; and the discussions on arthritis, amputation surgery, rehabilitation of the amputee, and blood transfusions have been enlarged. The discussions on poliomyelitis and bone tuberculosis have been shortened, and the references following each chapter have been updated.

We are grateful to the teachers of orthopedic nursing for their helpful suggestions, to Dr. Howard Hogshead for the material on amputees, to Dr. Merlin P. Strottmann for the material on rheumatoid arthritis, and to Dr. Elmer DeGowin for his elaboration on blood transfusions. In addition, we acknowledge the assistance of those others who have provided illustrations and helpful criticism.

C. L.
M. G.

v

Preface to first edition

This textbook on orthopedic nursing is presented in an attempt to bring together in one volume the background of medical information and nursing techniques necessary to assist the nurse in caring for the orthopedic patient. It is not intended to be encyclopedic, and the lesser known entities have been passed over briefly or omitted entirely where the judgment of the authors considered it permissible. The book is not, of course, intended to take the place of a comprehensive reference text on the subject of orthopedic surgery.

Principles remain constant, only techniques vary. Recognizing this, the authors have sought to place emphasis upon established principles of knowledge and procedure, realizing that such variations as occur in different parts of the country are so manifold that no textbook of this size could take cognizance of all of them. With the foundation in principle well laid, it was thought that the student's own natural ability to adapt to various life situations could be counted upon. The adjustability aim of the *Curriculum Guide* clearly supported our thinking in this matter.

Gratitude is due to the members of the Joint Orthopedic Nursing Advisory Service, and in particular to Jessie L. Stevenson, without whose invaluable assistance the material herein would have been less comprehensive.

Acknowledgement is likewise due to the students, the head nurses, and the faculty of Denver Children's Hospital and the University of Virginia Hospital for suggestions and assistance which they gave in working out many difficult nursing problems.

R. F.
C. C.

Contents

Calderwood's
Orthopedic nursing

Chapter 1

Introduction for the teacher and the student

Principles of nursing care applied to the orthopedic patient

Orthopedic nursing has been defined as the application of the principles of body mechanics to all nursing. If this is true, no textbook on the subject can rightfully be without a discussion of the elementary principles of body mechanics and their application to all nursing.

In the past the principles of proper body mechanics and body alignment have been referred to as the orthopedic aspects of nursing care. This assumption is questionable, and perhaps it is presumptuous to allocate to one medical specialty the principles which, like cleanliness and adequate nutrition, belong to all branches of healing. It is far better to think of these principles as being fundamental to the care of every patient, and as such they are principles of good nursing care. However, there is little doubt that in the clinical specialty of orthopedics more emphasis is placed on this subject than in any other branch of medicine or nursing. It seems logical, therefore, to begin a textbook of orthopedic nursing with a discussion of the fundamental principles upon which the

prevention, as well as the treatment, of orthopedic conditions is based.

The definition given—that orthopedic nursing is the application of the principles of body mechanics to all nursing—sometimes presents an unfamiliar concept to nurses working in highly specialized orthopedic services in hospitals. Analysis of any equipment or apparatus used in the care of the orthopedic patient, however, will reveal that its fundamental purpose is the maintenance or restoration of proper body mechanics. Student nurses have often looked askance at a sharply angulated turnbuckle cast, puzzled by the abnormal position of the patient in the cast. It seems to be the very reverse of good body mechanics! Nevertheless, the overcorrected position that the cast maintains is one step toward recovery of a normal spine, and it may be impossible to apply the principles of body mechanics to the patient until a period of overcorrection has been maintained.

In the past those of us in orthopedic nursing were absorbed almost entirely in the care of patients with affections of the musculoskeletal system. Indeed, we who were teaching the subject to student nurses often prefaced our lectures with a definition of orthopedic nursing as the care of patients with disease or dysfunctions of the musculoskeletal system. There was little carry-over of our knowledge of orthopedic nursing to patients in other divisions of the hospital. For instance, little attention was given to the musculoskeletal system of the patient on the medical or surgical ward. All too often a patient recovering from a cerebral accident and hemiplegia was allowed to lie in an unphysiologic position that contributed to a condition of permanent deformity. It must be admitted, however, that the same oversight occurred on orthopedic wards. Not infrequently, patients with osteomyelitis developed flexion contractures in uninvolved joints, such as the hip or knee, from long-continued positions of flexion. Furthermore, it was not uncommon to have patients who had lain on Bradford frames over a period of months develop drop foot because no support had been provided for the feet on the frame. Certainly, it is lamentable to be so absorbed in the care of a patient with an existing deformity that one fails to see the forces at work to bring about other deformities, but in the past we were often guilty of the oversight.

Sir Robert Jones spoke very truly when he said: "It can never be realized too widely that deformity is an unnatural and preventable affliction, which treatment may alleviate or cure, but which a more complete understanding could abolish."* At the present time it is most heartening to see that nursing educators are emphasizing a more complete understanding of the causes and prevention of crippling. Nursing instructors, clinical instructors, and teachers of the sciences are striving to overcome the old specialistic tendencies of nurses by including the principles of body mechanics in the subject matter they teach. One has only to read the more recent nursing textbooks on clinical subjects to see how well these principles have been integrated into all branches of nursing. It seems altogether unlikely that they will ever be forgotten or overlooked again. Nevertheless, the subject will bear "enormous repetition, representation and illustration in all possible forms."* It is, in fact, scarcely possible to overemphasize the need for proper alignment and the importance of recognizing the limitations of joint motion in all phases of nursing activity.

POSTURE AND BODY MECHANICS

Student nurses who are given the benefit of an initial posture analysis by an orthopedic specialist early in their careers are fortunate. They are still more fortunate if their postural weaknesses can be pointed out to them in the presence of someone equipped to help them overcome these weaknesses, such as an instructor in physical education, if there is one on the faculty, or perhaps the hospital physical therapist. The advice the orthopedist gives the student can be interpreted to her by the physical education teacher, who will be able to follow her progress later both in the classroom and on the wards. Corrective exercises, if prescribed, will often bring about noteworthy improvements in the student's posture if she understands their purpose, is adequately supervised in their performance, and is faithful in the practice of them. It is indispensable that

---

*Jones, Sir Robert: Notes on military orthopedics, London, 1917, Cassell & Co., Ltd.

*Holmes, Oliver Wendell: Medical essays: scholastic and bedside teaching, Boston, 1892, Houghton Mifflin Co.

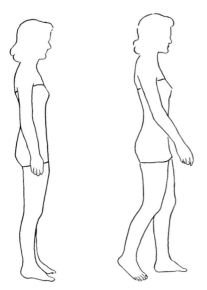
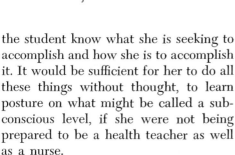

Fig. 1. Good standing and walking posture. Note position of the head, normal curves of the spine, the flat abdomen, and relaxed position of the knee joints.

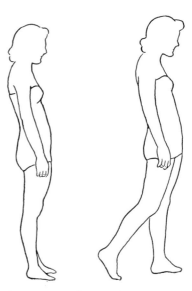

Fig. 2. Poor standing and walking posture. Note forward position of the head, rounded shoulders, increased lumbar lordosis, flat chest, protruding abdomen, and hyperextended knees.

the student know what she is seeking to accomplish and how she is to accomplish it. It would be sufficient for her to do all these things without thought, to learn posture on what might be called a subconscious level, if she were not being prepared to be a health teacher as well as a nurse.

It is important, too, that every nurse know how to select a shoe for duty wear, so that she may purchase shoes intelligently, undisturbed by the rhetoric of the shoe salesman. The characteristics of a good shoe and the proper fitting of the shoe should be so well known to her that she will not be confused by imposing trade names, fancy prices, or an engaging array of built-in gadgets.

We know that learning is not conceded to be effective until behavior is altered in some way because of it. Probably no nurse completes her nursing course today without being able to recite the points a plumb line should pass through

for proper body stance. No doubt most of them will be able to write for the state board examination, if it is required of them, some of the criteria of good posture: that the sternum should be the most forward portion of the body, that the head is to be held up and the chin in, that the lower abdomen should be flat and retracted, that the curves of the spine should be maintained without exaggeration, that the knees should be in a relaxed position (not hyperextended), and that the feet should point straight ahead. However, the nurse is probably capable of writing these gems of wisdom with feet wrapped tightly around the chair rungs, chin glued to a caved-in sternum, and a back round as a barrel hoop.

Whether or not the student can interpret good posture to herself in a kinesthetic sense is conjectural. Secretly she may still be convinced that slouchy posture is easier and more comfortable for her and that good posture is a posi-

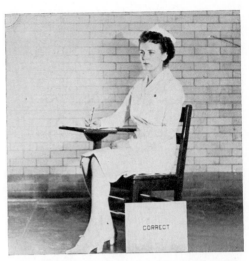

Fig. 4. Good sitting posture. (From Stevenson, Jessie L.: Posture and nursing, ed. 2, New York, 1948, Joint Orthopedic Nursing Advisory Service.)

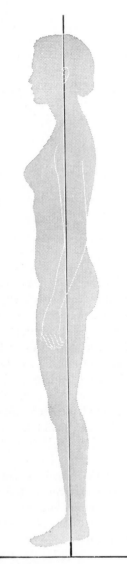

Fig. 3. The points a plumb line should pass through for proper body stance. To check correct posture hang a weighted cord so that it falls down the center of a long mirror, and stand sideways to the mirror. The cord should pass through the ear, shoulder joint, hip joint, slightly behind the patella, and reach the floor just anterior to the external malleolus.

tion leading to fatigue and strain. Since she has only theoretic knowledge—with which her own experience is perhaps not in accord—it is questionable that she will be able to describe good posture in simple language for the benefit of the patient who is rising from bed after long recumbency. Even if she can do this, there is still the question of whether she will be able to confidently accompany her verbal description with a graphic example by reference to her own body alignment, and unless she can do this her knowledge remains academic. If she herself does not understand the necessity for good posture and does not apply it to her everyday living, she will hardly be able to transmit her knowledge to others in a vitally effective manner, and she will not be able to present a convincing object lesson in her own activities.

The cosmetic appeal for good posture probably does as much as any other factor to motivate the student. Most young women can be approached through this channel. Because the stu-

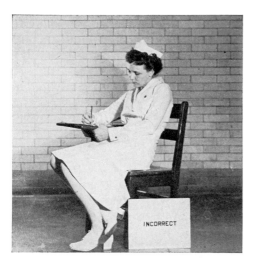

Fig. 5. Poor sitting posture. (From Stevenson, Jessie L.: Posture and nursing, ed. 2, New York, 1948, Joint Orthopedic Nursing Advisory Service.)

dent nurse is young and resilient, she seldom feels the result of the day's mechanical misuse of her body—certainly not seriously enough to keep her from dancing half the night in shoes with four-inch heels. It is difficult, if not impossible, to project her imagination forward to the day when the aches of approaching middle age will be upon her. Most students, however, are tremendously interested in their waistlines. Their hips are a constant source of speculative consideration as they rip the cellophane off a candy bar, and any exercises given for the reduction of this particular anatomic overload usually bring about some definite display of interest and earnestness. The young student firmly intends to carry out her exercises faithfully morning and evening. If she has the hardihood to do it, so much the better for her; but persistence in this endeavor is in the lap of the gods. Meanwhile, a concept of posture is being built upon a realization of the cosmetic benefit that results from her occasional tensing of the abdominal muscles and

contracting the gluteal muscles. She has only to look in the mirror to observe the effects. This may be the beginning of an attempt to create a more efficient set of corset muscles that will be helpful to her in many activities associated with the care of patients, although it must be admitted that this will probably not be her first consideration in acquiring them. Nevertheless, the first step is an important one.

Over fifty years ago physical educators and doctors interested in problems of the lower portion of the back were pointing out the importance of the trunk muscles in strenuous activity. The rectus abdominis muscle, the obliquus abdominis muscles, and the gluteus muscles were spoken of as an inner girdle that surrounded and supported the underlying pelvic structures. When this group of muscles was in good tone the likelihood of strain in the normal back became much lessened. Adequately developed trunk muscles made possible many feats of physical activity that otherwise could not be undertaken without possible inefficiency and strain. It is now well recognized that a soft flabby middle section of the body is a liability to anyone engaged in active physical work. A nurse should learn early to use the internal girdle that is her own, whether or not she elects to wear an external one.

Practice of nursing procedures can easily include concurrent practice in correct body mechanics. Once the student has learned to carry out procedures using correct body mechanics, it becomes a conditioned skill that she will be likely to carry with her into similar situations on the ward. The carry-over to the patient will not be automatic. The situation facing the beginning student is very complex, and there are many things for her to remember in the early days on the ward. She will need guided instruction. None of this material on body mechanics can be given in one gigantic dose; it must be given in suitable small doses and repeated often. That is why it is so important for all teaching personnel, supervisors, head nurses, and staff nurses who will come in contact with the student to be well-grounded in the subject and convinced of its importance.

It is not the purpose of this book to consider the subject of body mechanics in detail. Many excellent books and articles are now available for the student or teacher who wishes to make a study of the subject. Only a few simple suggestions for the student's guidance will be included here. Analysis and discussion of these suggestions might be included in the student's course in anatomy and physiology in the section on the erect and moving body.

1. In bending to retrieve an article

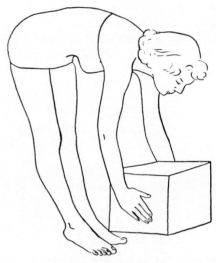

Fig. 7. Incorrect position for working at lower levels. Note parallel feet and hyperextended knees. Working or lifting in this position places strain on the back muscles.

from the floor, to lift, or to bathe a patient in a low bathtub, flex both knees and hips, keep the back straight and the shoulders in the same plane as the pelvis, keep the feet apart, and assume the foot-forward position. Do not bend at the hips with the knees straight or with the back rounded, for this will put the strain of any lifting on the back (where the muscles of extension are relatively inefficient) rather than on the stronger, more massive muscles of the thighs and buttocks. Avoid rotatory movements of the spine in lifting, and never lift an impossible load in an attempt to keep from asking for help. Avoid lateral twisting movements when reaching for objects above the head or out at the side.

2. Prepare for strenuous activity when it is required by setting the pelvis, i.e., by retracting the abdominal muscles and contracting the gluteal muscles. ("Up in front, down in back" and "Pull and pinch" are instructions sometimes used to give this concept to the student.)

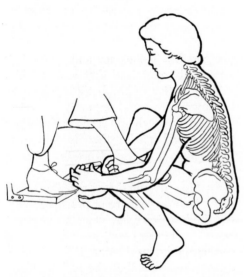

Fig. 6. Correct position for working at a lower level. Note flexed position of the hips and knees, the foot-forward position, and the placement of shoulders in the same plane as the pelvis. (Courtesy National Advisory Service for Orthopedics and Poliomyelitis, and Alfred Feinberg, artist, College of Physicians and Surgeons, Columbia University.)

3. Carry heavy burdens close to the body.

4. When moving a patient in the bed, avoid lifting or pushing movements if possible. Stand on the side toward which the patient is to be moved and exert the pull toward your own body.

5. Sit with hips well back in the chair, the ischia and thighs bearing the weight, the feet flat on the floor, and the trunk

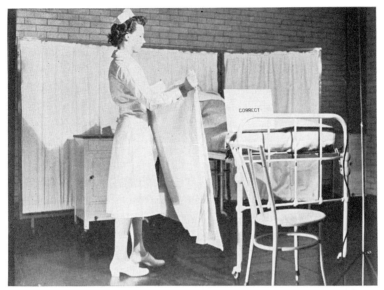

Fig. 8. Position of ease in removing linen from bed. (From Stevenson, Jessie L.: Posture and nursing, ed. 2, New York, 1948, Joint Orthopedic Nursing Advisory Service.)

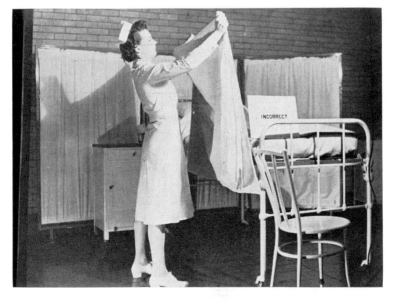

Fig. 9. Position of strain in removing linen from bed. (From Stevenson, Jessie L.: Posture and nursing, ed. 2, New York, 1948, Joint Orthopedic Nursing Advisory Service.)

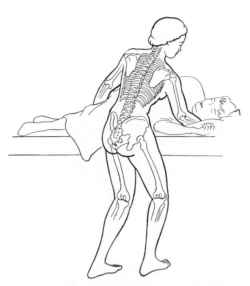

Fig. 10. When working at the bedside, assume the foot-forward position, face your work, flex knees and hips slightly, and maintain the shoulders in same plane as the pelvis. Protect the small muscles of the back while making the large muscles of the thigh work. (Courtesy National Advisory Service for Orthopedics and Poliomyelitis, and Alfred Feinberg, artist, College of Physicians and Surgeons, Columbia University.)

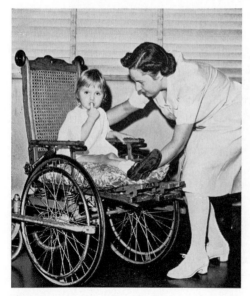

Fig. 11. Correct position for lifting.

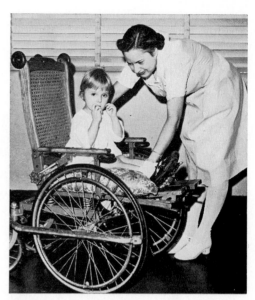

Fig. 12. Incorrect position for lifting. Note hyperextended knees.

in the same position assumed in standing.

6. When lying in bed approximate standing posture horizontally as nearly as possible. If lying on the back, avoid multiple pillows under the head, for they will depress the chest and force the chin forward. Pillows should support the spine and the shoulders as well as the head. Support to the feet should be provided to prevent drop foot and pressure on the toes from bedclothes. If lying face downward, provide relaxation and comfort for the spinal muscles by a flat pillow extending from the lower border of the ribs to the pelvis. While lying in this position, support the feet by a pillow placed under the lower leg or allow them to hang over the edge of the mattress.

FUNDAMENTAL JOINT MOTIONS

It is desirable for the beginning student nurse to learn to use certain anatomic terms having to do with the position of the body. These words have sometimes been erroneously referred to

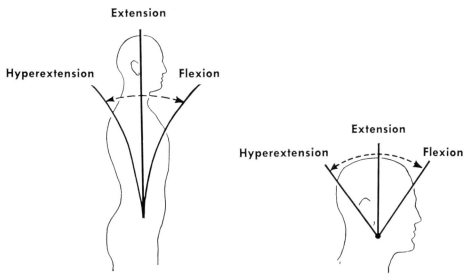

Fig. 13. Flexion, extension, and hyperextension of the spine.

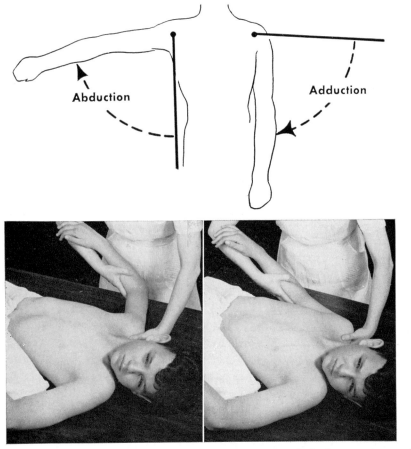

Fig. 14. Abduction and adduction of the shoulder joint. Note method of supporting paralyzed arm. (Photographs courtesy Iowa State Services for Crippled Children.)

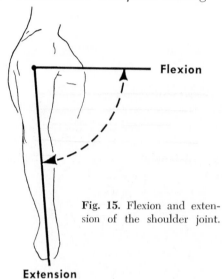

Flexion

Extension

Fig. 15. Flexion and extension of the shoulder joint.

as part of an orthopedic vocabulary, but the student first learns them in anatomy and should carry them from that course to the study of nursing. They should be familiar to her long before she has seen an orthopedic patient. The joint motions illustrated in Figs. 13 to 24 are almost indispensable for understanding the simplest and most fundamental body mechanics of the bed patient. Many others will be learned, but it is urged that these, at least, become part of the working vocabulary of every nurse.

Text continued on p. 16.

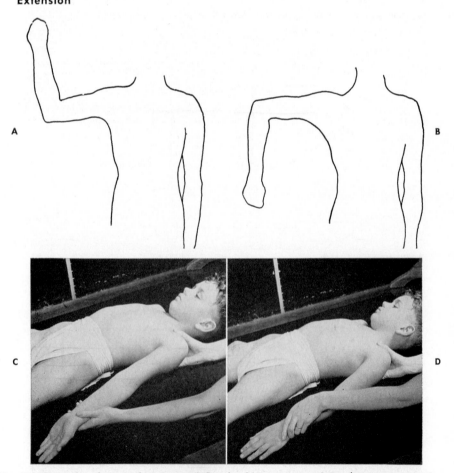

Fig. 16. External and internal rotation of the shoulder joint. A, Abduction with external rotation. B, Abduction with internal rotation. C, Adduction with external rotation. D, Adduction with internal rotation. (Photographs courtesy Iowa State Services for Crippled Children.)

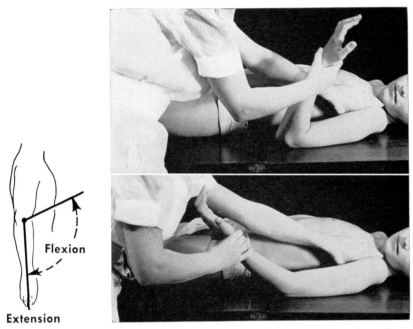

Fig. 17. Flexion and extension of the elbow. (Photographs courtesy Iowa State Services for Crippled Children.)

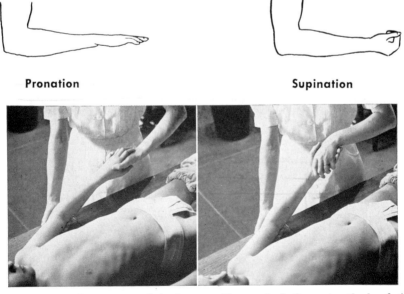

Fig. 18. Pronation and supination of the forearm. Note method of grasping the hand. (Photographs courtesy Iowa State Services for Crippled Children.)

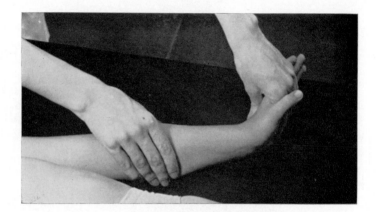

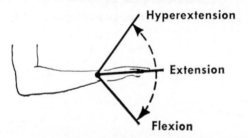

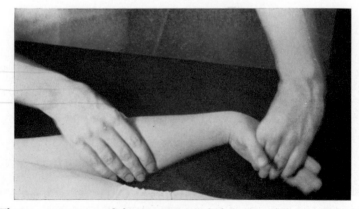

Fig. 19. Flexion, extension, and hyperextension of the wrist. (Photographs courtesy Iowa State Services for Crippled Children.)

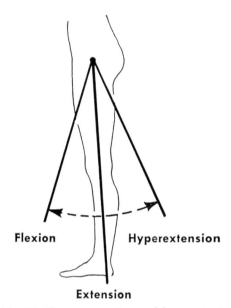

Fig. 20. Flexion, extension, and hyperextension of the hip.

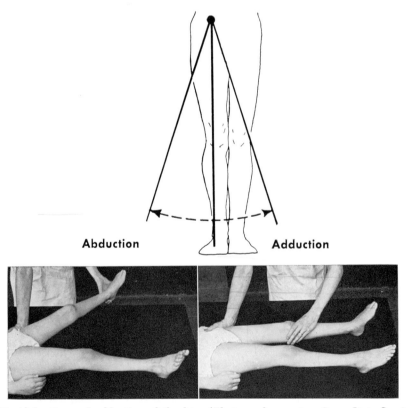

Fig. 21. Abduction and adduction of the hip. (Photographs courtesy Iowa State Services for Crippled Children.)

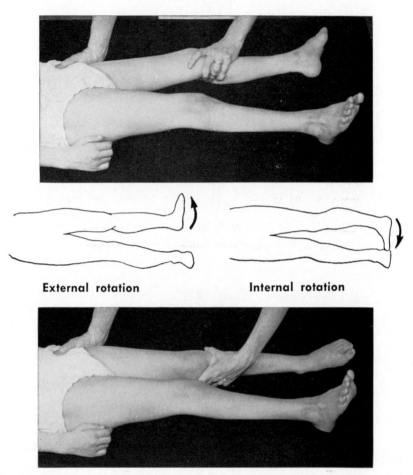

External rotation   **Internal rotation**

Fig. 22. External and internal rotation of the hip. (Photographs courtesy Iowa State Services for Crippled Children.)

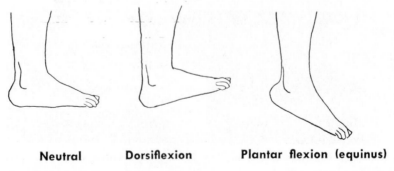

Neutral   **Dorsiflexion**   **Plantar flexion (equinus)**

Fig. 23. Dorsiflexion and plantar flexion of the foot.

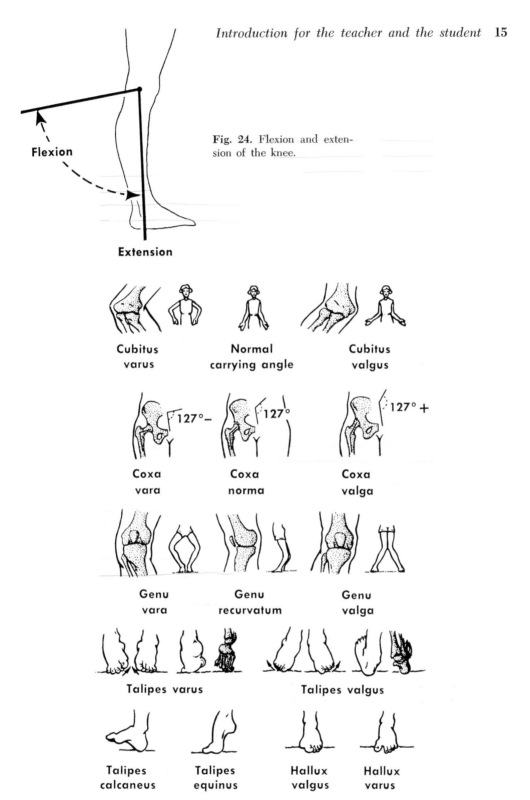

Flexion

Extension

Fig. 24. Flexion and extension of the knee.

Cubitus
varus

Normal
carrying angle

Cubitus
valgus

Coxa
vara

Coxa
norma

Coxa
valga

Genu
vara

Genu
recurvatum

Genu
valga

Talipes varus

Talipes valgus

Talipes
calcaneus

Talipes
equinus

Hallux
valgus

Hallux
varus

Fig. 25. Common orthopedic deformities. (From Manual of Orthopaedic Surgery, American Orthopaedic Association, 1960.)

BODY ALIGNMENT FOR
THE BED PATIENT

To prevent deformities the nursing care of the patient confined to bed must include maintenance of proper body alignment plus frequent change of position. Unaffected joints should be taken through a full range of motion at least once daily. The inactive patient, whether confined to bed or wheelchair, is prone to develop joint contractures and deformities in a relatively short time. Figs. 26-33 illustrate good and bad body alignment that is of special importance for the patient with muscle weakness or paralysis.

Supine position. Fig. 26 illustrates a poor back-lying position. Note the equinus position of the feet and the external rotation of the lower extremities. The left limb is externally rotated, and the knee and hip joints are held in a flexed position. The adducted position of the arms and the forward position of the head with the chin on the sternum decrease the chest capacity. The wrist drop position, one commonly assumed by the patient with arthritis, places the hand in a poor functional position. If this picture is tilted so that the patient assumes the standing position, one immediately recognizes the poor posture and the possible handicapping deformities.

Fig. 27 illustrates a good back-lying position. The patient is lying on a firm, nonsagging mattress. The footboard holds the covers off the toes and maintains the feet in a walking position midway between dorsiflexion and plantar flexion. The small pillow or bath blanket placed under the calves of the legs lessens the pressure on the heels, a likely spot for decubitus ulcers. This arrangement also provides for a relaxed position of the knee joint and avoids pressure on the popliteal space. The trochanter roll is made by folding a sheet or bath blanket

in thirds lengthwise and in half crosswise. The smooth folded edge is placed under the buttocks of the patient, and the outer end is rolled under firmly against the thigh. This roll assists in maintaining a neutral position of the extremity. The leg is held with the kneecap and toes pointing forward, the position desirable for walking when the patient is ready for ambulation. A small pillow or folded pad placed under the lower portion of the back gives support to the normal lumbar curve. This nursing measure will add considerably to the comfort of the patient forced to lie on his back for indefinite periods.

The arms may be abducted and internally rotated with the forearm supported on a pillow. This position may be changed by placing the abducted arms in a position of external rotation, as illustrated in Fig. 28. The wrist is maintained slightly dorsiflexed in a functional position with the fingers flexed. If the wrist is to become ankylosed, the fingers and hand are more useful when the wrist is fixed in this cock-up position. It should be remembered also that the hand is most useful when the thumb is in a position to oppose the fingers, that is, in a grasping position.

If one pillow is used for the head, it should be placed so that the lower edge is well under the shoulders. This helps to keep the chest forward and avoids flexion of the cervical spine. If three pillows are used, the first pillow must be placed well under the back so that the head and shoulders are supported in proper alignment.

Prone position. When the patient is turned to the face-lying position and no support is placed beneath the ankles, the feet are forced to remain in an equinus position (plantar flexed). Fig. 29 shows a markedly increased hyperextension of the lumbar spine. It is apparent that the patient would be more comfortable with

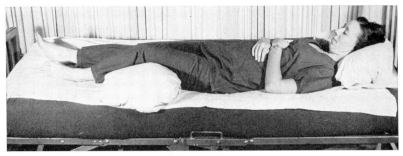

Fig. 26. Poor body alignment in the supine position.

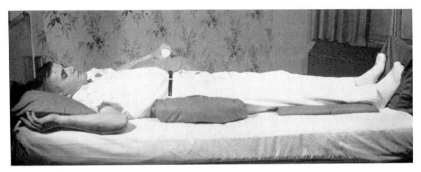

Fig. 27. Good body alignment in the supine position.

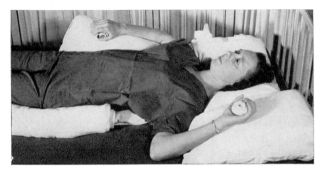

Fig. 28. Positions of rest for the arms. The right arm illustrates a position of abduction with internal rotation. The left arm illustrates a position of abduction with external rotation. Note the position of the wrist and fingers.

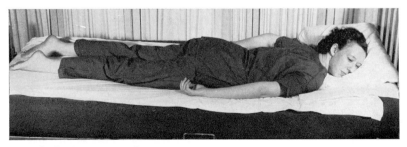

Fig. 29. Poor body alignment in the prone position.

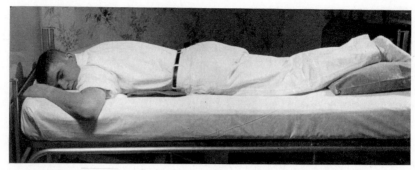

Fig. 30. Good body alignment in the prone position.

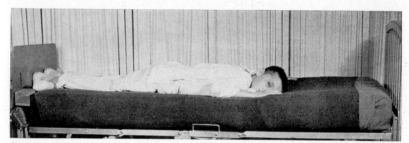

Fig. 31. The footboard with blocks provides a space at the foot of the bed, making it possible for the patient's feet to extend over the end of the mattress.

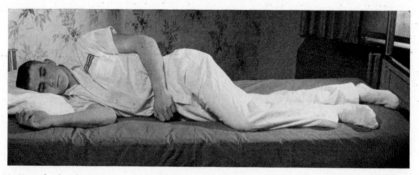

Fig. 32. Poor body alignment in the side-lying position.

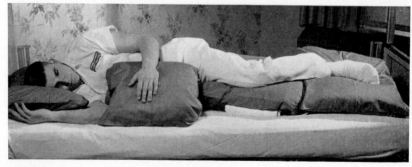

Fig. 33. Good body alignment in the side-lying position.

a support placed beneath the abdomen and with the pillow beneath the head removed. When a patient is in the face-lying position, the pillow beneath the head causes hyperextension of the cervical and lumbar spine.

When the patient is in the prone position, the pillow previously used to support the head may be used to support the feet. This prevents drop foot and also provides for slight flexion of the knee joints. The same result may be obtained by having the feet extend over the edge of the mattress with a small roll placed beneath the ankles. Some persons are more comfortable with a thin pillow beneath the abdomen. This support protects the breasts and prevents an increased lordosis of the lumbar spine. Other patients, however, can be made comfortable without this pillow and still maintain good body alignment. The abducted and externally rotated position of the arms (spread-eagle position) is restful and permits full expansion of the chest. Usually no pillow is needed beneath the head.

Side-lying position. Fig. 32 illustrates a poor side-lying position. Note the adducted position of the uppermost leg and the adducted position of the arm allowing little room for chest expansion.

When the patient is turned to the side-lying position, the uppermost leg should be supported with pillows to prevent an adducted position of the extremity as well as pressure on the lower limb. When the patient is permitted to lie with the leg in adduction, additional strain is placed on the hip joint and the region of the lower back. This is especially bad for the patient who has involvement of the hip joint or back. A pillow is used to support the uppermost arm to avoid pressure on the chest. The wrist and fingers are maintained in a functional position.

POSTURAL PROBLEMS OF THE BED PATIENT

From the study of physiology the student will remember that, in order to move joints, muscles must contract or relax. For maintaining the upright posture, however, they must have a constant slight contracture. This constant slight contracture is called muscle tonus or tone. To maintain the body in a standing position a higher degree of muscle tonus is required than is required for lying in bed. After a day of bed rest one often feels a weakness out of all proportion to the minor illness one has experienced. From this common observation the student can easily understand that when bed rest is continued over a considerable period of time muscle tone may be greatly depleted. Lack of muscle tone, even in healthy subjects, produces wasting of the muscles, often referred to as disuse atrophy. Muscles with diminished tone may become permanently stretched from being held in a lengthened position, or they can become contracted by being held in a shortened position, thus producing so-called myostatic contractures. In terms of the patient's well-being these things may mean a longer convalescence, discomfort on assuming the upright position, and possibly a persistent deformity.

Even two weeks of bed rest in faulty positions may be sufficient to bring about contractures of important muscle groups. When a joint is held in a certain position without change for such a period of time, it has the tendency to stay in that position.

Drop-foot deformity. Of particular significance in nursing is the fact that the tendon of the muscles of the calf tends to shorten if the foot is allowed to rest in an unsupported position, whereas the muscles in the anterior portion of the leg become stretched. Even a mild degree of this muscular imbalance can cause the patient many long weeks of painful concern with his feet.

Conscientious nursing care can do much to eliminate this unnecessary sequela of illness. Adequate support for the feet (including the toes) should be furnished during confinement in bed; exercises to maintain muscle tone (prescribed by the physician) should be intelligently supervised; and a sensible shoe rather than soft scuffs or felt house slippers should be provided when the patient is allowed out of bed.

Knee flexion contractures. Another set of muscles that tend to contract quickly is the hamstring group of the posterior thigh, whose tendons pass under the knee. Flexion of the knees continuously supported by pillows may bring about contractures in that area in a surprisingly short time. The nursing measures to counteract this are quite simple and obvious. Pillows under the knees must be used with caution and with constant awareness that the position of the knees must be altered from flexion to extension at frequent periods during the day and night.

Hip deformities (flexion, adduction, and external rotation). Let us consider the problem of the patient with an acute condition of the abdomen that requires prolonged semisitting in a Gatch bed.

Such a patient may be in danger of flexion contractures of hips and knees as well as of drop foot. If he sits in a slumping position on the lumbar spine with his chest caved in and his shoulders sagging forward, pulled down by the weight of his arms, pain and muscle spasms are likely to occur in the muscles of the back, particularly those muscles which lie between the scapulae. Dr. Jessie Wright, author of *Protective Body Mechanics in Convalescence*, tells us that the muscles most likely to lose tone in this position are the abdominal muscles, the gluteal muscles, the quadriceps muscles, the tibial muscles, and the interscapular group—all muscles which will be of great importance to the patient when he becomes ambulatory again.

Even though the patient's condition after surgery is such that he must be kept in the sitting position, certain measures can be used that will afford him greater comfort and also minimize the aftereffects of his illness. If the nurse understands the principles of sitting posture, she will know that the weight of the body should be borne on the ischia and the thighs. Therefore she will see to it that the hips are back as far as possible in the angle of the bed in order to prevent the patient from slumping down and sitting on his sacrum or lumbar

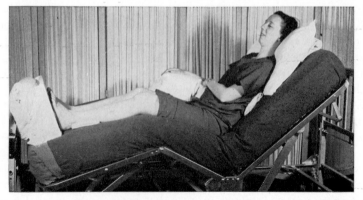

Fig. 34. Fowler position. Support beneath the left arm has been omitted to show the position of the body.

spine. The angle of the bed and the angle made by the flexed hips should be approximated. Although flexion of the knees is necessary to relax the spinal extensor muscles, the knees must be extended fully several times during the day. The back should be supported in its entirety, and pillows must not be allowed to bunch up under the shoulders and head, thereby forcing the spine out of its normal curves. Recognizing the dangers of prolonged outward rotation at the hips that so often accompanies such bed posture, the nurse will improvise a simple piece of equipment for overcoming this tendency, such as a sandbag, a pillow, or a trochanter roll made by anchoring a sheet folded lengthwise under the patient's hips and rolling it firmly against the thigh and knee. For the feet, if the customary type of footboard does not suffice, she may be able to devise a sling made of a bath blanket or sheet folded in a huge triangle and fastened to either side of the bed so that the feet may rest against it. Pillows placed under the forearms will eliminate the pull on the shoulders. When it is finally permissible for the patient to lie flat in bed for certain periods during the day, the nurse will be alert to the necessity of restoring full extension to hips and knees to overcome the results of long-continued flexion in those joints.

The development of a sacral decubitus always presents a grave situation, particularly in a thin, elderly patient or in one in whom dehydration and pyrexia persist over a long period. The potential danger of pressure areas is always in the mind of the nurse caring for such a patient. She knows that they must be averted at all costs. This is one preventive feature of which no nurse is uninformed or neglectful today. Sometimes, however, the problems involved in preventing a breakdown of the skin in the threatened area are so manifold that the nurse forgets the rest of the patient's problem entirely. Perhaps he is turned on his side and allowed to lie a great portion of the time with his legs adducted and his hips and knees flexed. The danger of decubitus is overcome, but if no one thinks to place pillows between the thighs for alignment of the extremities, by the time he is ready to sit up and walk he has a dislocation of the hip that lay adducted and unsupported for so long. A crippling condition results, which will require many months, or even years, to remedy. This outcome is no hypothetical possibility; it has happened often enough to make it essential that the student be taught the important part she plays in the prevention of such disasters. She should be well aware of the response of the musculoskeletal system to disease, to fever, and to disuse. The necessity for good body alignment in bed will become more reasonable and immediate to her as she gains in comprehension of these matters.

Deformities of the upper extremity. Another group of muscles that develop contractures because of faulty or unphysiologic positions in bed are the muscles at the axillary level, particularly the pectoral group. Patients lying in bed tend to be very limited as far as activity of the upper arms and shoulders is concerned. Many ambulatory patients, too, are somewhat restricted in this respect. The muscles that bring the arms away from the side and those that rotate the arms outward are used so infrequently that considerable disuse atrophy occurs in them. The patient with a debilitating illness is likely to lie in bed for many days in the "coffin position" (arms held closely to the sides of the body, elbows flexed at right angles, and wrists crossed and dropped). There is usually no reason at all why he must lie this way; he does it out of apathy or from lack of knowledge that it may be harmful to him. The skillful nurse will find reasons for making the patient use his arms in positions of abduction and outward rotation. She will have him reaching upward toward the head of the bed, combing his hair, or fastening his gown at the back of the neck. At other times she will provide for him to lie with his arms in a position opposite to the one he tends to assume constantly, that is, with the upper arm away from the body, the elbows extended, and the hands turned palm upward. By doing this she may be able to prevent the troublesome bursitis and synovitis that have sometimes followed long-continued restriction of motion in the shoulder, and she will certainly be able to prevent the tightness in the axilla that so frequently follows long illness. If, however, the patient has lain for a long time at home in a restricted position, such activity must be resumed by degrees and with caution.

These are some of the mishaps of poor bed posture, but there are others that may cause the patient discomfort, if not actual disability, after a period of bed rest. A sagging bed, for instance, can be the cause of insidious deformity, even though the nurse is careful to arrange the patient in positions of good body mechanics and is conscientious about teaching him his part in his own recovery. A depression in the mattress at the hip level may bring about contracture of the hip flexor muscles that may make the upright position of full extension at the hips next to impossible.

A patient who is gravely ill sometimes receives less attention to body mechanics than do others on the ward. It is said, and with some reason, that the problem of keeping such a patient alive takes all the nurse's strength and energy and that effort should not be dissipated on minor details, but it is a mistake to forget that the desperately ill patient

may recover. Indeed, one of the primary purposes of nursing is to help the patient get well if it is at all possible. No nurse wants a patient to recover from his original illness only to find that he has another handicap as a result of his stay in bed. Our concern for the horizontal man must not allow us to forget the vertical one.

Many deformities develop in patients with debilitating illnesses because they lie in bed over long periods of time in positions of adduction and flexion. The student should understand that flexion is one of the ways the patient learns to relieve discomfort in his back, his hips, and his knees. Sometimes he assumes these positions to keep warm when he has insufficient circulation or covers. Proper nursing care should overcome at least some of these discomforts. Sometimes making the patient comfortable may be as simple as giving support to the lower portion of the back, a little gentle massage perhaps, or an extra blanket, or a hot-water bottle.

Change of position is important. Any position, however adequate it may be as far as posture is concerned, will need frequent alteration. Human beings are not static, nor were they ever intended to be; movement is the very sine qua non of life itself. Sometimes these necessary alterations—from one type of good bed posture to another one equally good —will require all the ingenuity of which the nurse is capable.

In all these considerations, as in all treatment, we must face the irreducible and stubborn fact that patients are human beings; they are not dolls; they do not stay where you put them. They have their likes and dislikes about these things. Although we know that positions of good alignment usually produce more lasting comfort for the patient, nevertheless, if he has been so long in poor alignment that he has become accustomed to it, a little teaching and persuasion may be necessary. The student must understand that deformity cannot be corrected in a day and that zealousness should be tempered with patience and understanding. The patient's confidence and courage cannot be sacrificed in the attempt to overcome the results of neglect. Overdetermination, nagging, or sharpness demonstrates the fractional approach to the patient's total problem.

As the student goes through the clinical services she will become increasingly aware of situations in which her knowledge of elementary body mechanics is of importance. She may see a baby in the obstetric nursery whose head seems habitually to rest a little to one side with the chin pointed in the opposite direction. The baby may normally lie that way part of the time, but is he lying that way all of the time? And does he resist having his head turned the other way? Again, sometimes a patient is observed in an oxygen tent with two or three pillows under his head but with no support whatever to the back or shoulders. As a result the chest is concave and sunken. The student knows, of course, that the oxygen is being given to support a failing respiratory system. The incongruity of this in the face of such a sunken and depleted chest capacity should be apparent to her at once. But it will not be apparent unless instruction is given.

Charcot, the great French neurologist, once said that it was the mind that was truly alive and saw things but it would hardly see anything without instruction. This wise observation might well serve as a professional axiom for all teachers of student nurses. The difference between a trained observer and an untrained observer is never more important than it is in these instances. Unaided observation has but little value for the young student.

Prevention of crippling, of course, includes far more than attention to bed posture. Disease and accident are the causes of a large percentage of crippling conditions today. The nurse's function in the prevention and control of disease will be emphasized in all phases of her education, but the part she can play in accident prevention may not be so apparent to her unless it is given considerable thought and analysis both in the classroom and at the bedside.

Not long ago one of the largest insurance companies in this country undertook a challenging task: to determine the causes and kinds of home accidents that occur each year. Accidents in the home cause a high percentage of fatalities yearly. Besides the fatalities there were still to be considered the innumerable disabilities—temporary and permanent—and the resulting economic losses that they engendered. It seems that the results of such a study and others like it might form the subject matter for a unit of study in our nursing, community health, or sociology courses. When the situations in the home and hospital that are most likely to result in accidents are brought to the student's mind, her horizon for observation is enlarged immeasurably. A clear comprehension of what constitutes individual responsibility for community health and betterment is not the least of the lessons she has to learn.

GENTLENESS, A FUNDAMENTAL SKILL

If one could be arbitrary at the beginning and point out a single attainment indispensable for the nurse in any service, selecting it as a major objective for integration into all activities that she performs, one might be tempted to begin with the practice of gentleness. There is little argument that this is basic and a prerequisite for every new skill she will attempt to master. Gentleness, as it applies to all the healing arts, is too often taken for granted. It is taken for granted that we, as decent human beings, will treat the people under our care with gentleness. Certainly, it is true that no nurse worthy of the name would consciously mistreat a suffering person, but the acceptance of this as a foregone conclusion that does not need interpretation and emphasis is a questionable assumption. True, there are so many other things to be learned with great effort—methods, techniques, and manual skills—that it seems we must take some things for granted. Gentleness, we are likely to feel, should be natural and unlearned. So it is that we seldom carry this feature into the foreground of the nurse's mind, taking it for granted that it is there already. Yet this is a habit and an attitude that needs developing. Paradoxically enough, we even need to create respect for it in the student's mind. We know that gentleness in the use of the hands is very important. When prompted by kindness and understanding it has no counterpart in virtue. But these are overworked words—gentleness, kindness, understanding. We become supercilious in the use of them. They are adjuncts to the nurse's skill, felicitous for her if she happens to be blessed with them, but not indispensable for a successful career. Little emphasis is placed on acquiring them as part of one's necessary equipment for nursing.

The practice of gentleness, however, can be a conscious habit, a habit that makes the nurse use her voice and her hands with gentleness consciously because she knows it is good treatment. This is thoughtful objective gentleness, based not on compassion alone but upon the knowledge that sickness is an unremitting source of human fear, and, because she realizes this, the emotional components of the patient's illness are as important to her as other common symptoms she has been taught to observe and record.

Habitual gentleness is based upon understanding, experience, and an ability to identify oneself with the human race. It is cognitive as well as conative, based on intelligence as well as emotion. It seems that this is too frequently lost sight of in our nursing. Gentleness, whether it is in the handling of a patient with an acutely inflamed joint, the patient tense with fear of an oncoming treatment, or the patient pale with apprehension over a suspected malignancy, is a priceless possession. But it cannot be taken for granted that nurses will have this as a gift of God because they have elected nursing as their profession.

Biographers of Sir Robert Jones, the famous British orthopedist, have written often, and with deep appreciation, of the cordial spirit with which he received and handled his patients. They describe his methods of supporting a limb during examination—gently and with great skill in avoiding movement that would cause pain. Part of this skill, the cordial spirit, certainly was from the heart, but much of the rest of it must have been painstakingly learned. Both characteristics are greatly needed by nurses, particularly by those of us working with orthopedic patients.

CARE OF CHRONICALLY ILL PATIENTS

It has been said that ward aids and practical nurses give more satisfactory care to chronically ill patients than professionally trained nurses. If this is true, we need to examine our teaching methods rather carefully to determine what it is that we do not give our students to fit them for this type of nursing. A nurse never goes through a professional career without meeting over and over again the problem of the patient who has been ill a long time—a patient exhausted in courage, short in patience, unreasonable, fearful, and demanding.

Many of these problems will be discussed in other chapters of the book, particularly those having to do with the care of the arthritic patient and the care of the aged patient. Nurses working with the chronically ill are urged to read again Florence Nightingale's *Notes on Nursing*, particularly those passages having to do with the patient who has been confined to a bed or chair for a long time. No one has ever written of this matter with greater feeling and common sense than Florence Nightingale.

There are certain recurring problems regarding chronically ill patients which the nurse should bear in mind whether the patients are young or old. The very act of entering a hospital, for instance, may be a source of profound apprehension and fear to the patient. Perhaps he has had prolonged care in the home, care that he himself directed, wisely or unwisely. Every innovation that hospital nurses make is viewed with disfavor and suspicion, often because of the threat it offers to his comfort, but often, too, because the patient has come to take a negative attitude regarding any suggestion of change in his care. The student should realize that many of the most characteristic reactions of such patients come from a single source—fear. The nurse must recognize that she is the exciting cause of this reaction and accept the challenge to eliminate it in the patient's mind.

Again, all of us who have been in orthopedic nursing for very long have seen patients forcibly taken out of our hands after a day or two of preliminary treatment by what we justly call unreasonable, shortsighted relatives. Perhaps a large number of these withdrawals are unpreventable. But let us look to ourselves and to the initial treatment we give to cherished children or sheltered individuals.

One relatively uncomplicated situation is the case of the young girl admitted for treatment of a curvature of the spine. She herself is not disturbed by her back —not yet. But the threatened separation from her mother, her family, and her schoolmates is a break in her life that looms frighteningly on the horizon. The mother's face wears lines of worry. The family is in moderate circumstances; they have enough to live on decently but nothing put away for such an emergency as this. The very thought of having their beloved child on a charity ward, with dozens of other children of whom they know nothing, is abhorrent. They have debated long about this step. They trust their doctor's judgment, but is he, after all, quite sure? Might she not outgrow it as a neighbor assured them a friend's child had done? Might it not have been just a bit better to have taken old Mrs. Cutter's advice and to have sent Barbara to the chiropractor down the street for a course of adjustments before they began this prolonged treatment?

Into this confusion of fears and doubts comes a nurse who tells the mother: "You'll have to go now. We must take care of Barbara before supper." Or, "Will you step out of the room while we take care of your daughter?" (The student reading this will say, "That stupid nurse should not be allowed to practice.") That is what she should say; that is a hopeful response. Perhaps the student who makes that comment will know what should have been done: the sharing of the treatment with the mother, the explanation that should accompany each step to reassure her and to send her away confident that she has chosen the wisest, safest course for her daughter. Perhaps this nurse should have taken mother and daughter to look in upon a ward where other girls with curvature of the spine are wearing apparatus similar to that which Barbara will wear. The cheerfulness with which these young patients have accepted treatment will do much to allay the mother's fears. But will the student know this if we as teachers have not helped her in understanding the problems that lie behind such situations?

This is a very simple example. The nurse will be confronted by many more complex problems than this every day. Perhaps she will not recognize their complexity for many years unless she is guided to it. Perhaps the urgent, immediate problem will dominate her thinking forever unless we can help her to see beyond it.

The problem is resolved by the golden rule; it is just that simple, commonplace, and undramatic. It means that we must teach the student nurse to understand that her habitual response to these situations must be the response to a patient who is also an individual, a human being like herself. If she does this, she has understood and practiced democracy as truly in her sphere as though she went out on a soapbox and campaigned for it.

CONTINUITY OF CARE BETWEEN HOSPITAL AND HOME

There is another aspect which must be considered when continuity in nursing is discussed. It is the continuity that should exist between nursing care in the hospital and that in the home. All of us are aware of this necessity; indeed, neglect of it is so shortsighted an attitude that it could not escape attention for long. Yet there are still gaps that need to be filled in, gaps which the discerning student will not fail to draw to your attention. The intention to make continuous the treatment given in the hospital with that given in the home is sometimes blocked by lack of a functioning setup to accomplish this. Information sent to the family physician may not include instructions for actual nursing care. Sometimes there is an amazing lapse of time between the patient's dismissal and the relay of instructions for home care, so that the public health nurse is delayed in making her first visit because she does not know the patient is at home. Sometimes certain restrictions in hospital rulings prevent any instructions to public health nursing groups at all.

Ideally, the public health nurse should be informed of the patient's imminent dismissal before he leaves the hospital. If this were done, she could go into the home to assist the family in arranging equipment for the patient's return. She could plan to visit the home on the day the patient is dismissed and be on hand to aid the family in carrying out some of the instructions received at the hospital when taking the patient home.

Many hospitals have written forms that are mailed out in triplicate before the patient is dismissed: one to the public health officer, one to the physician in charge of the patient, and one to the public health nurse. Student nurses should be led to see how vital communications of this nature are to the patient's welfare. Provision for interchange of information should work both ways: the student should understand that the public health nurse may be able to impart much important information concerning the patient's attitude and progress during his stay at home in case he must return to the hospital. Fortified with this vision, the student will be less likely to think of illness only in terms of the patient's stay in the hospital.

Rehabilitation

Rehabilitation as we know it envisions a total effort toward the restoration of physically handicapped persons to a useful life. Total effort means surgical correction, functional restoration through exercise, special education, vocational training, and finally, employment. A team of doctors, nurses, physical and occupational therapists, social agencies, educators, vocational directors, and agencies of employment combine their efforts to meet this responsibility. Rehabilitation, for the sake of discussion here, will refer to that segment of the total which concerns the medical responsibilities. Obviously, all handicapped persons are not equally capable of complete rehabilitation.

Hospitals in increasing numbers are establishing rehabilitation centers where effort can be concentrated on the purely physical elements of restoration. This includes medical direction of physical therapy, occupational therapy, brace fitting, and on-the-spot work training. A pattern of treatment that will eventuate in maximum rehabilitation is available for many known physical defects, such as those that result from paraplegia, amputation, poliomyelitis, and cerebral palsy. The Army rehabilitation centers in World War II have shown how special exercises after acute trauma can hasten recovery. Graduated exercise programs, including heavy resistance exercise, are now commonplace therapy after operations on bones and joints. The field is so broad that it would be impossible to outline the details here, but discussion throughout this book will include rehabilitation as applied to specific conditions.

DEVELOPMENT OF HEALTHY ATTITUDES TOWARD HANDICAPPED PERSONS

There has been enough irresponsible sentimentality bestowed on the handicapped person. We must make certain that the nurse understands the difference between a shallow response of this nature and a realization of the responsibility she must assume for her own emotions. Threaded through her orthopedic nursing is the urgency of conditioning the handicapped individual

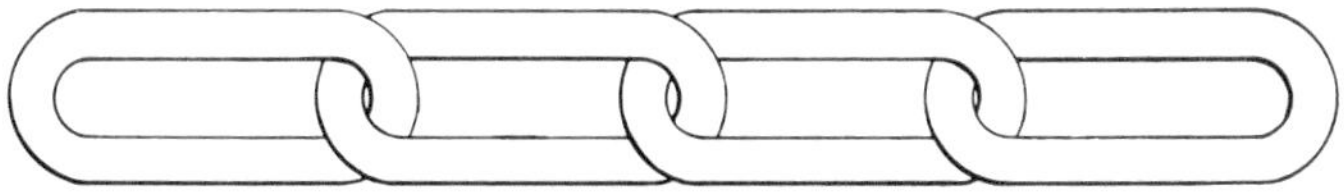

Medical care	Physical rehabilitation	Vocational training	Employment
Hospital	Physical therapy	Vocational counselor	Regular employment
Doctor	Occupational therapy	Vocational testing	Self employment
Nurses	Physiatrist	Vocational training	Home bound
	Psychiatrist		Sheltered workshop

Fig. 35. Concept of total rehabilitation.

physically and mentally, not only to be capable of doing things for himself but also to be willing to help himself. This urgency is the golden thread that must run through the whole fabric of nursing the handicapped as well as through teaching the patient's family. If there is a tendency on the part of the nurse to protect her patient, to indulge him, and to care for his wants so solicitously that he has no need or inclination to do anything for himself, there is an urge a thousand times more potent in the hearts of the family of the patient, an urge that seems good and natural to them. Reeducation of handicapped children of such parents sometimes acquires the nature of cruelty when viewed subjectively. We have all heard nurses called cruel and unfeeling. We have heard parents who try to create a sense of self-reliance in their crippled child by a little healthy neglect called cruel by their neighbors.

I once saw an 11-year-old boy with cerebral palsy who was brought to a hospital by a mother who had cared for him in every exquisite detail since birth. He could neither walk nor talk beyond a few guttural noises. A year later, after an expensive course of treatment that included muscle reeducation and intensive training in self-help, that boy left the hospital walking, unsteadily but still walking, on crutches. The mother had been told repeatedly by the nurses and doctors that all this expensive treatment must be carried on faithfully at home if she had the child's welfare at heart. However, they had little hope. He was an only child, his father and mother were indulgent and emotional, and they adored him with what seemed excessive affection.

Two months later, across the street from me, I saw this boy walking on crutches, appearing as unsteady as a drunken man, making his way, his eyes fastened fiercely on the mailbox at the corner, which I guessed was his goal. Half a block away I saw his mother. She took on a sort of nobility to me that afternoon—walking slowly, no doubt conscious of every staggering unbalanced effort of her son, but walking half a block behind him. God knows what emotions of apprehension and agonized fright were in her heart. When he got to the mailbox, he stopped, turned around triumphantly, and waited for her to catch up with him. She came unhurried and, in attitude at least, calm and unperturbed.

In regard to the overprotected handicapped person, there is the matter of teaching him not only to take care of his own wants insofar as he is able but also to take responsibility for his mistakes and misdeeds equally with his normal brothers and sisters. If the patient has had the benefit of this training at home, the student nurse will recognize the importance of doing nothing to undermine it because she is sorry for him and thinks that she understands his problems better than his parents or family do. Perhaps, however, the individual has not been taught these things at home. Perhaps the student has noticed tyrannical traits in the patient when his family visits him. In her quiet way she can do much to teach both patient and family. The incomparable experience in communal living that is given this overprotected person in the orthopedic ward is not the least of the benefits he will receive in the hospital. Sharing his pleasures with the other patients, himself sharing theirs, and assuming his part in responsibility for misdemeanors will perhaps be new to him, but the nurse should recognize the opportunity to use these as the first step in his long fight for social and emotional security. The wise nurse points up and makes purposeful these problems of everyday living in the ward. Properly directed, the experience should be highly beneficial to the crippled person. It should help him adjust to other handicapped individuals and to normal companions. It should prepare him to live with greater harmony in his own family group. It should serve also to overcome a crippled attitude of mind—a more serious disability, after all, than a crippled spine.

THE REHABILITATION TEAM

In rehabilitation the nurse always works as a member of a team. The team is composed of all those who are in some way contributing toward the total recovery of the patient, whether it be physical, psychologic, social, spiritual, or vocational. The team, always working under the captaincy of the orthopedist, may consist of the hospital nurse and her assistants, the public health nurse, the psychologist, the physical and occupational therapists, the teacher, the social worker, the speech clinician, the vocational counselor, the parents or family, and, last but not least, the patient himself.

When working with a team it is of course extremely important that the common objective be clearly recognized. It is equally important to learn how to work with people. It may often be necessary to subordinate one's own ego for the good of the whole group. The complete rehabilitation of a patient may require more of one group of workers than it does of another at certain stages of the program, but there are actually no stellar roles except that played by the patient.

Rehabilitation teamwork demands that the nurse, particularly the hospital nurse, learn perspective. The period of time that most rehabilitation patients spend in the hospital is only a small episode compared with the long years they may have been or will be disabled. Proper perspective requires that the nurse look both backward and forward. There was a time, before the disability occurred, when the patient lived as a member of a family and a community. There was the illness or accident that changed him from a normal person to one with a handicap. There was the period before he decided, perhaps with considerable anxiety and dread, to submit himself to treatment. Then there is the brief but intensive period of treatment in the hospital where nurses, occupational and physical therapists, and others work with the surgeon on some reconstructive problem that in itself is only a beginning. When it is over he will return to his home, his family, and his community to continue the treatment that was begun in the hospital. There will be a new group of helpers for him then, perhaps the social worker, the public health nurse, and the public health physical therapist. Other therapists in a sheltered workshop may be necessary to round out his functional recovery. It is a long road, and on it the rehabilitation patient meets many people.

The more awareness the hospital nurse has of the road the patient has traveled before she sees him and of the distance he must go before he will have made the maximum recovery he hopes for the more intelligent and unselfish will be her contribution to the rehabilitation team. It will be apparent that many pairs of hands will be required to assist the patient toward his goal.

It is sometimes extremely difficult to work harmoniously with other groups when one is under pressure. Often it seems that there are endless conflicts in aims and method, and one is inclined to feel that there is a great deal of pulling in opposite directions. It is vital for the efficiency of the program that these conflicts be resolved as soon as they occur. Frequent conferences between groups with opportunities to discuss troublesome problems are bound to pay dividends in easier working relationships. Fundamentally the aim of all the workers, nurses, and therapists is the same: to assist the patient in his fight for complete recovery and rehabilitation.

What can the nurse, herself, do to promote better working relationships with other clinical groups?

First, and most important, she can develop a cordial spirit for these other people who are working in the rehabilitation area. This area is, in a sense, the nurse's house; she is the mistress. The other persons who work there are acutely aware of this fact, and they would like to feel that they are welcome there as part of the rehabilitation family.

Second, she must seek to learn as much as she can about the work of other clinical groups; that is, she should know the aims of treatment, the problems, and many of the skills and techniques that enter into the general care of the patient. It will be necessary for her to encourage the patient to carry out correctly the instructions agreed upon by the team. Without this follow-through, the relatively brief periods the patient spends with the special therapist may be of little lasting value. The nurse must supervise the patient's intelligent and conscientious practice of the exercises given him, or he may sometimes be tempted to use slipshod methods, knowing that the therapist is not there to observe him. Furthermore, nurses must work with these other groups and with the social worker to plan a coordinated home program to fit the needs and capabilities of the patient. Instructions given to family or patient at the time of discharge should be a joint responsibility, and conferences on this subject should be held frequently so that no overlapping or omissions will be likely to occur.

Third, the nurse should prepare the patient to go to the occupational or physical therapy departments, to the school, or to the speech therapist by caring for his basic needs. He should be clean, and he should have had an opportunity to use the bedpan or urinal before he goes. If he is scheduled for walking exercises, his braces should be correctly applied and his crutches placed beside him. If he has had an enema that has not been fully expelled, the therapist should be notified before he is sent to the department. Furthermore, he should be sent to the department on time, and if some unavoidable emergency makes this impossible, the department should be notified so that the therapist is given an opportunity to rearrange her schedule with as little time loss as possible.

Finally, it must be assumed that each worker on the rehabilitation team is trying sincerely to do his or her part toward the patient's full recovery. Yet, unless effort is put forth to view the recovery program in its entirety, it may resemble a kind of jigsaw puzzle with each worker concentrating on her own phase of the work to the exclusion of the others. The central theme, the unifying pattern, is the patient. He is the focal point. The pieces of the jigsaw must be fitted together for his benefit so that lines of cleavage are not too evident, and they must be fitted together with tolerance, understanding, and mutual respect to give satisfaction and dignity to the workers themselves.

The whole truth, Steindler once wrote, cannot come from a solitary voice. Similarly, planned rehabilitation does not come from a solitary pair of hand. The nurse who recognizes this fact and wholeheartedly accepts it will take her place on the rehabilitation team with increased benefit to her patient and greater happiness to herself.

PROBLEMS OF REHABILITATION

The basic principles and practices used in giving nursing care are most applicable and essential to rehabilitation

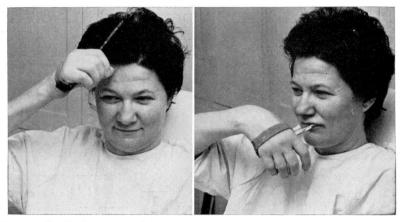

Fig. 36. By using the leather holder, this patient with quadriplegia is able to comb her hair and to brush her teeth.

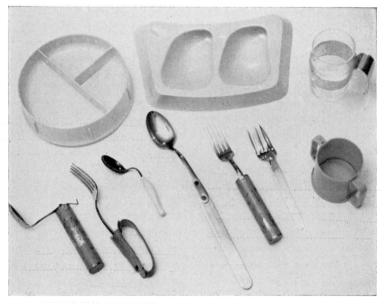

Fig. 37. Mechanical aids that facilitate self-feeding for the person who has weakness or paralysis of the muscles of the upper extremity. Suction-cup dishes that adhere to the table and have divided compartments make getting food on the spoon easier. Padded or enlarged handles may make it possible for the disabled person to grasp the eating utensil.

nursing. In fact, they are the essence of rehabilitation nursing.

Good hygienic care is very important for this patient. It is not only conducive to good physical health but also has value in sustaining morale and a feeling of well-being. The rehabilitation patient is encouraged and taught to take care of as many of his personal need as possible.

Longer periods of time must be allowed for these activities, and an infinite amount of patience is required of the nurse who works with and encourages the disabled patient to manipulate his own toothbrush or to manage his own brace. What mechanical aids can be used? Can the patient with weakness of the upper extremities be taught to feed

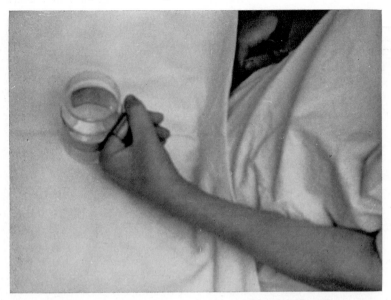

Fig. 38. This glass holder enables the person who is unable to grasp objects with his fingers to drink from a glass.

himself and to light his own cigarette? One no longer concentrates on doing for the patient, but one thinks in terms of how he can do it for himself.

Maintaining a state of good nutrition is an important aspect of the care of the rehabilitation patient. A strenuous exercise program increases his food requirements. The paralyzed patient needs adequate intake of protein to prevent breakdown of the skin and underlying tissues. The individual with an arm or hand disability may experience fatigue when feeding himself and consume an inadequate diet unless help is offered. The overweight patient must not be forgotten. Extra pounds may make ambulation impossible. At mealtime, the nurse who understands what the rehabilitee is being taught by the occupational therapist can help him practice self-feeding. If he can learn to feed himself, mealtime can become a sociable hour. This is important for the handicapped person attempting to find his place in family and community life. Equipping a dining room with tables that accommodate

wheelchairs provides a more normal situation for practicing the activities of daily living.

Prevention of decubitus ulcers is another important aspect of rehabilitation nursing. Many of these patients have one or more paralyzed extremity. Frequently, incontinency is a problem. One or both of these factors make the maintenance of a healthy skin a real challenge to nursing personnel. Frequent change of the patient's position (every 2 hours) is important to relieve pressure. Protection of the bony areas with foam rubber and the maintenance of a clean dry bed are necessary nursing measures if pressure areas are to be prevented. This sounds simple, but to maintain this kind of nursing care 24 hours a day requires the vigilance of all nursing personnel, constant teaching of new personnel, and last but not least, an adequate amount of nursing help.

Regardless of the cause for the illness or disability, the importance of preventing deformity is apparent very early in the nursing care. Emphasis is placed on teaching the handicapped individual and his family how joint deformity can be prevented. The maxim "an ounce of prevention is worth a pound of cure" was never more applicable than to the prevention of secondary joint deformity. Those of us who have seen patients spend weeks (to say nothing of the pain endured) receiving treatment directed at the correction of contractures can appreciate the importance of their prevention. Applying knowledge of proper body alignment, providing for frequent change of position, and maintaining a normal range of joint motion is necessary if deformity is to be prevented.

During the bath procedure the nurse may carry out simple passive exercises of the involved extremity or extremities and thus help maintain a normal range of motion. As she bathes the axillary region she moves the arm away (abduction) from the patient's side. Bending and straightening the elbow provides for flexion and extension. The movements of the wrist, plus closing and opening the hand for finger flexion and extension, can be accomplished nicely as the extremity is bathed and dried. Raising and lowering the leg and bending the knee provides for flexion and extension of the hip and knee joints. Moving the leg toward the edge of the bed helps maintain the motion of abduction, and rolling the limb in provides for internal rotation. Simple dorsiflexion of the foot during the bath procedure will help prevent tightening of the heel cord (Achilles tendon). These joint motions carried out by the nurse who knows how to support and move a paralyzed extremity can be most helpful in preventing joint contractures.

In addition to exercises of the involved extremities directed by the nurse or therapist, the disabled patient is taught and encouraged to do simple exercises of the uninvolved extremities early in the course of his care. These exercises are valuable in improving circulation, in maintaining muscle strength, and in preventing tightness of tendons and limitation of joint motion.

As the nurse works with the patient she may ask herself, "Is this patient able to plantar flex his foot? Is he able to turn his foot in (inversion) and to pull his foot up (dorsiflexion)?" This activity is valuable in preventing drop foot and tightness of the heel cord.

Can the patient tighten the quadriceps muscle? This muscle located on the anterior portion of the thigh enables one to brace and extend the knee and it is important in maintaining erect posture. The quadriceps-setting exercise is taught with the patient in the supine position and with the limb in extension. He is instructed to contract the muscles on the anterior portion of the thigh so that the kneecap is drawn upward toward the thigh. He maintains the muscle contraction for 5 seconds and then allows the muscle to relax for 5 seconds. The physician may request that the patient do this exercise for 5 minutes every hour during the waking day. Straight leg-raising is another exercise frequently prescribed to strengthen the quadriceps muscle. In the supine position, with the knee in extension and the foot in a neutral position, the patient lifts the limb off the bed. At first this is difficult, but with practice the limb is raised to form approximately a 45-degree angle with the body. This position is held for several seconds, and the limb is lowered slowly.

If tightness of the hamstring muscles (flexion contracture) is to be prevented, the knee joint should not be supported continuously in a flexed position. The position of extension must be secured at frequent intervals.

Does the patient lie or sit with his limb in a position of external rotation? A sandbag or trochanter roll placed along the lateral aspect of the thigh will remind and encourage him to maintain his limb in a neutral position.

Does he like to have the backrest elevated, or does he sit in a chair for long periods? To avoid flexion contractures of the hips, he needs to lie (on a firm mattress) with the hips in full extension.

Can he abduct and externally rotate his arms to tie his gown strings and to

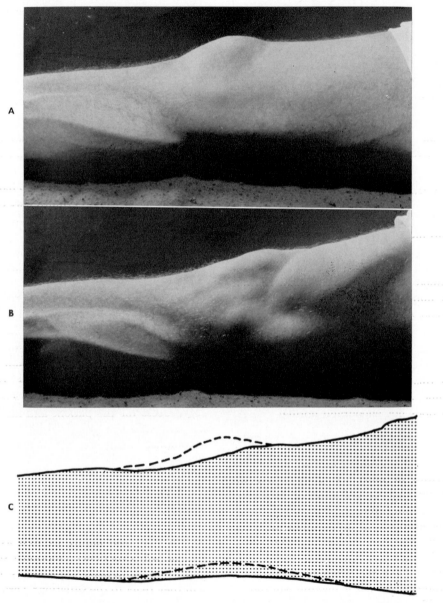

Fig. 39. Quadriceps-setting exercise. **A,** Relaxed thigh and knee joint. **B,** Quadriceps muscle located on the anterior thigh is tightened and shortened, moving the patella proximally. **C,** Movement of patella proximally and pressing of popliteal space against the mattress. (**A** and **B** from Gould, Marjorie L.: Nursing care—internal derangement of the knee joint, Am. J. Nursing **56:**577-582, 1956.)

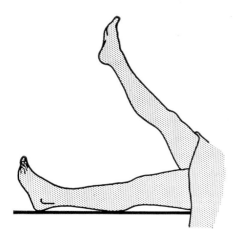

Fig. 40. Performing straight-leg-raising exercises develops the strength of the quadriceps muscle. (From Gould, Marjorie L.: Nursing care—internal derangement of the knee joint, Am. J. Nursing **56:**577-582, 1956.)

comb his hair, or have his pectoral muscles become too tight?

Is full extension of the cervical spine attained at intervals throughout the day and night, or is the patient lying with marked flexion of the neck? Frequently, patients like this position because it facilitates their seeing about the ward. However, the nurse needs to remember that this position, held for long periods of time, is not conducive to good posture and does not encourage normal respiratory expansion.

There is no better place than the ward for the rehabilitation patient to practice activities of daily living. Whether the task be that of learning to brush his teeth, getting from the bed to a chair, or doing exercises in preparation for walking on crutches, the nurse who keeps herself informed concerning the plan of treatment and the progress that the rehabilitation patient is making can render valuable assistance to her patient and to her co-workers on the rehabilitation team.

It is essential that members of the rehabilitation team have knowledge of re-sources—local, state, federal, and private—that may be utilized in the field of rehabilitation. During the past few years many facilities have been made available, and as the need is recognized and as the number of personnel trained in this area increases, assistance to the disabled person will increase many times. The worker who keeps himself informed of available resources will be able to offer the patient valuable assistance as he travels the road of rehabilitation.

Teaching the patient and his family is an important aspect of rehabilitation. The patient learns that good skin care is essential to prevent pressure areas. He learns that his position must be changed and that wrinkles and crumbs may cause breaks in the skin. He inspects his skin for redness or blisters that may come from shoes or braces. He knows that poor position results in deformity and that lack of exercise means stiff joints. He recognizes the necessity for adequate intake of fluid for the prevention of kidney stones, and he learns how to care for his catheter properly. He practices applying his brace, dressing himself, and taking care of his personal needs. To be successful rehabilitation must be a learning process for the patient and his family. The disabled person must learn to accomplish many of the activities of daily living by new methods.

The nurse on the rehabilitation team has a better opportunity than any other member of the team to know and understand the patient and his family. She recognizes that the family as well as the patient will experience emotional strain and will need to make adjustments. How will they react to the situation? Throughout this period of adjustment a trained clinical psychologist will be of value to the family and patient in resolving their problems and apprehensions. However, the rehabilitation worker recognizes that

Text continued on p. 40.

EVALUATION OF DAILY LIVING ACTIVITIES
OCCUPATIONAL THERAPY

Name_____Birth date_____Age_____Sex____

Address/Hospital No._____

Diagnosis_____Date onset_____

Vocation_____Handedness_____

KEY
(Scores indicate skill accomplished within a reasonable time)
0—Cannot be accomplished
1—Can be accomplished with human aid
2—Can be accomplished with adaptation of environment (low bed, special toilet
    seat, handrails, ramps, etc.)
3—Can be accomplished with use of mechanical aids (splints, braces, prostheses,
    crutches, wheelchair, etc.)
4—Can be accomplished without aids, adaptation, or assistance
*—Not practical (time, too much supervision required)
N.A.—Not applicable to this patient

Date and √ form on initial test.
Any changes in status from initial test should be dated.

HOME SITUATION
Note suggestions for adaptation next to each line or check when so indicated. In special
instances, diagram of layout will be advisable.

Location: City_____Rural_____

Travel: Own car____Hand controls____Taxi____Bus____

Apartment: Floor____Rooms____Elevator____Self-service____None____Walk up_____

Private house: Floors____Rooms____Stairs____Elevator____Self-service____None_____

Entrance: Door____Step____Railing:____right____left____none____Ramp____

Bathroom: Door____OK for wheelchair____Tub____Shower over tub____Stall shower___

Note type of floors: Bedroom____Living room____Kitchen____Bath____

Information unavailable (explain)

Assistive devices

An up-to-date chart (pp. 36 to 39) of the rehabilitee's accomplishments pertaining to activities of daily living can be most helpful to the nurse. It provides her with a better understanding of what she can expect from the patient pertaining to self-care as well as goals that he is working toward. (Courtesy Occupational Therapy Department, State University of Iowa Hospitals, Iowa City.)

I. BED ACTIVITIES	0	1	2	3	4
1. Moving in bed: Roll to right___ to left_____					
2. Turn onto abdomen_____					
3. Come to sitting position _____					
4. Sit erect in bed (LSP)_____					
5. Sit on edge of bed (SSP)_____					
6. Adjust blanket, sheets, etc._____					
7._____					

II. WHEELCHAIR SKILLS					
1. Bed to wheelchair; wheelchair to bed_____					
Method_____					
2. Propel chair_____					
Number of feet_____					
3. Lock/unlock brakes_____					
4. Raise/lower footrests_____					
5. Open, close, and pass through door_____					
Type of door_____					
6. Pick up objects off floor_____					
7. Transfer to/from straight chair_____					
At table_____					
Standing free_____					
8. Transfer to/from easy chair/couch_____					
9. Transfer to/from toilet_____					
Method_____					
10. Transfer to/from car_____					
11. Get from wheelchair to floor, from floor to wheelchair_____					
12._____					

III. PERSONAL HYGIENE					
1. Comb/brush hair_____					
2. Set hair_____					
3. Brush teeth or clean dentures_____					
4. Apply toothpaste to brush_____					
5. Shave/put on cosmetics_____					
6. Care for fingernails/toenails_____					
7. Use handkerchief_____					
8. Give self bed bath_____					
Unable to reach_____					
9. Dry thoroughly with towel_____					
10. Use of shower_____					
11. Get into/out of bath_____					
12. Toilet_____					
Method_____					
Flush toilet_____					
Use of toilet paper_____					
Adjust clothing_____					
Use urinal/bedpan_____					
13. Manage catheter:					
Independent care_____					
Clamp off/unclamp_____					
Empty SP bag_____					
14. Feminine hygiene _____					
15._____					

Continued on next page.

IV. DRESSING   0   1   2   3   4

1. Put on/remove bra_____
   How? What method_____
2. Put on/remove shorts, panties _____
   Method_____standing, on bed, seated
3. Put on/remove slipover garments_____
   Method_____standing, on bed, seated
4. Put on/remove button shirt _____
   Method_____standing, on bed, seated
5. Put on/remove slacks or pants_____
   Method_____standing, on bed, seated
6. Put on/remove socks or hose _____
   Method_____standing, on bed, seated
7. Put on/remove shoes_____
   Method_____standing, on bed, seated
8. Lace/unlace shoes_____
9. Tie/untie laces_____
10. Hook/unhook garters/suspenders_____
    Front_____
    Back_____
11. Fasten/unfasten buckle_____
12. Button/unbutton_____
    Little_____
    Big_____
    Circle location—front, side, back
13. Fasten/unfasten snap_____
14. Fasten/unfasten zipper_____
    Circle location—front, side
15. Fasten/unfasten hooks and eyes_____
16. Tie/untie necktie_____
17. Fasten/unfasten safety pin_____
    Small_____
    Large_____
18._____

V. APPARATUS

1. Put on/remove braces _____
2. Lock/unlock braces _____
3. Put on/remove splints, feeders, slings _____
4. Put on/remove corset_____
   Type of lacing _____
5. _____

VI. EATING

1. Eat with fingers/sandwich_____
2. Eat liquids with spoon_____
3. Eat with fork/cut with fork_____
4. Cut with knife_____
5. Butter bread_____
6. Drink from glass, cup, paper cup_____
7. Pour liquid from milk carton/pour liquid from
   bedside pitcher_____
8. Open carton of milk_____
9. _____
10._____

VII. AMBULATION	0	1	2	3	4
1. Walks_____					
2. Stand and work at table_____					
Regular table_____					
Stand-up table_____					
3. Walks with package_____					
4. Get up from floor when falls_____					
With crutches_____					
Without crutches_____					
5._____					

VIII. UTILITIES					
1. Write:					
Legibly_____					
Name and address_____					
Copy paragraph_____					
2. Turn pages of book/magazine_____					
3. Cut with scissors_____					
4. Open a package of cigarettes_____					
5. Light a match/lighter_____					
6. Pick up change_____					
7. Make correct change_____					
8. Telephone:_____					
Standing_____					
From wheelchair_____					
Hold receiver_____					
Dial_____					
Use coins_____					
9. Wind watch_____					
10. Open/close windows_____					
11. Open/close drawers_____					
12. A.D.L. Board check-out_____					
Height of board_____					

Numbers accomplished

_____   _____

_____   _____

_____   _____

SUMMARY

Therapist's signature _____

the patient and his family need to be realistic about his disabilities. False hopes must not be fostered. They must realize that certain handicaps do exist but that remaining abilities and capacities can be defined, guided, and developed. The regime of treatment should be such that the patient is given the opportunity and motivation to do as much for himself as is humanly possible. This includes the privilege of making his own decisions and taking responsibility for his own acts. Day-by-day improvement may seem very small. Discouragement and an attitude of futility must be combated from the beginning.

ADL: Briefly then, the ordinary activities required for daily independent living must be painstakingly relearned by the patient. These will include sitting, bending, turning, getting out of bed, walking, climbing stairs, putting on clothes and braces, and all types of personal care. The program to develop these skills is highly complex. Experience and a high degree of skill are required to teach them effectively. Nurses should know what system of rehabilitation is being employed so that they may constantly encourage and instruct the patient in his struggle for physical independence.

FAMILY AND JOB ADJUSTMENTS

The other factors in the total rehabilitation of patients, particularly those concerning family, social, and job adjustments, are fully as important as the physical aspects of the task. The advancement made since World War II in this matter has been heartening. Many new types of jobs have been discovered in which handicapped patients can contribute almost as much as a physically normal person. Sheltered workshops and shops attached to hospital wards have been set up in some communities and are used by local industries for piecework, such as construction of radio and airplane parts. Weaving, watch repairing, typing, printing, metal and leather crafts, painting, and wood carving have always provided occupation for patients with severe orthopedic handicaps and have, in many instances, provided a means of earning a livelihood. Factories in many communities have sent small machinery to hospital workshops to be assembled by handicapped patients. Watch and radio repairing are within the grasp of all but the most severely affected patients.

Family acceptance of the severely handicapped person, accompanied by an understanding of his need to live his own life as much as is possible, is probably the most important factor in the total rehabilitation program. All of the splendid work accomplished in the hospitals and workshops can be nullified in the home if oversolicitousness, rejection, or pity is evident to the patient. Nurses will need the help of social workers and social agencies to work out the problem of family adjustments for these patients.

The problem of caring for an occasional disabled patient is indeed a most perplexing one for the nurse. But if she is fully cognizant of the dangers and armed with knowledge of means to overcome them, she will be able to play an important part in his early physical rehabilitation. Indeed, her efforts may be fundamental in that they actually may keep the patient alive. If she is also imbued with a determination to help the patient become as independent as it is humanly possible for him to be, she will no doubt be able to secure assistance from others more skilled than she to aid the patient at various stages of his progress.

OCCUPATIONAL THERAPY IN ORTHOPEDICS

Occupational therapy may be defined as any activity, physical or mental, which is definitely prescribed and guided for the distinct purpose of contributing to and hastening recovery from disease or injury. Briefly speaking, it is remedial activity. Therefore, the goal of an occupational therapist for an orthopedic patient is restoration of physical function. This is specific for each patient in the restoration of joint motion, in the regaining of muscle strength, or in the promotion of coordination. The general aim with all patients is the development of work tolerance, socioeconomic adjustment, and prevocational testing.

Certainly, the psychologic manifestations of the orthopedic patient must not

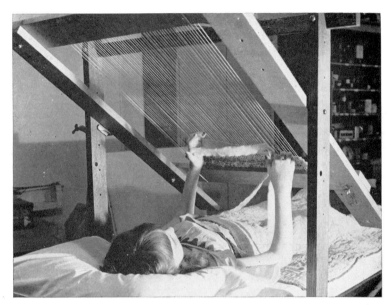

Fig. 41. Adjustable rug-weaving frame for use by the bed patient. This type of activity not only appeals to the patient but also provides valuable exercise for fingers, wrists, elbows, and shoulders afflicted with arthritis.

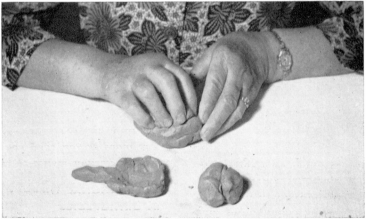

Fig. 42. Using modeling clay for finger mobilization. Sponge rubber may also be used to strengthen finger muscles.

be overlooked. The tendency of a patient to withdraw from society or to dwell on the pain and problems he has is not a healthy attitude. The occupational therapist substitutes an activity for inactivity, thus preventing this regression and promoting a good adjustment.

The media used in accomplishing these objectives are varied. Too frequently there is a wrong impression created when a patient busy with a craft is observed. The craft is noticed; the activity is not. The *occupational* of occupational therapy is not the project the patient is concerned with, nor is it his vocation or avocation upon leaving the

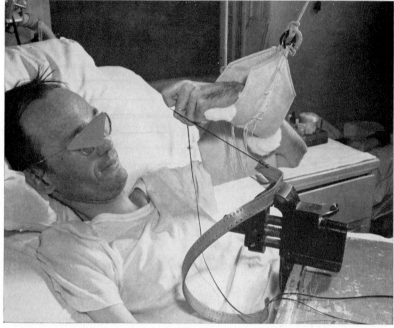

Fig. 43. Arrangement of belt-making equipment for the bed patient. This activity provides muscle-strengthening exercises and joint motion for the fingers and arm.

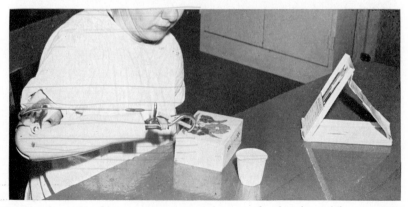

Fig. 44. Patient with upper extremity amputation learning to perform fine movements with prosthetic appliance.

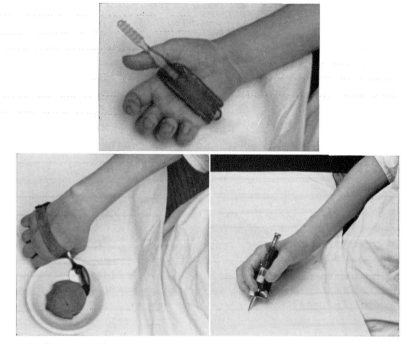

Fig. 45. The leather holder with a pocket for holding a spoon, pencil, or other utensil is helpful for the person who has lost the use of the small muscles of the hand but still has some shoulder and elbow motion.

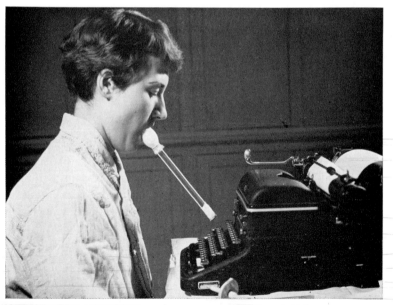

Fig. 46. The handicapped person with paralyzed upper extremities may learn to use the typewriter by utilizing a mouth stick. The stick is made of plastic material and has plastic-covered padding, which facilitates holding it in the mouth and provides protection for the teeth.

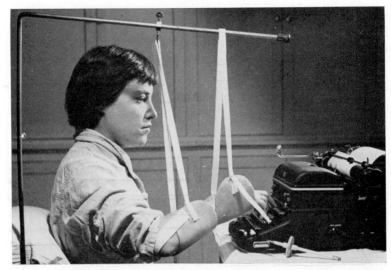

Fig. 47. The disabled person who possesses the use of her fingers but has weakness or paralysis of the arm and shoulder muscles may find this supension sling helpful in performing activities of daily living.

hospital, but rather it is the *occupation or activity of mind and body.* Use of the arts and crafts is a valuable method employed by the occupational therapist, but it is only one of many. Adapted recreational activities and self-help training in dressing and feeding skills are other important means. Writing, use of the telephone, manipulation of doors, latches, and dials, and similar activities for daily living are taught to the handicapped patient. The media used are selected with the patient in mind at all times. The referring physician's aim and the patient's involvement, interest, background, age, sex, and many other factors must be carefully reviewed.

Occupational therapy plays a coordinating role in the total rehabilitation of a patient. It bridges the gap from total hospitalization to life outside the hospital by enabling the patient to realize his own abilities and to carry out the practical actions learned in physical therapy. It prevents the disability that often comes from disuse; it encourages the development of latent abilities; it trains the patient in prevocational skills; and it develops work tolerance.

DIVERSIONAL THERAPY

The importance of the diversional aspects of occupational therapy should be more evident to the student than it is. Emphasizing the principles learned in her mental hygiene classes may be necessary in order to create an awareness of its value in the care of the handicapped person. She should have some conception from this course, and perhaps from her own experience, of the mental hazard that accompanies too little to do and too much time to think. Under the pressure of her ward work, in the midst of the many duties imposed on her during a busy period in the day, values sometimes become confused, and diversional therapy takes on the aspect of a frill or luxury treatment. This is where the nurse's thinking must be directed toward a broader concept of what it means to the handicapped person to be given something to make or to do to fulfill the essential drive toward productivity which, consciously or not, every human being possesses. To underestimate this need, to adjudge it secondary to the patient's need perhaps for a daily bath, is an abysmal misconception. Baths can be frills. The need for productive activity is a fundamental need. Therapeutic treatment that is part of the rehabilitation of the handicapped person's physical capacities is hardly less important, and its scope needs to be made known to the student early in her orthopedic nursing course.

EDUCATION FOR THE CHILD WITH A HANDICAP

In order for the nurse to evaluate the place of community activity in the care

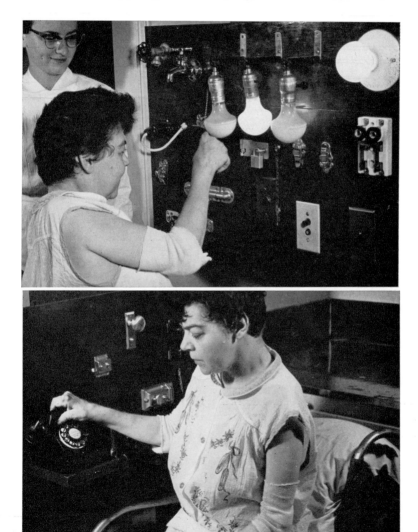

Fig. 48. The person with shoulder, elbow, or hand disability finds these boards most helpful in practicing and mastering activities essential to everyday living. The boards may be raised or lowered and contain such articles as light switches, water faucets, doorknobs, lock, and telephone.

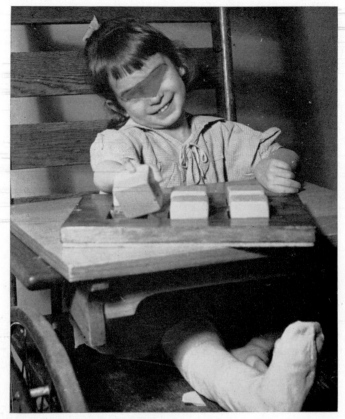

Fig. 49. Patient with spastic cerebral palsy using educational toys for eye-hand coordination exercise.

of crippled persons, she should be guided toward the existing community agencies for the rehabilitation of the handicapped. She should understand that education for the crippled child is imperative, perhaps more so than for his normal brother. Many roads to self-sufficiency and self-support are available to the normal person that are barred to the handicapped one, and so he must be better prepared to fulfill the more limited type of service of which he is capable. The student should understand that the newest concept of vocational guidance and placement emphasizes the versatility rather than the limitations of crippled individuals. Perhaps the student may one day imbue some earnest civic group with a great urge to help the handicapped, not to buy the twenty-second iron lung for the state but to take upon themselves the education of some homebound child. Services are generally available for the homebound child with two-way radio telephonic class communication as well as home teacher service provided by the public school system.

PHYSICAL THERAPY

Physical therapy or physical medicine may be defined as that science which deals with the management of disease by means of physical agents such as light, heat, cold, water, electricity, and mechanical agents.

From ancient times the principle of physical therapy has been employed, but

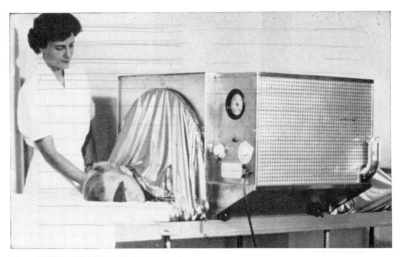

Fig. 50. Fever cabinet.

not always on a scientific basis. The practices of lying in the sun, rubbing a bruised muscle, and bathing a wound in a woodland stream have led through the years to the development of present methods of treatment. These have an important function and are well recognized in most outstanding hospitals today.

Thermotherapy

Heat therapy includes fever therapy and paraffin treatments.

Fever therapy. The fever cabinet is used to produce a mild elevation (100° to 101° F.) of the patient's body temperature. The treatment usually consists of 30 minutes in the cabinet, during which time the temperature and pulse are recorded at frequent intervals. During the course of treatment the patient is carefully watched, cool cloths are applied to his head, and he is encouraged to sip cold water.

Fever therapy is used to assist in the treatment of chronic atrophic arthritis. Moderately longer and higher fevers have proved successful in treating some patients with acute atrophic arthritis. The combined use of chemotherapy and artificially produced high fever has yielded satisfactory results in the treatment of gonorrhea and syphilis.

Paraffin. Melted paraffin to which mineral oil or white paraffin No. 72 oil has been added is very satisfactory as a method of applying heat. The melted paraffin is kept at a temperature between 124° and 132° F. If the paraffin is completely melted and has a little scum on the surface, the temperature is correct. The dip pack is very satisfactory for treating a hand or arm afflicted with arthritis. The extremity is dipped into the paraffin six to ten times until a thick coat (½ inch) is obtained. This, carefully wrapped in a bath towel or bath blanket, will hold the heat 20 to 30 minutes. The paraffin can also be painted on the involved area. If alternate layers of paraffin and gauze are used, the resulting pack will hold heat for more than an hour.

Paraffin is used chiefly for arthritis, bursitis, fibrositis, or when contractures of the hand have developed. Following the paraffin treatment the treated area is well prepared for massage and exercise. Paraffin-dip treatment can easily be carried on at home by heating the paraffin in a double boiler and using the scum test as a temperature guide.

Light therapy

Light therapy includes ultraviolet and infrared radiation.

Ultraviolet radiation. The ultraviolet radiation is in the range of the light spectrum from 1 to 390 milliamperes. It can be produced by several artificial sources including the hot quartz mercury lamp, cold quartz lamp, or the

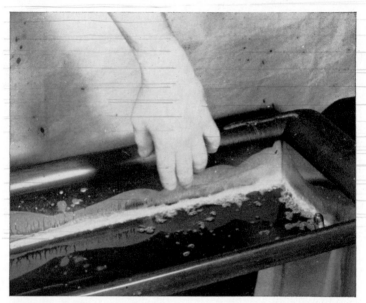

Fig. 51. The hand has just been dipped ten times into the melted paraffin.

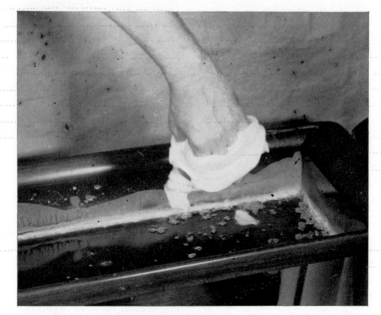

Fig. 52. The paraffin glove is being removed. This may be put back into the paraffin bath and remelted.

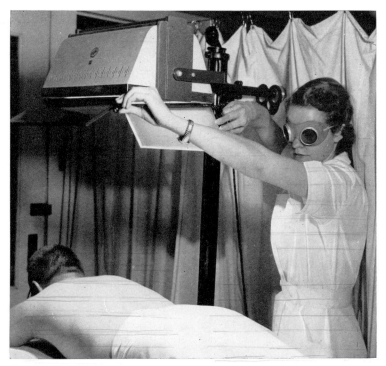

Fig. 53. Ultraviolet lamp being opened for an exposure to the back.

carbon arc. The dosage is governed by the minimal erythema dose (M.E.D.). This is defined as the shortest exposure at a certain distance that will produce a perceptible reddening of the skin within 6 to 8 hours and disappear within 24 hours. Care must be taken to cover the eyes of the patient with moistened pledgets of gauze or cotton, and the operator must wear goggles. Conjunctivitis could result from neglect of these precautions.

The aforementioned erythema with resulting increase in local circulation and the well-known bactericidal effect of ultraviolet radiation govern its indications. It is extensively used in the treatment of decubitus ulcers, infected superficial wounds, and many skin diseases. It has been shown to produce antirachitic effects also.

Infrared radiation. The infrared lamp is a simple way to apply local heat. There are various kinds and sizes of infrared lamps. The energy output that reaches the patient depends on the wattage of the lamp, the distance from the lamp to the patient, the angle at which the rays strike the patient, and the total area radiated. Infrared radiation includes the light radiation from 770 to 220,000 millimicrons. The amount used in physical medicine usually ranges from 1,200 to 1,500 millimicrons. This includes no bactericidal rays. The main effect consists of heating the local area.

Infrared radiations are used in the treatment of arthritis, bursitis, fibrositis, muscle strain, and muscle spasm. It is a convenient way to apply heat at home.

Infrared treatments should not be given following large doses of deep irradiation, because serious burns sometimes result.

Electrotherapy

Electrotherapy includes electrical stimulation and diathermy.

Electrical stimulation. Each electrical stimulation machine will give a variety of currents in combination, but the main currents used are galvanic and faradic. Galvanic current stimulates the muscle and therefore causes a response in patients whose nerves have been damaged. Faradic current stimulates the nerve and can only stimulate a muscle with a normal nerve innervation. These currents and their various combinations and derivatives can be used as testing devices to determine whether or not the nerve to the muscle is normal. If it is damaged the extent of the damage and the rate of nerve rejuvenation can be determined. Electrical stimulation approaches voluntary activity, producing approximately the same metabolic effects, and has proved valuable as a form of exercise to avoid muscle atrophy.

Diathermy. Shortwave diathermy is used to generate heat in the body tissues by means of the resistance offered by the tissues to the high-frequency currents forced through them. Diathermy can be administered by wrapping cables around the part to be treated or by applying the drums to the area. A padding of toweling ½ to 2 inches thick is used between the skin and electrodes to absorb perspiration and prevent burning. Physiologically, the effects of shortwave diathermy are synonymous with the effects of any other type of heat. The only difference is that the hyperemia produced by shortwave lasts longer and penetrates the deeper layers of tissue.

Diathermy is used for treatment of chronic sinusitis, mild inflammation of bone, joint, and muscle, chronic osteomyelitis, and various forms of arthritis and bursitis. High-frequency currents are also used surgically. Fulguration and

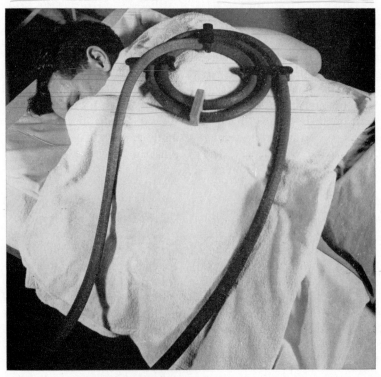

Fig. 54. Diathermy coils wound to produce heat on the upper back. No bare coil may be allowed to touch the patient's skin or another coil.

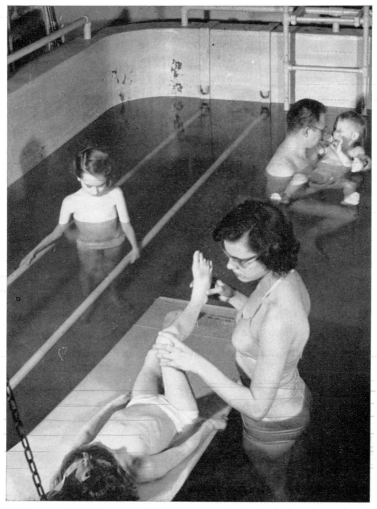

Fig. 55. By the use of this canvas table routine stretching exercises as well as underwater exercises and walking practice can be given in the pool.

electrodesiccation are used to destroy warts and small skin blemishes. Electrocoagulation is used to remove large tumors and to stop bleeding.

Hydrotherapy

Hydrotherapy consists of the use of therapeutic pools, the Hubbard tank, whirlpools, contrast baths, sprays and douches, and hot packs.

Therapeutic pools. To be most useful a therapeutic pool should be 12 to 15 feet wide and 20 to 24 feet long. It should have walking bars and proper depth to permit walking practice for the patients. The temperature of the water depends on the amount of activity the patient will perform, the age and diagnosis of the patient, and the length of time the patient will be in the water. If the program is one essentially for exercise, the water could be between 80° and 95° F. If a heating effect is desired, the temperature could be up as high as 102° F.

Therapeutic pools have proved very

valuable in treating patients convalescing from poliomyelitis and children with cerebral palsy. The buoyancy of the water makes it possible for a child to use a weakened muscle through a greater range of motion. Patients can use the walking bars in the pool earlier than out of the pool because of the buoyancy of the water. The heat of the water raises the pain threshold so that the patient can tolerate stretching exercises more easily. The buoyancy and the heat encourage relaxation of the cerebral palsy patient, and he can perform his exercises with more ease. In addition to the physical and physiologic benefits from a therapeutic pool, the psychologic lift to the patient is very valuable. He just feels better after he has been in the pool and looks forward to the next treatment.

Hubbard tank. The shape of the Hubbard tank is such that it permits exercise movements of the arms and legs that are not possible in an ordinary tub. The water temperature is usually kept at about 99° to 100° F. for exercise and 102° F. for fever. Although a Hubbard tank is not as satisfactory as a therapeutic pool for exercise, it is frequently employed. Since it is not necessary for the therapist to be in the pool to care for the patient as it is in a therapeutic pool, the Hubbard tank may be more practical as far as the personnel are concerned. The tank may also be used in place of the fever cabinet to induce fevers of less duration. Sometimes a whirlpool agitator is placed in the tank.

Whirlpools. The temperature of the water in the whirlpool is maintained between 100° and 110° F., usually 105° F. The air pressure coming into the water gives a swirling, gentle massaging action to the water. Whirlpools are especially valuable in treating patients with fractures or muscle transplants after removal of splints. The whirlpool

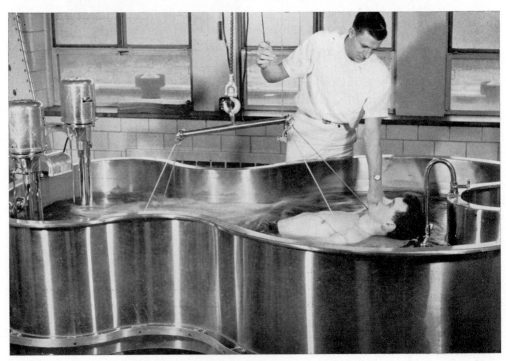

Fig. 56. The patient is lowered into the Hubbard tank by a hydraulic lift.

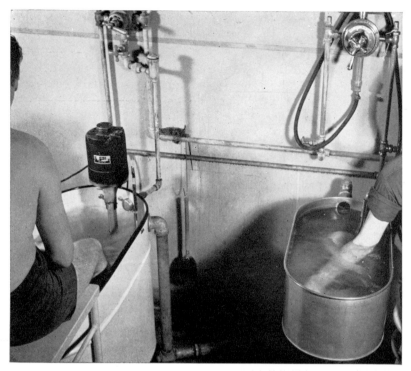

Fig. 57. Leg and arm whirlpools.

treatment makes it much easier to clean dry scaly skin from affected areas, increases circulation to the part, and tends to relieve pain and stiffness. Whirlpools are also used in the treatment of burns and amputations that are not completely healed. In these cases a mild antiseptic solution is often added to the water. Children can be put into the whirlpool tank for general heating to the entire body prior to stretching and exercises. Whirlpool treatment for patients with arthritis has proved very helpful in relieving pain.

Contrast baths. In contrast baths the patient's feet or hands are moved alternately from hot to cold tubs of water. The temperature in the hot tubs ranges from 100° to 105° F. and in the cold tubs from 65° to 70° F. Immersion should begin and end in hot water—4 minutes in hot water and 1 minute in cold water. Seven to nine immersions are usually given. The treatment is generally used for arthritis and peripheral vascular disease and as a preliminary to massage and exercise for sprains and contusions.

Sprays and douches. There are many kinds of sprays, douches, ablutions, and affusions used in various hospitals. They are beneficial because of the heating effect or the alternate heat and cold as in contrast baths. They are also used as a refresher after prolonged heat treatment.

Hot packs. There are many ways to make and apply hot packs in a hospital and at home. One of the most convenient methods is one in which a very heavy turkish towel (or two turkish towels sewed together) is heated in boiling water and then quickly wrung out so that as little steam as possible escapes. The pack is then wrapped inside a 40-inch square of wool blanket. In this pack the patient's skin is not touched by the hot towels but only by the dry wool with the steam coming through it. There is no danger of burning the patient if he is carefully dried off between the application of packs. While one set of packs is on the patient, another set should be boiling. The first set is left on 3 to 4 minutes, and then the second is applied. Three or four sets are usually needed. These packs are easily applied to almost any area of the body, either by laying the pack on the area or by wrapping it. They have been found very beneficial in treating various areas with muscle

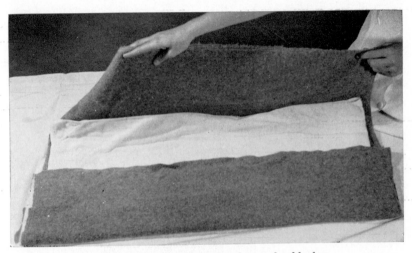

Fig. 58. A steaming hot towel being folded inside the dry woolen blanket.

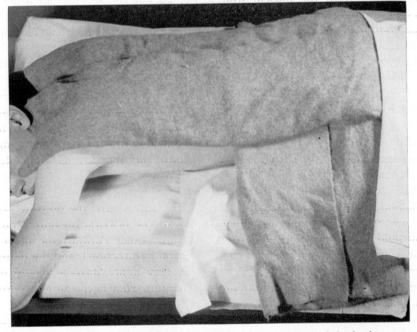

Fig. 59. Hot packs applied to the back for pain in the lower portion of the back.

spasm, strains, sprains, arthritis, and bursitis. Many hospitals prefer hot packs for heat to any of the other available methods.

Mechanotherapy

Mechanotherapy includes massage and therapeutic exercises.

Massage. Massage is the term applied to the systematic and scientific manipulation of body tissues for remedial and restorative purposes. For effective application of massage it is essential that one has (1) a fundamental knowledge of muscle, joint, and nerve anatomy of the affected part, (2) a knowledge of the desired effects, and (3) a skillful technique and understanding of the various strokes.

Physiologic effects of massage on the skin include a sedative effect on the peripheral sensory nerves, with a resulting reflex stimulation of motor nerves, a temporary hyperemia, and a cleansing of the epidermis. The main effect on the muscles is the hastening of the removal of metabolites from the muscle which helps relieve fatigue and spasm. Massage will not build up muscle strength. Only active exercise can do that. Depending on the intensity of the stimuli, massage can produce either a sedative or a stimulating effect on the nervous system. It has been shown that massage definitely increases the pain threshold; this is apparently related to the counterirritant phenomenon. Since the lymph circulatory system is entirely dependent upon external pressures (normally, muscle contraction and joint movement), massage has proved valuable in moving lymph fluid in patients with edematous conditions. Massage has a minimal effect on venous or arterial flow. The pumping action of the heart is a much more adequate means of circulating the blood. More recent literature indicates that massage produces no significant change

in red or white blood cell count or in the hemoglobin. Massage cannot rub away excess fatty tissue. A very heavy abdominal massage given to animals produced multiple hemorrhages in the area but no change in the amount of adipose tissue. Massage is highly effective in stretching excessive fibrous tissue in subcutaneous areas.

The massage technique is generally based on the following four strokes. Effleurage consists of stroking the surface of the skin. The amount of pressure is varied to make it a light or heavy stroking. Petrissage is the kneading of the soft tissues. Friction is applied by rotary movements of the skin over underlying tissue. The thumb or fingers are kept in firm contact with the skin, and the movement is between the skin and superficial tissue and the underlying structures. Tapotement consists of a percussion-type movement against bodily tissues. This type of massage has very little place in the treatment of pathologic conditions because it is too heavy.

To get the best results from a massage the patient should be in a comfortable relaxed position. The part to be massaged must be supported and completely uncovered, and the rest of the patient's body carefully draped. The operator should be in a comfortable working position. Once the massage is started, the therapist's hands maintain contact with the part being massaged until the massage is completed. The stroking pattern generally follows the muscle groups. The rhythm should be slow and steady; the pressure gentle but firm. The heaviest pressure is on the upward stroke (toward the heart, centripetal in direction), and the return stroke is very light. Massage should never be painful. Pain is the prime contraindication for massage. Cold cream is generally preferred as a lubricant, although cocoa butter is often used for burned or scarred areas, and talcum powder is used over hairy surfaces. Any baby oil, olive oil, or mineral oil may be used. Considering the physiologic effects of massage, it is used in the treatment of patients with arthritis, fibrositis, edema, traumatic conditions such as sprains and strains, fractures, burns, amputations, and various areas of muscle spasm. Massage should not be given to anyone with any acute inflammatory process, skin eruption, malignancy, or fever.

Therapeutic exercise. The aim of therapeutic exercise is to achieve a maximum body function for each particular individual. Therapeutic exercises classified according to type of exercise are passive, active assistive, active, and resistive.

Passive exercise. The motion involved in passive exercise is performed by some outside force. It may be a gentle relaxed motion just carried to the patient's tolerance or a stretching motion carried beyond the patient's tolerance to prevent muscle contractures or to achieve joint mobility.

Active assistive exercise. The patient performs this exercise with the assistance of the operator. The division of labor should be such that the patient is doing all within his capacity and the therapist gives just the very minimum of assistance or completes the range of motion that the patient cannot achieve alone. An assistive exercise is often given in such a position as to eliminate gravity, since the weight of the extremity is often too much resistance for the muscle.

Active exercise. The patient performs the movement wholly by himself with no aid from outside forces.

Resistive exercise. The patient performs the exercise and is resisted by the therapist or an apparatus. At the start the resistance is at a minimum, and it is gradually increased as the strength of the exercised muscle increases. To gain strength in a muscle as rapidly as possible resistance should be sufficient to

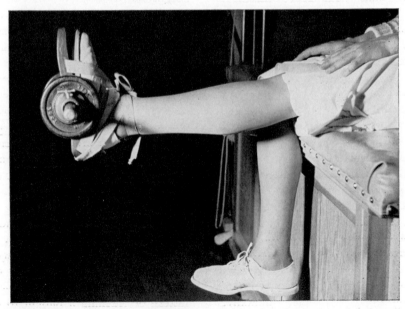

Fig. 60. Resistance exercise for the quadriceps muscle. Starting position for this exercise is sitting with the legs over the edge of the table with a rolled towel placed under the knee for proper support. The leg being exercised is then raised to the position shown, held there for a few seconds, and slowly lowered.

fatigue the muscle after ten repetitions of the exercise. For a patient with a weak muscle manual resistance by the therapist is sufficient. As soon as the patient is able to perform the arc of motion against weight, an apparatus may be used. Regulation apparatus, such as a quadriceps boot, back and abdominal resistance harness, DeLorme exercise table, and various pedaling and pulley devices, are used in a physical therapy department. This equipment can be adjusted easily to the proper amount of resistance. For home exercises relatively simple devices, such as weight bags, pails with sand, scale weights, or window-sash weights, can be adapted to provide resistance. As in any form of exercise, the muscle will perform most efficiently if a warm-up period is given prior to the maximum effort required. A satisfactory pattern for exercise is as follows: (1) ten repetitions with 25% maximum weight, (2) ten repetitions with 60% maximum weight, and (3) ten repetitions with 100% maximum weight.

To obtain satisfactory results from any exercise it must be performed regularly for a relatively long period of time. In most cases this program can only be started in the hospital and must be carried on at home.

The scope of therapeutic exercise is indeed broad. It includes coordination exercises for patients with multiple sclerosis and cerebral palsy; muscle-strengthening exercises for those with many orthopedic and neurologic disorders; exercises to prevent a deformity, such as range of motion activity for the patient with arthritis; to correct a deformity, such as a clubfoot; and to maintain mobility of joint and muscle, such as stretching for patients with poliomyelitis. Exercises are given for an esthetic effect, as in the treatment of patients with postural defects, and to give relief from pain, as in patients with pain in the lower portion of the back. Exercises are given to teach a patient to relax. Respiratory exercises will increase a patient's vital capacity. In England much work has been done with breathing exercises for patients with asthma. The patient has been able to increase his ability to breathe during an attack and in many cases to prevent an attack. Exercises given for peripheral vascular disease will improve the efficiency of the circulatory system.

Let us briefly follow a patient in his attempts to ambulate after four months in traction because of a hip fracture. During the past several weeks the therapist has had the patient perform a series of arm-strengthening exercises in preparation for his ambulation. The first step will be the tilt table, where the patient is strapped across the knees and abdomen and gradually brought from the horizontal to the vertical position. He may have crutches to take some of the weight off his feet. When the patient tolerates the tilt table in a vertical position for several minutes, he is advanced to parallel bars, where he learns the proper gait and can practice balancing himself. The bars are more stable than crutches, and the patient develops confidence in his walking ability. When he can walk several lengths of the parallel bars, he is fitted properly with crutches. Once he learns the proper gait and develops some skill and endurance in handling crutches, he is taught to get in and out of a chair, to climb up and down stairs, to walk backward and sideways, and to open and close doors. A person on crutches can learn to be very independent and capable of taking care of himself in almost any circumstance. This pattern of teaching a patient to be ambulatory is in evidence at many stages every day in a physical therapy department.

STUDY QUESTIONS

1. Select several pictures from a magazine and study the body alignment. Do they represent good or poor body alignment? What criteria of good posture can you cite to support your opinion?
2. Does the furniture in your room (bed, chair, and desk) promote good body alignment and prevent undue fatigue?
3. Cite principles of body mechanics you will use when doing the following activities: moving a patient to the side of the bed, giving back care to a bed patient, and assisting a patient with a tub bath.
4. Describe the normal motions at each of the following joints: ankle, knee, hip, and shoulder.
5. Be prepared to describe or demonstrate good back-lying position, good side-lying position, and good face-lying position.
6. Explain in detail the nursing care you will provide for the bed patient to prevent drop foot, flexion contracture of the knee, flexion contracture of the hip, external rotation of the hip, adduction of the shoulder joint, and wrist drop.
7. Discuss some concrete ways in which the nurse and physical therapist may assist each other in the care of orthopedic patients.

REFERENCES

Barckley, V., and Campbell, E. I.: Helping the handicapped child achieve emotional maturity, Am. J. Nursing 59:376-379, 1959.

Bier, R. I.: Rehabilitation on a shoestring, Am. J. Nursing 61:98-100, 1961.

Brown, F. G.: Who said care of long term patients is routine? Am. J. Nursing 62:58-61, 1962.

Buchwald, E., Rusk, H. A., Deaver, G., and Covalt, D. A.: Physical rehabilitation for daily living, New York, 1952, McGraw-Hill Book Co., Inc.

Buck, L.: Nursing care during the long rest period, Am. J. Nursing 61:91-92, 1961.

Covalt, D. A., and Buchwald, E.: Aids to ambulation, Am. J. Nursing 53:1085-1088, 1953.

Deaver, G. G.: Rehabilitation—a philosophy, Am. J. Nursing 59:1278, 1959.

Dock, W.: The evil sequelae of complete bedrest, J.A.M.A. 125:1083-1085, 1944.

Fash, B.: Kinesiology in nursing, New York, 1952, McGraw-Hill Book Co., Inc.

Fisher, S. H.: Role of the psychiatrist on a rehabilitation service, Arch. Phys. Med. 37:347-348, 1956.

Fox, V., and Spain, R. W.: The long-term patient: a new challenge to nursing, Nursing Outlook 4:559-561, 1956.

Hartigan, H.: Nursing responsibilities in rehabilitation, Nursing Outlook 2:649-651, 1954.

Hauser, E. D.: The child's posture, Am. J. Nursing 55:1338-1341, 1955.

Holmes, Oliver Wendell: Medical essays: scholastic and bedside teaching, Boston, 1892, Houghton Mifflin Co.

Howorth, M. B.: Posture in adolescent adults, Am. J. Nursing 56:34-36, 1956.

Hurd, G.: Teaching the hemiplegic self-care, Am. J. Nursing 62:64-68, 1962.

Institute of Physical Medicine and Rehabilitation: Rehabilitation monographs I-VIII and X, New York University, Bellevue Medical Center, 400 East 34th Street, New York 16, N. Y.

   An evaluation of rehabilitation (I)
   Psychiatric aspects of rehabilitation (II)
   Bladder and bowel training for patients with spinal cord disease (III)
   Manual of procedures of the children's division (IV)
   Braces, crutches, wheelchairs (V)
   Self-help devices for the arthritic (VI)
   Survey of 95 custodial patients in a municipal hospital (VII)
   A manual for training the disabled homemaker (VIII)
   Activities of daily living (X)

Jerome, M. M.: Rehabilitation of the bed patient, Am. J. Nursing 59:1279, 1959.

Jones, F., Benz, G., Mereness, D., Kleffner, F., and Jensen, D.: Principles and technics of rehabilitation nursing, ed. 2, St. Louis, 1961, The C. V. Mosby Co.

Jones, Sir Robert: Notes on military orthopedics, London, 1917, Cassell & Co., Ltd.

Madden, B., and Affeldt, J.: To prevent helplessness and deformities, Am. J. Nursing 62:59-61, 1962.

Mercita, Sister M., and others: Rehabilitation, Nursing Outlook 10:581, 1962.

Morrissey, A. B.: Rehabilitation in hemiplegia . . . major nursing functions, Am. J. Nursing 62:58-61, 1962.

Morrissey, A. B.: Psychosocial and spiritual

factors in rehabilitation, Am. J. Nursing **50:** 763-766, 1950.

Morrissey, A. B.: Rehabilitation nursing, New York, 1951, G. P. Putnam's Sons.

Morrissey, A. B.: The nurse and rehabilitation, Am. J. Nursing **54:**1354-1355, 1954.

Morrissey, A. B., and Sherman, N.: The tilt board—an aid to rehabilitation, Am. J. Nursing **56:**1146-1147, 1956.

Morrissey, A. B., and Zimmerman, M. E.: Helps for the handicapped, Am. J. Nursing **53:**316-318, 1953.

National Society for Handicapped and Adults: Self-help clothing for handicapped, 2023 West Ogden Avenue, Chicago 2, Ill.

Olmsted, L.: The orthopedic nurse specialist in the hospital, Am. J. Nursing **45:**838-841, 1945.

Peszczynski, M.: The rehabilitation potential of the adult hemiplegic, Am. J. Nursing **63:** 111-114, 1963.

Phillips, E.: The role of the nurse in rehabilitation, Canad. Nurse **52:**810-818, 1956.

Rusk, H. A.: Rehabilitation belongs in the general hospital, Am. J. Nursing **62:**62-63, 1962.

Rusk, H.: A.: Rehabilitation medicine, ed. 2, St. Louis, 1964, The C. V. Mosby Co.

Rusk, H. A., and Taylor, E. J.: New hope for the handicapped: the rehabilitation of the disabled from the bed to the job, New York, 1949, Harper & Brothers.

Rusk, H. A., and Taylor, E. J.: Living with a disability, Garden City, N. Y., 1953, Blakiston Co., Inc.

Schroeder, C.: Accepting the handicapped pupil, Nursing Outlook **11:**372-373, 1963.

Smith, G. W.: A stroke is not the end of the world, Am. J. Nursing **57:**303-305, 1957.

Stevenson, J. L.: Posture and nursing. Published and distributed by the Joint Orthopedic Nursing Advisory Service, 1790 Broadway, ed. 2, revised, 1948.

Talbot, H. S.: A concept of rehabilitation, Rehabilitation Literature, **22:**358-364, 1961.

Taylor, W.: Rehabilitation of the ambulatory patient, Am. J. Nursing **59:**1280, 1959.

Van Kaam, A. L.: The nurse in the patient's world, Am. J. Nursing **59:**1708-1710, 1959.

Ward, M. M.: Self-help fashions for the physically disabled child, Am. J. Nursing **58:** 526-527, 1958.

Ward, M. M.: Toilet seats for disabled children, Am. J. Nursing **57:**483-485, 1957.

Wellvard, F.: The meaning of rehabilitation, Canad. Nurse **52:**904-910, 1956.

Whitehouse, F. A.: Stroke—some psychosocial problems it causes, Am. J. Nursing **63:**81-87, 1963.

Wiebe, A. M.: Orthopedics in nursing, Philadelphia, 1961, W. B. Saunders Co.

Williams, M., and Worthingham, C.: Therapeutic exercise in body alignment and function, Stanford, 1953, Stanford University Press.

Winters, M. C.: Protective body mechanics in daily life and nursing, Philadelphia, 1952, W. B. Saunders Co.

Wolff, I. S., and Wilcoxson, H.: The public health nurse and the patient with long-term illness, Am. J. Nursing **56:**614-618, 1956.

Wright, J.: Protective body mechanics in convalescence, Am. J. Nursing **45:**699-703, 1945.

Chapter 2

General features
of orthopedic nursing

Nursing care of patients in casts

To preserve the efficiency of a cast and, at the same time, to maintain the patient in cleanliness and comfort taxes the ingenuity of the best nurse. This skill is one of the most essential of orthopedic nursing, and doctors frequently judge the competency of the nursing staff by the care they give to patients in casts. No one way of caring for these patients can be arbitrarily defined, and nurses are learning new and better methods daily. The directions given here are offered solely to the perplexed nurse who has not had sufficient experience in these matters to assume the care of patients in casts to her own and the doctor's satisfaction.

The efficiency of the cast (that is, its ability to maintain the position for which it has been applied over the period of time necessary for the accomplishment of the doctor's purpose) is the nurse's responsibility. Yet she must be constantly aware that the patient inside the cast is her first concern. One thing she must understand clearly from the outset is that the patient's every complaint must have her prompt attention, even though his complaint seems trifling and she may privately consider him a chronic complainer. The patient who seldom complains will be given solicitous attention when he reports a burning sensation over common points of pressure, such as the heel, the malleoli, or the sacrum. It is the constantly complaining patient who may be overlooked, so that when the cast is finally removed a sloughing sore appears over an area he told the nurse about at one time. It is the old "wolf-wolf" story in an orthopedic version.

OBSERVATION OF CIRCULATION

Nurses have been warned repeatedly about the dangers of impaired circulation in an extremity upon which a new cast has been applied, and it seems as though the subject could be passed over with a word. However, the alarming number of accidents that occur year after year in the hospital wards because of neglect of this extremely serious matter does not justify an optimistic attitude. It is as important to inspect fingers and toes that have been recently encased in plaster as it is to take a pulse after an operation. Circulatory impairment is as important to watch for as are signs of hemorrhage. The rapidity with which it may progress from bad to worse is difficult for the inexperienced nurse to comprehend. A paralysis of such seriousness that the patient may never again be able to use his hand or foot may be produced within a 24-hour period.

Nurses should be familiar with the blanching sign. This is particularly important in caring for patients who have casts applied to the leg or arm. The nail of the thumb or great toe is momentarily compressed and the return flow of blood to the nail is observed. The compressed area should refill with blood immediately upon the release of pressure; that is, the nail should turn from white to pink at once. It must be emphasized, however, that some blood often remains in the fingers or toes even after circulation is impaired, and the nurse may be misled to believe that the circulation is satisfactory because blood does return, although somewhat sluggishly. Doctors warn us that the anemic area must flush rapidly with blood and that the fingers or toes should be warm and of good color. Inspection should be made every 10 to 15 minutes if there is any sign of impaired circulation.

Frequently the physician will cut a hole in an arm cast near the radial artery, so that the nurse can take the pulse of the patient frequently through this opening to ascertain whether the circulation to the hand is normal. The order on the chart will usually read simply: "Take the patient's pulse every 10 minutes." This does not mean that the nurse is to take his pulse to assure herself of the patient's general condition, as she does in other patients postoperatively, but rather to keep an accurate check of the circulation in the extremity in the cast. Misunderstanding this order, nurses have been known to take the pulse religiously every 10 minutes on the un-

affected wrist, not realizing the special significance of the order in orthopedic cases. Such an order should indicate to the nurse the grave necessity the physician feels of checking circulation in that arm. Failure to feel the pulse under the cast is warrant for notifying him at once. Symptoms of coldness, pallor, blueness, edema, loss of motion, numbness, pain, and a slow return of blood to the part on blanching are cardinal. In addition, it is important that the nurse be able to see all the fingers and toes. Nor should she be satisfied with 12 or 24 hours of close watching. The extremity must be watched during many succeeding days. A feeling of security is not justified merely because the patient is conscious and in apparent good condition after the operation.

CARE OF THE CAST

Supporting the wet cast. The care of the patient as an individual is primary, but the cast is important also. The doctor has spent considerable time and thought on the cast. He sends the patient from the operating room to the ward, often with some concern as to the treatment the cast will receive. The doctor should expect the nurse caring for the patient to know how to protect the cast. It has cost both time and money, and its importance in the patient's recovery is considerable.

The care of the cast begins before the patient returns to the ward from the plaster room. It begins with the preparation of the bed. A firm mattress is a necessity. Boards spread, preferably lengthwise, under the mattress are essential when the cast is the body type, or a hip spica, enclosing the legs and the body. Pillows should be ready to support the wet cast. These pillows need rubber or plastic covers to prevent dampness and mustiness that will result from absorption of moisture from the

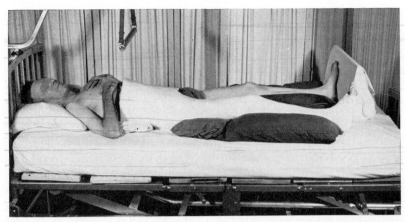

Fig. 61. Correct support for the patient in a hip spica cast in the supine position. The pillows beneath the limb enclosed in plaster provide support for the thigh and avoid pressure on the heel. The small pad that supports the lumbar region prevents the anterior portion of the cast from pressing on the abdomen, and the pillow for the head, placed well down under the shoulders, maintains good alignment of the cervical spine. Boards beneath the mattress provide a firm surface for the cast. Note the trapeze, which facilitates nursing care of the patient in a hip spica cast.

plaster. They also need to be pliable and easily adjusted to the coutour of the patient's body. If the patient is to have a body cast, three pillows laid crosswise on the bed are usually satisfactory. For a hip spica cast it is best to arrange one pillow crosswise at the level of the waist with two laid lengthwise for the single leg in the cast. If both legs are to be encased, two more pillows will be needed for the second leg of the adult patient. A pillow for the head and shoulders will be necessary if the patient has not had an anesthetic. Under no circumstances is the damp cast to be lifted directly onto the hard bed when the patient is returned from the plaster room. One of the chief causes of pressure sores in orthopedic patients is allowing an incompletely set cast to lie unsupported on a hard surface. The cast will become flattened over the bony prominences, particularly the back of the heel and the sacrum, and damage to the underlying soft tissues will be unavoidable.

Some doctors prefer to have one sand-bag placed under the groin on the affected side and another under the heel. These are used to prevent excessive weight on the damp cast. It is essential that no sharp break in the pillow alignment under the cast be allowed that might cause the cast to sag at some strategic point, particularly at the junction of the leg and body sections of the hip spica cast.

The patient must be lifted carefully onto the bed, not simply rolled or dumped onto it. Much damage to casts occurs at this point. The nurse supervising this procedure must use only the palms of her hands, and not her fingers, to lift the cast. Fingers may make indentations in the soft plaster if it is not sufficiently set. This is particularly important in handling the foot and leg section of the cast. Support should be given all along the cast, particularly under the hip and knee, to prevent any cracking.

Drying the cast. If the patient has not been anesthetized, the cast is usually left uncovered for several hours. Many phy-

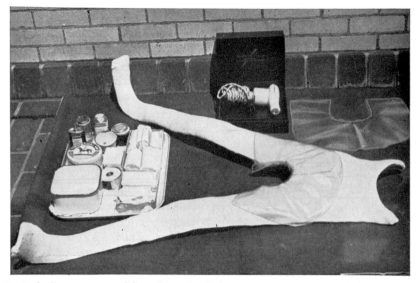

Fig. 62. Bedside cast tray and hair dryer for daily use on casts. Anterior shelf is covered with stockinet and protected with waterproofing.

sicians prefer that casts be dried in this way, that is, by natural evaporation. If, however, quick drying is essential, as it often is when the patient is to leave the hospital shortly, it can be started as soon as the cast is set. However, a cast should never be baked until it has set, for the temperature may be raised to the point where setting proceeds slowly. After the cast has set it is usually satisfactory to use some form of external heat for drying it. Heat lamps or a cradle on which a low watt incandescent lamp is suspended at a safe distance from the patient and the cast may be used for this. Cages of wire encircling these lamp bulbs are desirable, and a distance of at least 15 inches from the cast to the light is usually considered safe. The cradle should not be covered with bedclothes because the moisture will go back to the cast as the confined space under the bedclothes becomes saturated. Escape for the moisture-laden air is essential. Another method for drying casts is provided by specially constructed cast dryers that usually allow

for circulation of air around the cast as well as for heat. These are excellent for drying casts evenly and quickly. A hand dryer, such as is used for hair drying, may be employed and is especially good for small areas of plaster that have become dampened through mishaps. Intense heat is never recommended because it tends to cause the outer layers to dry too swiftly while the underlying layers remain moist.

During warm weather it has been frequently observed that, with the early setting and drying process, the cast becomes very hot, so much so that it is sometimes necessary to provide the patient with ice bags and electric fans to prevent heat exhaustion. If the cast is left entirely uncovered, the air will greatly hasten evaporation and hardening, and the heat of the cast will be transitory.

It may be wise to insert here something about the basic chemistry of plaster of paris, so that the nurse may know exactly what is happening in the cast as it sets and hardens. In the excellent pamphlet on plaster casts prepared by the Curity Research Laboratories, Edward Atkinson says: "The crystalline substance, gypsum, is dihydrated calcium sulfate, having the chemical formula $CaSO_4 \cdot 2H_2O$. In its natural state, gypsum contains about 21 per cent of water of crystallization, water (H_2O) which is combined in the crystals of calcium sulfate ($CaSO_4$). When gypsum crystals are pulverized and heated to about 250° F., all but about 6 per cent of this water of crystallization is driven off into the air. The calcined gypsum which remains is plaster of Paris.

"If water is added to plaster of Paris, the reverse action takes place—the plaster takes up sufficient water to replace the moisture driven off by the heating process and crystals of gypsum are again formed."*

The writer comments that what we call a plaster of paris cast is in reality a gypsum cast: "As soon as water is added to pure plaster of Paris, gypsum crystals begin to form. During the formation of these gypsum crystals the potential full strength is determined according to the closeness with which the crystals interlock during their formation." The maximum strength is obtained only after all excess water has been evaporated from the cast's surface. When this is accomplished and the cast is wholly dry, it is strong and firm and able to withstand sudden stresses.

Turning the patient. The time of the first turning of a patient in a new cast is frequently dependent on the physician's order, but in orthopedic hospitals a standing order usually exists that all patients be turned by the evening of the day the cast is applied. This is done,

first, for the comfort of the patient and, second, so that the cast may be dried on its posterior surface. The first turning of a patient in a body cast or a hip spica cast requires more help than will be needed subsequently when the cast has become rigid and firm through drying. To turn a patient with a new cast without assistance endangers the cast and should not be attempted if it can be avoided.

With a crew of three people an adult patient in a hip spica cast can be turned without much risk either to the patient's comfort or to the integrity of the cast. The patient is gently pulled toward the side of the bed that corresponds to the leg in plaster. With patients who have recently been operated upon and are apprehensive of pain all three of the crew should stand at this side of the bed. It is possible to effect this moving by exerting a pull on the pillows beneath the cast. When the patient is pulled to this side, two of the crew should go around the bed, where if necessary a fresh drawsheet may be started and the pillows may be arranged to receive the cast when the patient is turned.

Dry pillowcases may be necessary if the ones in use are damp. When the pillowcases do not need changing, it is sometimes possible to pull the pillows partially through from under the cast without allowing the cast to drop from them.

Turning should always be done on the side not enclosed in plaster or toward the side that has not been operated upon if the cast is a double spica. The patient is thus turned on his normal leg and toward the nurses who are assisting him. One nurse remains on the side of the bed toward which the patient has been pulled in order to overcome any sense of insecurity he may have from a fear of falling. The other two nurses turn the patient toward them from the oppo-

*Atkinson, E. W., Curity Research Laboratories: Plaster casts: their preparation in the hospital, Walpole, Mass., 1937, Lewis Manufacturing Co., Division of The Kendall Co.

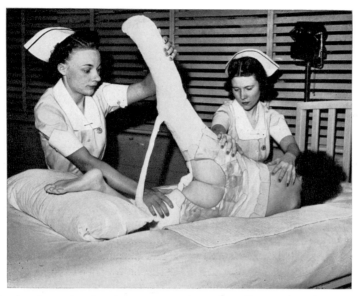

Fig. 63. Turning the patient in a hip spica cast. Note the pillow in place for foot support. The abduction bar should not be used as a handle when lifting or turning the patient.

site side. The patient is told exactly what is to be done, and he is instructed to place the arm on which he is turning above his head. With adult patients it may be easier to have the patient keep his arms close to his sides. To avoid pressure on the arm on which he is turning a folded towel should be placed between the arm and the cast. The pillow beneath the patient's head should be removed during the turning. In turning, care is taken to move in unison. One nurse places her hands on the shoulder and hip of the patient, and the other supports the thigh and foot of the extremity in the cast. The nurse on the opposite side assists with the turning by pulling the shoulder through as the patient is gently eased onto his face.

Pillows along the entire length of the cast must be in readiness in order to avoid lifting the patient once he is turned. Lifting the cast is exceedingly hard on the patient and endangers the soft cast. In addition, it is an unnecessary strain to the nurse's back that can be avoided with foresight. After the patient has been turned the nurse should observe his position to see that the toes of the leg in the cast do not jam against the bed. A pillow laid crosswise on the bed will provide support for both feet. If there is wide abduction in the cast, the toes of the foot in plaster may hang over the edge of the mattress. Another point to observe is the position of the body section of the cast. If there are too many pillows under the patient's head and shoulders, the plaster may press into the back just below the ribs. If the pillow under the abdomen is not placed correctly, the cast edges may press into the soft tissues of the chest and abdomen.

Later, when the cast is completely hardened, one or two nurses may turn the patient with a minimum of difficulty. Patients soon learn to assist with turning to such an extent that little help is needed from the nurse or attendant. When the cast is dry, pillows are needed only for the patient's comfort and may be dispensed with except at points of pressure. A support for the heel so that

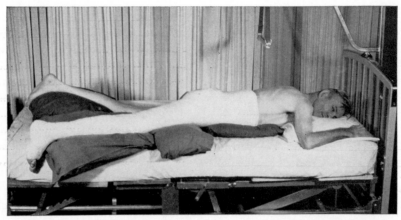

Fig. 64. Correct support for the patient in a hip spica cast in the prone position. The extremity enclosed in plaster is supported by pillows to prevent strain on the cast at the groin area. There is enough abduction to permit the foot enclosed in plaster to extend over the edge of the mattress. The thin pillow placed crosswise at the top edge of the cast prevents undue pressure on the abdomen, and one pillow for the head maintains good alignment of the shoulders and neck. Note the position of the normal extremity.

it does not rest on the bed is usually considered essential, and patients are usually more comfortable with a pillow beneath the body portion of the cast as they lie prone. When this pillow is in place, the patient's chest will be the forward portion of the body, which is always desirable for good body alignment.

When the patient is turned the first time, the cast will still be damp on its posterior surface and will usually be rather compressed against the back. Some method of quick drying should be used at this time, and the patient's back should be given meticulous care. The buttocks will be blue and creased and will need particular attention. The skin around the cast edges and immediately beneath the cast can be reached with the fingers, and this area can be rubbed and gently stretched away from the cast to increase comfort and circulation. Any rough edges on the posterior surface of the cast must be cared for at this time. Insufficient room for defecation should be noted and reported. The stockinet lining may be pulled down snugly in-

side the cast and attached over its edges by securing it temporarily with small pieces of transparent mending tape or adhesive tape, although the latter will not adhere well to the moist surface of the cast. It is too soon to finish the cast permanently. This will have to be tended to the following day. If the patient is a child, however, some thought must be given to the protection of the buttocks region. It is never safe to hope the child will get through the night without soiling his cast. Waterproof material may be tucked under the cast as securely as possible and will usually suffice for the night without being fastened with tape. A scratcher bandage may be inserted under the cast at this time if the patient complains of an itching sensation. The patient should be urged to lie prone as long as he can. Encouragement from the nurse may often prolong this period to from 45 minutes to an hour. When this rest period is completed, he is again turned with the precautions described.

If the surgeon has ordered a window cut over the abdomen or chest, it is usually wise to wait until the cast is dry before having this done. There is a tendency for the cast to break or buckle if the window is cut too early. The surgeon, of course, should be consulted in this matter.

Finishing the cast edges. Perhaps the most common method of finishing cast edges is by using adhesive tape. To prevent the tape from rolling the cast must be thoroughly dry. This usually requires 24 to 48 hours, depending on the thickness of the cast and the humidity of the air. Petals of tape cut round or oval and about 1½ inches in diameter are excellent to bind cast edges or to apply waterproofing. Curved edges of adhesive tape do not roll as easily as square edges. When the tape is applied, it is important that the edges be pressed securely against the plaster to prevent the tape from rolling and sticking to the bed linen. Plaster of paris strips may be moistened and placed over the adhesive tape to hold the petals of tape in place and to maintain a smooth tape-covered cast edge.

Another satisfactory method of petalling cast edges is to fold a length of 2-inch wide adhesive tape lengthwise and cut it through at a 45-degree angle. The diamond-shaped pieces are then unfolded and applied to the cast with the single point on the outside and the double points on the underside of the cast. This method is more economic in the use of time and materials than the use of circle petals.

If a stockinet has been used to line the cast, the ideal method of finishing the cast is to pull the stockinet out over the edges and secure it with a plaster splint. This can be done at the bedside. The splint is cut to the size needed and immersed in water to moisten. It is then placed in the desired position to secure the stockinet. If the cast is hard and dry, it is advisable to roughen the surface prior to the application of the splint. Roughening of the dry plaster cast plus rubbing will make the plaster splint adhere to the cast surface.

Before the cast edges are finished all rough spots or irregularities likely to

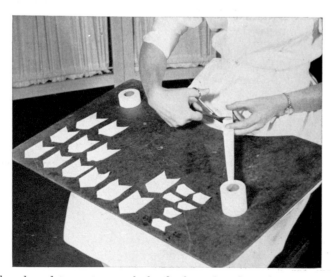

Fig. 65. Lapboard used in cutting petals for finishing the edges of a cast. Note the position of the tape strip. It is folded so that the sticky sides are out and then cut diagonally toward the center fold.

cause pressure areas or irritation of the skin must be removed. Also, before the cast is finished around the buttocks enough room for the patient to have proper care after voidings and defecations must be ensured. If the cutout space seems unnecessarily small, the physician should be consulted before it is bound. Most doctors are eager to give nurses enough room for proper care of these patients, and usually the insufficient space cut out is an oversight rather than a design. An exception to this may occur in the care of patients in whom adductor tenotomies have been performed and whose incisions are very close to the perineum.

Protection of casts. The protection of casts from soiling and moisture is one of considerable interest. The ingenuity of a generation of nurses has been taxed by this troublesome problem. The impossibility of protecting it properly made such men as Dr. V. Putti and Sir Robert Jones declare that plaster of paris could be used for home treatment only with the greatest risks and danger. However, the modern nurse can devise many methods of protecting casts that are also simple enough to make home care of patients in casts not only safe but also quite satisfactory.

To protect the perineal region against body excretions, a waterproof material such as oiled silk or oiled rayon is often used. Inexpensive plastic materials also provide excellent protection when they are properly applied.

Waterproof material is cut in strips from 4 to 5 inches in width and tucked under the cast around the curved area at the buttocks. It is secured on the outside of the cast with either adhesive tape, mending tape, or a single layer of plaster of paris. Oiled paper, the type used in every kitchen, is a cheap and fairly satisfactory waterproof material. Parents taking home children in casts should be told of this and encouraged to apply it to the cast to protect it from soiling and dampness. Oiled paper does not have the durability of other waterproof fabrics and must be changed frequently.

For protecting the entire cast various methods are used. Shellac and varnish may be painted on the cast with a brush and will dry quickly. White lacquer makes a particularly good surface, which has the additional advantage of looking

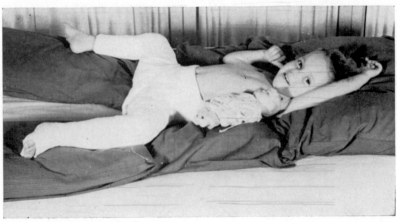

Fig. 66. Supine position in hip cast, illustrating Pliofilm strips tucked about the perineum. A piece of Pliofilm may be tucked over the diaper, which is being used as a perineal pad. This will help prevent wetting of the cast.

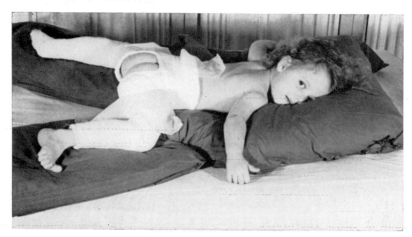

Fig. 67. Hip cast illustrating position of Pliofilm to protect cast from wetting or soiling. The Pliofilm is applied in strips, with the outer end secured with tape or plaster of paris. The strips have been pulled out to permit air to get to the posterior aspect of the cast.

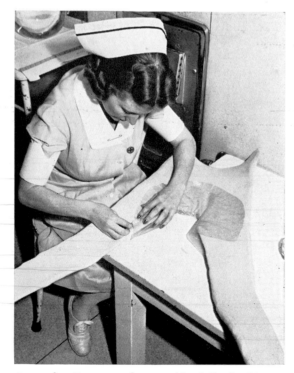

Fig. 68. Basting waterproof pattern around removable shell of a hip spica cast. Pattern is a double semicircle of Pliofilm cut out to fit cast opening and basted together on concave edges before it is applied to the shell.

extremely good. None of these finishes, of course, will provide perineal protection for the cast, in that they do not protect the inside of the cast from excreta. They do, however, make it possible to remove pencil and crayon marks and other soilage from the outer surface of the cast and are particularly useful in caring for young children.

Casts cannot be washed, for water will soften them. The life of the cast will be shortened and its efficiency lessened, and mold will almost inevitably appear on the surface of a frequently dampened cast. It is usually considered permissible to remove very minor stains from casts with a cloth squeezed almost dry and rubbed over a cake of Bon Ami. If the area is large, this must be followed by some form of artificial heat or sunlight to dry the cast as quickly as possible. Shellac, varnish, or lacquer must not be used to waterproof casts until they are thoroughly dried, preferably not until 48 hours have elapsed. Waterproofing the entire cast before it is dry prevents the proper evaporation of moisture beneath.

Old stockings or underwear may be used to cover casts in the home and provide excellent protection for leg casts on children. In some clinics all casts are covered completely with stockinet before the patient is discharged. Outer stockinet is sewed to that which has been used beneath the cast as a lining. Unquestionably, this method does preserve the cast more satisfactorily than any other, but it entails a considerable amount of time, more than is usually available in the modern hospital.

It has been suggested that the waterproof material used to protect casts be applied in strips rather than in a solid piece. The reason for this is obvious because a curving surface is to be bound. The material is tucked under the cast so that it folds back very tightly, thus forming a dam against excretions, but too much material must not be used under the cast or it will become wrinkled. Tape should be applied in such a fashion that the oiled silk can be easily slipped out from under the cast without entirely detaching it.

Placing the patient in a cast on the bedpan. Even with the most artful padding and waterproofing, the nurse's worries are not over. She must still be extremely cautious when placing the bedpan so that the buttocks are not higher than the head. Inevitably, this situation will cause urine to flow backward inside the cast, and the drying out of the cast afterward is no small problem. Elevating the head of the bed slightly and placing another pillow under the back while the patient is voiding will prevent this accident. Unless a patient is in shock or hemorrhaging, it is almost always permissible to elevate the head and shoulders for use of the bedpan. Sharp angulation at the groin must be avoided to prevent breaking the cast. A second precaution that may be taken is that of placing a folded diaper or gauze pad on the posterior aspect of the bedpan. This padding will absorb moisture and prevent the lining of the cast from becoming wet with urine.

To place an adult patient on the bedpan one of two methods is usually employed. The patient is turned onto his good side, the bedpan is placed so that the fleshy part of the buttocks contacts the posterior section of the pan, and pillows or blankets are arranged to support the legs and back on the same level as the buttocks. The patient is then returned to the back-lying position. By the other method, with an overhead trapeze to support himself, the patient may be placed on the pan without turning. The nurse elevates the hips with one hand while she slips the pan under them with the other.

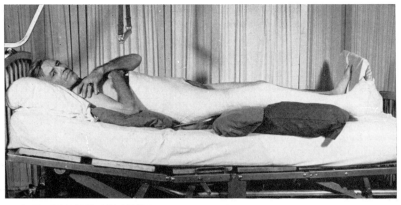

Fig. 69. Placement of patient with hip spica cast on the bedpan. To avoid strain on the cast at the groin area, pillows have been placed beneath the limb enclosed in plaster and beneath the lumbar and hip regions. The head of the bed has been elevated slightly to help prevent soiling or wetting the posterior aspect of the cast.

With the small child in the hip spica cast the problem is more complicated. A Bradford frame hung on hooks in the crib or supported on boxes may be used. The frame is prepared with a two-piece covering, so arranged that a space is left under the buttocks. A bedpan is kept constantly under this space. Most orthopedists object to diapers for infants in hip spica casts, because the diaper serves to spread the urine over the cast and thereby soften it. Many ingenious frames have been reported in orthopedic literature for keeping the child off the bed, with the bedpan beneath the buttocks at all times, but the suspended Bradford frame is probably as efficient as any of the newer types of apparatus.

If the frame is not used, the position of the patient must have considerable attention. The child may be supported on rubber-covered pillows, with the body on a slant in the crib. If a diaper is used, it is advisable to fold it in the shape of a perineal pad and to apply it in such a manner that the diaper does not rest on the cast. The waterproof material used around the groin and buttocks should cover a generous area.

Sometimes no stockinet is used for lining the spica cast, and the plaster is applied directly over the sheet wadding and padding. In these cases it is not unusual to find young children busily pulling handfuls of sheet wadding out from under the cast. To prevent this and to add to the comfort of the patient small towels may be used to slip under the cast anteriorly and posteriorly. If the cast is rather tight, a tongue depressor or comb may be used to push the towel under the cast, but great care must be taken not to injure the child's skin. These cast towels may be changed daily. Older patients who complain of itching will derive comfort from a long flexible feeler that may be wrapped in cotton and dampened in alcohol. Fly swatter handles or corset stays serve this purpose nicely. A wide muslin bandage, single thickness, may be stretched inside the cast. This is the old Lorenz scratcher, a device that has never lost its usefulness.

CARE OF THE PATIENT'S SKIN

Good powers of observation are necessary in caring for the patient in a cast. All visible skin must be inspected daily for signs of abrasions or irritation. All areas that come in contact with cast edges must have particular attention, for cast sores are very frequently encountered at these places. Fingers moistened sparingly with alcohol should explore under the cast as far as it is possible to reach. If beginning abrasions or skin blemishes are noted, they should be inspected frequently during the day. Sometimes collodion-based or tar-based emollients are prescribed to protect the skin at these points against further irritation. Nurses should learn to inspect casts with the sense of smell as well as with the senses of sight and touch. It is not enough, however, for the nurse merely to sniff at the cast as she stands in an upright position. She must get her nose down to within an inch of the plaster and learn to smell discerningly. It takes experience to learn to detect abnormal odors, but sometimes even an inexperienced nurse will be able to locate the exact position of a musty odor that may be the only evidence of a sloughing area beneath a cast. It is sometimes possible to detect an underlying pressure sore by the temperature of the cast, for the cast tends to become much hotter over an area that is beginning to discharge. Eyes, nose, and fingers are of equal importance in cast care.

Each time the patient is given nursing care the waterproof fabric around the groin and buttocks should be pulled out from beneath the cast. The cast beneath this waterproofing should be inspected for soilage, dampness, and mold. Droplets of water adhering to the plastic material may indicate that the cast was not thoroughly dried before the waterproofing was applied. Time should be taken to dry this portion of the cast before the waterproof material is reapplied.

The waterproof fabric should be washed with hot soapy water, rinsed, dried, and powdered. It is then tucked neatly and smoothly under the edges of the cast. If this is done at least once a day, the life of the material will be greatly prolonged. It will also prevent the forming of small troublesome pimples on the skin that appear around the edges of the cast when the skin and cast are neglected.

Certain other areas of the patient in a cast are commonly vulnerable to pressure sores. The heel of the normal foot may become sore because the patient habitually pushes himself up in bed with that leg. The elbows sometimes become sore because the patient braces himself on them to see what is going on around him. These places can be cared for more easily than areas covered by casts and should never be allowed to reach the stage of skin breakdown.

The importance of providing support for the uninvolved extremity cannot be overemphasized. The patient's good extremity should be in excellent condition to withstand the strain that will be put upon it when he becomes ambulatory. Provision for support should be made in the form of footboards, boxes, pillows, or sandbags. Bed exercises when prescribed will do much to maintain muscle tone in the feet.

CLEANING THE CAST

Adhesive stains that remain after the waterproofing has been changed several times can be removed with benzine applied sparingly on a damp cloth and rubbed briskly over the area. The orthopedic nurse should take pride in keeping casts as spotless as she possibly can.

With all the best care we can give, however, accidents do occur, particularly with small children. Knowing how to repair damage is a satisfactory accomplishment and seems like nothing short of a miracle to the onlooker.

The outside of the cast may be easily

repaired. Bon Ami, carefully applied with a damp cloth, will remove the most superficial stains. For the larger areas of soilage, the pattern method of repair is recommended. From a plaster bandage of suitable width a double thickness is cut to fit exactly over the soiled area. This pattern is swiftly immersed in water so that it is barely moistened through when it is lifted from the pan. The pattern is applied directly over the soiled area and is carefully rubbed into the cast. It must be well incorporated by rubbing, or it will peel off later like an onion skin. Some orthopedists advise that the cast be roughened slightly with a nail file or scissors before the pattern is applied. A generous sprinkling of baby powder rubbed into the moistened plaster will remove the odor that may accompany soilage.

A more troublesome problem is encountered when the inside of the cast becomes soiled. To remedy this, the stockinet lining of the cast may be carefully detached from the area around the buttocks or groin with either a razor blade or sharp scissors. The stockinet can then be pulled down and the soiled area trimmed off. Stockinet stretches to a considerable degree and is not at all difficult to manage. The clean edge is then brought out over the cast edges and secured to the cast either with adhesive tape or a bit of damp plaster of paris bandage. Repeated soiling of this kind would deplete the available stockinet lining.

If stockinet has not been used to line the cast, small portions of the sheet wadding must be carefully pulled out, and the inside of the cast must be cleaned with a sparingly dampened cloth.

When new layers of plaster are used to refurbish casts, some drying agent, such as a light cradle, hair dryer, or sunlight, must be used before waterproofing is again placed on the area. It cannot be emphasized too often that mold will inevitably form on damp casts which are covered with waterproof material.

Another method of cleaning the inside of a cast is by the use of a single thickness of muslin bandage 6 to 8 inches in width. It can be run through the cast, moistened slightly, and pulled out further as it becomes soiled or saturated. Relatively few casts need ever become this badly soiled if intelligent care is given beforehand.

On the adult wards, where all this elaborate precaution seldom seems necessary, protection may be managed by small squares of waterproof fabric put in place only when the patient uses the bedpan. These squares may be washed and dried afterward. This requires less use of materials and is usually sufficient, particularly on an adult male ward. To risk such underprotection on a child's ward is usually dangerous to the cast, however. Nor should too much confidence be placed in the adolescent girl in a spica cast. Any patient in a cast is relatively helpless in taking care of his own toilet needs, and the nurse must understand this from the outset of her orthopedic work.

ARM AND LEG CASTS

Most of the admonitions mentioned earlier have to do with patients in the larger types of casts, but there are things that must be borne in mind about the patient in the foot or leg cast or in the arm cast reaching from the wrist to the shoulders. Paramount in importance, as has been stated, is the matter of circulation in the part. Arm casts should be supported in a sling if the patient is ambulatory, and it scarcely seems necessary to remind the nurse that a sling should support the arm and not allow it to drop forlornly at an angle of 120 degrees at the elbow. It must be remembered, too, that the hand and wrist should be supported and not permitted to hang in a wrist-drop position. The weight of an unsupported cast on the shoulder is considerable and will cause the patient discomfort that a well-applied sling can eliminate. In this connection the nurse should be reminded of the potential danger and discomfort of a sling tied in a hard knot over the back of the neck, so that the knot constantly presses on the cervical spine. A sling is more comfortable if it is pinned in two places neatly with two small safety pins dividing the stress of the weight.

Long leg casts should be supported on pillows when the patient is placed on a bedpan. Otherwise, the patient will be insecure and uncomfortable with his legs unsupported in space as his body is elevated to the level of the pan. The groin area of long leg casts in children needs protection with a waterproof material.

The bathing care of toes and fingers in casts is frequently a point of neglect. The patient may be well bathed otherwise and the toes or fingers overlooked. Applicators moistened in alcohol can be used to clean, refresh, and deodorize otherwise unreachable fingers and toes. Cast crumbs at these points are dangerous as well as annoying. They can be eliminated to a great extent by binding the edges of the cast around toes and fingers with adhesive tape if there is no stockinet to be taped over these edges.

ANTERIOR AND POSTERIOR SPLINTS

Quite frequently, hip casts are bivalved and made into removable shells so that the patient may receive the benefits of sun treatment, massage, or exercises. If these casts have been on the patient for some time, considerable cleaning may be necessary in order to

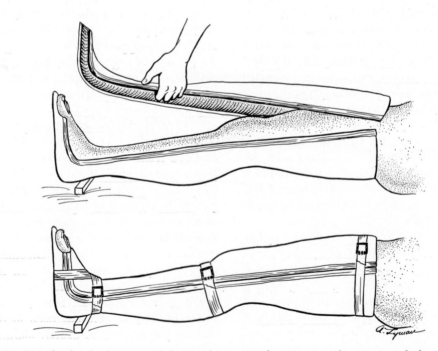

Fig. 70. The bivalved cast used frequently in convalescent care of patients with fractures, sprained ligaments, bursitis, poliomyelitis, arthritis, synovitis, and many other conditions, where protection is still necessary but access to the limb and joints is needed for daily treatments.

renovate them. A change of stockinet lining may be easily effected without disturbing the cast's padding. The cut edges may be bound with adhesive tape or the entire cast may be covered with stockinet that can be stitched on. Straps are used to secure the bivalved sections securely on the patient's body while he is being turned. If many such casts are in use on the wards, it is a good policy to keep circular pieces of waterproof material on hand for protection of the gluteal region. These are made in various sizes, half-circle in shape, and stitched on the sewing machine around the concave section. They may then be turned inside out and neatly fitted into the curved area of the perineal buttocks region. Simple basting stitches will secure them nicely to the stockinet-covered bivalved shell; or they may be attached with adhesive strips.

Frequently, posterior splints or bivalved casts are made to maintain the patient's extremities in good alignment. The splint illustrated in Fig. 70 is designed to maintain a neutral position of the foot and limb. The posterior shell provides support for the foot, preventing drop foot, and the bar placed at the ankle prevents external rotation of the limb. This type of support may also be worn to help prevent flexion contractures of the knee. It is held in place by an elastic bandage, or figure-of-eight straps placed about the ankle and knee. Nursing problems, however, are not eliminated with the application of the bivalved cast. If they are not applied correctly, the patient may pull his foot up within the splint, and the foot is then held in a definite drop-foot position. Pressure areas at the heel also must be prevented. Although these casts are lined carefully, the heel may be a constant source of trouble. Sometimes this can be prevented by placing a small piece of padding, felt or sponge rubber,

in the cast just above the heel space. This tends to relieve the pressure and helps to prevent blisters or pressure sores.

Bivalved casts may be aired daily and placed in the sunlight for drying. A rack to hold such casts is an excellent device to have on hospital sun decks. An ordinary clotheshorse will serve the purpose and will hold a number of such bivalved sections. Collapsible clotheshorses that can be stored away when not in use are also helpful in orthopedic wards during baths and evening care. There are seldom enough chairs to hold all of the orthopedic patient's paraphernalia (casts, sandbags, pillows, restraints, etc.). A clotheshorse placed between two beds affords a solution for this problem and adds considerably to the neatness of the ward during the working period.

CARE OF THE PATIENT WHEN THE CAST IS REMOVED

Nurses who have watched orthopedic surgeons apply casts have observed the comfortable support that such casts give the joints. Although we may have a private conviction that casts are clumsy things to handle, a well-applied cast is as perfect a fixation apparatus as can be devised for the human body. The patient himself may never realize this until he is removed from its support. Once out of his cast, he will become conscious of many aches and discomforts, and even minute changes in the position of the joints will cause him pain. Joint structures have become somewhat contracted, and muscles that have been immobilized are suddenly stretched. In addition circulation is sluggish, and coldness, mottling, and swelling are often present. If the primary trouble has been in the hip, the patient may be acutely alarmed because his greatest discomfort and stiffness now seem to be in the knee. This is a common occurrence and usually results from the fact that the quadriceps muscle group, which forms the bulk of the muscle at the front of the thigh, has suffered considerable disuse atrophy from the weeks spent in the cast. This muscle group is the main extensor of the knee and is absolutely essential in rising from the sitting position to the upright standing position. When attempting to rise, the patient will be much concerned with the weakness, instability, and pain he experiences in the knee. If he can be told that the cause of his discomfort is merely the result of disuse and is not a permanent deformity, he will be able to bear it with much more fortitude.

To minimize the patient's discomfort, support to the joints is necessary immediately after the cast is removed. Slight relaxation rather than complete extension is usually the goal in applying casts, and it is important that this position of relaxation be maintained after the cast is removed. The normal curve of the lumbar spine should be supported with a firm narrow pillow or with a sheet folded to make a firm pad measuring about 6 by 20 inches. Soft wide pillows do not give the correct anatomic support that is needed in this area. The knee should be slightly relaxed by placing a rolled towel beneath the head of the tibia. A footboard or box should be used to maintain the anatomic position of the feet, a 90-degree angle leg position, with the toes pointing toward the ceiling. Frequently outward rotation of the hip will be a troublesome feature that may need attention. Sandbags placed from the hip to below the knee may be used to overcome this, or a trochanter roll may be made of a sheet or bath blanket. This is done by folding he sheet lengthwise in quarters and then folding it in half crosswise. The folded end is then placed under the buttock and thigh to anchor it in position, and the opposite end is rolled firmly under until it forms a tight roll along the patient's hip and thigh. This is an effective method of overcoming outward rotation of the hip.

The boards that have been in use under the mattress should not be taken out because the cast has been removed. A firm bed is necessary to protect the patient from the aches that a sagging bed would cause him.

Some physicians feel that support should also be given immediately to the integumentary system after the cast is removed. If this is done, the edema that so often occurs after the removal of a cast can be somewhat lessened. All-cotton elastic bandages may be used and must be applied immediately after the cast is removed to be effective. Other physicians feel that elevating the limb for certain periods of the day may be sufficient to reduce the edema. If elevation is ordered, nurses should see to it that support is given along the entire limb from the buttock to the heel and that the knee is not acutely flexed.

After the cast is removed movement in bed is usually freely permitted, but certain precautions should be observed. Nurses should remember that considerable decalcification has occurred and that the bone is more brittle and vulnerable to stresses that would not affect it under normal conditions. Fractures brought about by minor stresses sometimes occur at this time and are sometimes disguised by the patient's general discomfort. In addition, muscles that are weakened need careful handling to eliminate unnecessary pain and discomfort. Nurses should be careful to lift a limb newly out of a cast by providing adequate support at contingent joints. Such a limb should never be lifted by grasping the muscle belly.

When plaster casts that have been on the patient a considerable period of time are removed, the skin will be noted to be caked with a yellow exudate that is partly dead skin and partly secretions from the oil sacs of the skin. It is generally conceded to be poor policy to try to soften the skin or forcibly remove the closely adhering exudate, particularly if a new cast is to be applied at once. If the patient is to remain out of the cast permanently or for a considerable period of time, the skin can be cleaned at the nurse's leisure and the patient's comfort, never forcing the caked matter off in such a way as to cause bleeding or rawness. There is plenty of time for this, and no one will be accused of neglect if this is allowed to take several days. Zeal in this matter is misplaced. If the patient is not to be put in a cast again at once, the use of olive oil packs on the skin, left on for 24-hour periods, is an easy and safe method of cleaning the skin. Cocoa butter may be used for gentle massage.

CUTTING CASTS

Cutting windows or holes in casts is usually considered a dangerous procedure, because the flesh under the opened area bulges out alarmingly after an hour or so and the patient's discomfort is only exacerbated. If the doctor in charge of the patient orders windows cut out, it is customary for him to request the nurse to apply a pad of felt over the area that has been removed and to use a snug bandage for eliminating this complicating edema. Sometimes a window is cut in the cast so that a surgical dressing may be applied, or the heel may be cut out to relieve pressure on a tender area. In any case the nurse must not discard the part of the cast that has been removed. These pieces are nearly always put back and held in place by a new roll of plaster.

Every nurse should know how to cut a cast if an emergency arises. The short curved-bladed plaster knife in common usage is not a difficult tool to handle. If a cast knife is not available, an ordinary shoe knife or a pruning knife may be used. Very heavy casts may be spread with a household pliers. A spoon handle may be inserted under the cast to protect the patient's skin from the plaster knife. The spoon is advanced as the cast is cut. Vinegar, dilute hydrochloric acid, hydrogen peroxide, or citrate of soda is sometimes used to soften the cast before it is cut, but most workers feel that water is equally satisfactory. The liquid is dropped on the line of cutting with a syringe of the Asepto variety.

When an arm or leg cast is to be split to relieve edema, it should be cut along its entire length. Splitting the cast only part way will often add to circulatory congestion. It is always a mistake to attempt to prevent or overcome swelling of toes or fingers by cutting the edges of the cast. Usually, the more the cast is cut or trimmed back, the greater the area that will swell. In emergencies, when it is impossible to reach the physician for orders and the edema is such that immediate attention is imperative, the nurse should split the cast along its full length and spread the plaster slightly. It is not enough to cut the plaster only, for frequently the underlying bandages or dressings may be the cause of the circulatory impairment or the pain. They should be loosened so that no constricting material binds the extremity. When a newly applied cast is split to relieve congestion, it may be taped together loosely until further instructions can be obtained from the physician.

It is never safe to postpone reporting circulatory congestion of an extremity in a cast. Night nurses sometimes feel that they can risk waiting until daylight or for the early morning rounds of the house physician. Although it is prompted by the best of motives, such a policy is dangerous. Irremediable damage may be caused by 2 or 3 hours of neglect.

INSTRUCTION OF PARENTS

What nurses have been taught or have learned through experience and the application of their ingenuity concerning the care of casts is no sacred professional secret. It must be shared with all those to whom the care of casts is confided. Parents must be given adequate instruction before taking children with plaster of paris casts away from the hospital, and this includes instruction in all the details that have been mentioned: close check on circulation of the exposed body parts, attention to complaints of pressure and burning, the manner of detecting odors in casts, the care of the skin under the cast, and the cleaning and protection of the plaster itself. If possible, the parents should observe the patient's bath and cast care completely. They must be told that young children often make a game of hiding things in their casts that may cause damage to the skin. They must understand why the patient is wearing the cast and must recognize when the cast has become inefficient to maintain the position essential to correction of the child's deformity. They must be taught to look for signs that the child is outgrowing the cast. If the parent is manifestly slow to understand such instructions and seems confused by the number of things to watch for, instructions of this nature may be written down and sent home with the child. On the whole, patients in casts spend only a small portion of their convalescence in the hospital. It is but a short interlude, and the excellent care the child experiences in the hospital will be absolutely negated unless a follow-up of some type is provided for him when he returns to his home. The nurse should have enough understanding and sympathy for the parent's economic status

not to suggest elaborate and expensive means of cast protection to a family of limited means. Ingenuity in improvising will be of untold value to the parent and will be a source of great satisfaction to the nurse when she sees later what it has accomplished.

Written instructions for parents on the care of patients in hip casts

Even though the plaster cast may seem extremely bulky and awkward, the patient has been placed in the cast for definite reasons, mainly to immobilize the hip joint and to maintain a corrected position. Consequently, if a definite position of the hip joint is to be maintained, the care of the patient must be such as to prevent softening or cracking of the cast. Equally as important, this care must provide for the general welfare of the patient and the prevention of cast sores or bed sores.

Skin care

Special attention should be given the skin of the patient in a cast.
1. Daily cleansing of the skin is desirable.
2. Reach up with fingers under the cast to eliminate plaster crumbs or other foreign objects.
   Feel and look for skin irritations at the cast edges.
   Do not permit youngsters to poke crayons or other small objects down in the cast. Such articles may cause severe pressure areas.
3. Turn patient every 4 hours during the day and encourage him to lie on his abdomen several hours each day. Frequently, a patient will find it possible to sleep in this position.
   If reddened areas appear on the sacral area, the patient must stay on his abdomen more.
4. Rub the back, especially around the edges of the cast and over the sacral area, with rubbing alcohol several times daily.

Check the following closely when caring for a patient in a plaster cast
1. Is there swelling or discoloration of the toes?
2. Is the patient able to wiggle his toes? Are they warm?
3. Does he complain of pain or numbness?

4. If the patient is a small child, does he fuss and seem unduly irritable?
(If for any reason you are in doubt concerning any of these things, consult your doctor.)

Drying the cast

If the cast becomes damp, it can be dried by exposing the area to the air or by using an ordinary hair dryer.

Cleaning the cast

If the cast becomes soiled from stool, it may be cleaned by using a damp cloth with Bon Ami.

Finishing the edges of the cast

To eliminate plaster crumbs in the bed and to provide a smooth nonirritating cast edge, adhesive tape may be used to bind the edges of the cast. To do this one must wait until the cast has dried. This usually requires 24 to 48 hours.

Protecting the cast from urine

On the baby or small child plastic waterproof material may be used to protect the cast around the perineum and buttocks. This material should be cut in 4 by 6 inch strips.

One end of the strip is tucked under the cast at the perineum opening and the material is folded back over the outer side of the cast.

The outer end of the material is secured with adhesive tape to the plaster cast.

Six to eight strips of the plastic material are needed to protect both the back and the front of a hip cast on a small child.

These strips may be pulled out at the perineum, washed, dried, and powdered daily. (The nurse will provide you with the plastic material and show you how to apply it.)

In addition to the plastic material a perineal diaper may be used on the child who is not toilet trained. Fold a diaper in the form of a perineal pad and place it across the perineum, tucking it under the edges of the cast in the front and in the back. The ordinary diaper may be applied over this.

It is essential that this pad and diaper be changed as soon as it becomes wet or soiled.

The small youngster or baby in a hip cast may be supported by placing plastic- or rubber-covered pillows so that the head and shoulders are slightly higher than the buttocks. This will aid in keeping the cast dry.

Placing the patient on the bedpan

Elevating the patient's head and shoulders by using pillows when he is on the bedpan will tend to keep the cast from becoming wet with urine running back from the pan.

A folded diaper, soft cloth, or gauze pad placed on the back of the bedpan will absorb any moisture and will help to keep the cast clean and dry. It must be removed with the bedpan.

Turning the cast patient

If only one leg is enclosed in the cast, turn the patient toward the normal leg (the leg not in the cast). Turn the body simultaneously to prevent undue pressure on the cast at the groin.

PLASTER ROOM TECHNIQUE

Several types of instruments are usually considered necessary for the application and removal of casts. Cast knives, cutters, and saws are needed for removing an old cast. Bandage scissors will be necessary for removing bandages under the cast, and a heavy pair of shears will be essential for cutting pieces of felt.

Sheet wadding, a thin unabsorbent cotton web covered with starch to hold it together, is commonly used for padding. Piano felt, cut in suitable sizes, is used to provide additional protection against pressure on bony prominences. Sponge rubber may occasionally be used for this purpose. Material will be needed for reenforcing the cast at points of stress, and aluminum strips, yucca board, and plywood are among the most popular of these. Tubular stockinet, which comes in many different widths, from 2 to 18 inches, is used for a cast lining. A deep pail for soaking bandages, a pan of splints, and a waste-water vessel, all of them lined with brown paper or old pieces of cloth to filter the waste plaster, will be necessary. Gloves and gowns should be at hand for the surgeon and assistants who are to apply the cast.

The temperature of the water that is used to soak the bandages should be between 95° and 105° F. Warmer or cooler water will delay the setting of the plaster.

Paper-wrapped bandages retain plaster satisfactorily when they are put on edge in water until the bubbling ceases. They may then be lifted vertically from the water with the ends firmly grasped in the palms. Bandages not so wrapped are usually submerged horizontally, with the nurse or assistant keeping her palms cupped over the end of the bandage to prevent loss of plaster. No compression of the bandage must take place at this time.

The bubbles of air in the water will rise until the bandage is completely saturated; that is, until the water has penetrated every part of the bandage. When this is completed, the bandage should be removed immediately, because the crystallization (setting) process will have begun.

The bandage is lifted from the water

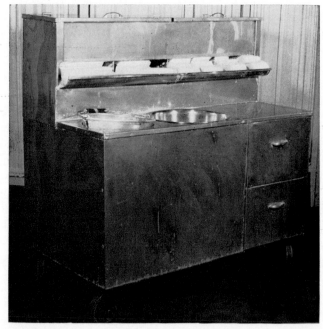

Fig. 71. The plaster cart may be taken to the operating room or to the bedside when plaster of paris is to be applied.

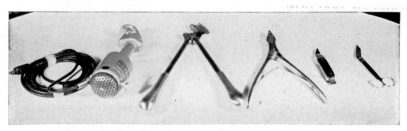

Fig. 72. Cast instruments: cast saw, cutter, spreader, knife, and bandage scissors.

and held horizontally with the ends secured in the nurse's palms. Water is expelled by gently compressing the bandage in a short twist—no more than is necessary to supinate the right hand a single time, keeping the left hand in pronation. The bandage should not drip when it is handed to the surgeon, but, on the other hand, it must not be wrung so dry that the surgeon will have difficulty incorporating it into a cast. The end of the plaster bandage is unrolled from 2 to 4 inches before it is handed to the doctor. Only a few bandages should be put in the water at one time. Change of immersion water may be necessary if a large cast is being applied. A waste basin lined with paper may be used to receive the plaster that is wrung from the plaster bandage when it is removed from the water.

By the time the cast application is over the plaster in the basins used for immersion will usually have settled to the bottom. The water above this plaster is poured into the sink, with the faucet wide open to assist in washing what plaster is still present in the water through the drain. If paper has been used to line the immersion basins, this is lifted from the container and deposited in waste containers. Garbage pails are used in some clinics, but improvised waste containers may be made of large discarded tin cans. Caution must be exercised in the care of all this equipment so that plaster is not allowed to gather in the sink and to clog plumbing fixtures.

Recently, a new substance, melamine polymer, has been used in making plaster of paris casts. A solution is made by dissolving this substance in warm water. The solution is then used to moisten the plaster rolls. The cast made by using this substance is lighter and stronger than the ordinary cast, dries much more quickly, and is water-resistant. The water-resistant quality makes it especially desirable to use for small children. However, this quality does not eliminate the need for protecting the cast. The sheet wadding or stockinet that lines the cast, unless protected with waterproof material, may become wet or soiled.

The unused solution should be discarded with care. It must not be poured into a sink unless there is an adequate plaster trap, and then it should be poured down the drain slowly, with a large amount of running hot water.

Traction, including nursing care of the patient

MODES OF TRACTION

The following brief classification of traction has been inserted to clarify the different methods of securing traction.

1. *Skin traction* is applied to the skin and soft tissues and thus indirectly to the skeletal system.

2. *Skeletal traction* is applied directly to the skeletal system. The Steinmann pin or Kirschner wire is used in applying traction to an extremity. Skeletal traction to the skull is secured by Crutchfield tongs, Vinke tongs, or other devices.

3. *Manual traction* means the application of traction to a part of the body by the hands of the operator. A student nurse, when assisting with the applica-

tion of traction or a cast, may be asked to apply manual traction. She should have a smooth firm grip on the extremity and should avoid sudden jerking movements. Occasionally, when nursing care is being given or when traction is changed, it is necessary to apply this type of traction to the extremity. Permission to substitute manual traction for the regular traction must be secured from the attending physician.

PURPOSE OF TRACTION

Perhaps the best way to begin studying the care of the patient in traction is to ask why a patient is placed in this apparatus. What is accomplished by exerting a pull on an extremity or a part of the body? As the student cares for patients on an orthopedic service she will discover varied reasons for the application of traction. Frequently she will find that when the physician wishes to immobilize an extremity traction is applied. The desired rest and immobilization for a patient with a tuberculous joint may be secured in this manner. Traction may be applied to the extremity of a patient with a fracture, first to lessen the muscle spasm and to reduce the fracture and then to immobilize and to maintain the corrected position. The patient with arthritis who has flexion contractures of the hip and the knee may have traction applied to correct or prevent the development of these deformities. The child with scoliosis may have traction as a form of treatment to lessen the deformity. Occasionally, the patient with back pain may be placed in traction to relieve muscle spasm, or traction may be applied to lessen muscle spasm about a joint.

PRINCIPLES PERTAINING TO TRACTION

Nurses sometimes believe that clumsy insufficient care is the best that can be given to patients in traction. However, a definite understanding of the purpose of the traction and its working principle will give the nurse confidence and enable her to care for the patient with greater efficiency and satisfaction.

Position of the patient. Often nurses will discover that more movement can be permitted than at first seems possible. The surgeon should be consulted about the amount of liberty permissible for these patients, for unnecessary restriction of motion should not be imposed upon them. Such restriction may cause aches and discomforts or actual numbness that might be avoided by allowing the patient such body activity as is compatible with good local immobilization of the affected part. However, the patient in traction is very seldom allowed the privilege of turning onto either the side or the abdomen. It is not possible to maintain any kind of efficient longitudinal traction unless the patient lies in the dorsal position. Lying on the side particularly causes the hips and limbs to sag out of alignment medially. Sitting up in bed also diminishes the effect of the traction and is usually not permitted except when the threat of hypostatic pneumonia exists, as it may in aged persons who are in traction for fracture of the hip.

Countertraction. Provision for countertraction must always be made when traction is applied. Countertraction can be obtained in two ways: pull may be exerted against a fixed point (such as the pelvis when a Thomas, Hodgen, or Keller-Blake splint is used), or pull may be exerted against countertraction in the opposite direction. This can be accomplished by elevating the bed under the part that is being placed in traction; that is, the foot of the bed is elevated for traction on the lower extremity, causing the body itself to exert countertraction in its gravitational pull away from the limb extension. Elevation of the bed should be from 8 to 12 inches. If a child or a thin adult is being subjected to many pounds of traction, this amount of countertraction may not suffice to keep the patient balanced against the traction being applied. Other methods must be employed. One of the most commonly used is the perineal strap made of tape webbing and padded at a central section for about 12 inches with flannel or silence cloth. This padded section passes under the groin, and the ends of the strap are fastened to the head of the bed. It serves the purpose well for some patients, but for an older child with a congenital dislocation of the hip, in which condition tight adductor tendons are the rule, pressure sores may form rapidly over this area. Head traction may be used, but it offers additional confinement to an already confined patient and is not resorted to unless it is absolutely necessary. Further elevation of the bed may be of assistance here, and of course, nurses must be most conscientious in aiding the patient to pull himself up in bed at frequent intervals during the day. The footplate or spreader must never be allowed to come in contact with the foot of the bed at any time, or traction on the extremity will become entirely useless.

Friction. Any friction created by ropes riding on the foot of the bed, ropes impinged by bedclothes, or heels digging into the mattress will lessen the efficiency of traction greatly. Orthopedic nurses must train themselves to observe these details and others which their experience and common sense tell them mitigate efficiency of the traction. A hard, thin pillow, covered with oiled silk and kept well powdered, does much to eliminate bed friction when it is placed under the limb in extension.

Continuous traction. In caring for patients in traction a safe rule to follow

is that traction cannot be released for any nursing procedure and that it must be continuous for 24 hours of the day. There are exceptions to this rule, but they must be given by the physician for a specific patient. Patients with arthritis who have had traction applied to prevent or correct flexion contractures of the joints are sometimes an exception to the rule and are frequently allowed to be released from traction for a few hours during the day. There may be others from time to time who have this privilege, but it is given only on the explicit order of the doctor in charge.

Line of pull. When evaluating traction, first, see that the pull extends in a straight line and, second, maintain the pull in line with the deformity. When flexion contracture of the joint is present, as is so often the case in patients with arthritis and tuberculosis of the joints, the nurse must realize that a straight pull on the contracted limb is impossible both mechanically and from the standpoint of the patient's comfort. Some support for the contracted extremity is necessary so that traction may be exerted in the line of the deformity. Pillows or a wooden box to support the calf of the leg will accomplish this and can be gradually diminished in height as the contracture of the joint lessens. The addition of boxes or pillows means, of course, that the pulley at the end of the bed must be at a higher level than the foot of the bed will usually permit. Some kind of upright bars on the bed with horizontal crosspieces will be necessary for this type of traction (Balkan frame).

Frequently in cases of contracture an overhead bar or frame with pulleys is used for suspending the calf and thigh, particularly if there is a flexion contracture at the hip level. Small canvas hammocks provide support for the leg and are suspended by weights to the overhead pulleys. A balance of weights is commonly used at the beginning of the traction period. The weights on the overhead frame are gradually diminished, and those on the leg pulley are increased as the muscle spasm relaxes and the joint becomes less contracted. The doctor in charge of these patients usually attends to this type of traction, because it presents certain responsibilities nurses are not prepared to assume. This type of traction is mechanically more correct for patients with flexion contracture of the joints than is the use of boxes or pillows for support in that the friction engendered by the latter

undermines the efficiency of the traction considerably.

TRACTION EQUIPMENT

Traction cart. A traction cart is a helpful device for orthopedic hospitals or wards and will save much time and effort when traction is to be applied. Any type of wheeled carriage can be used for the purpose. The cart may be stocked with various types of orthopedic equipment such as moleskin strips sewed or stapled to tape webbing, self-adhering traction strips, felt, stockinet, bandages (cotton elastic, muslin, and gauze), bandage scissors, a screw driver, tincture

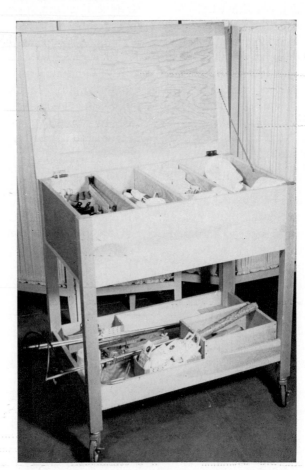

Fig. 73. The well-equipped traction cart is a timesaving device when traction is to be applied. Traction equipment can be taken to the bedside without delay or preparation.

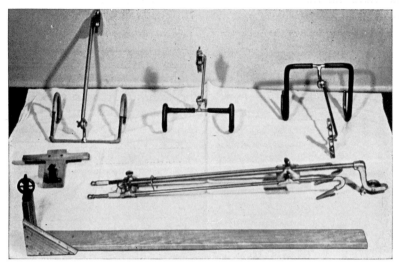

Fig. 74. Types of pulleys, commercial and improvised.

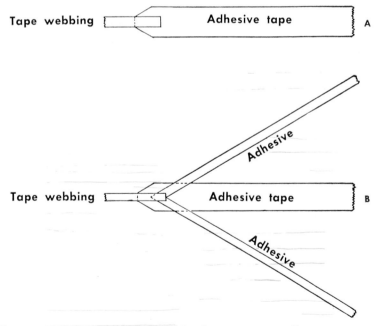

Fig. 75. Two types of adhesive tape patterns for skin traction. **A,** Adhesive strip is tapered off and a one-inch width of tape webbing is sewed or stapled onto the adhesive tape. This must be done firmly; otherwise separation will occur if considerable weight is applied. **B,** The three-tailed design is also stitched or stapled where the strips adjoin. The tape backing is left attached until the tape is used, but it is not sewed or stapled to the tape.

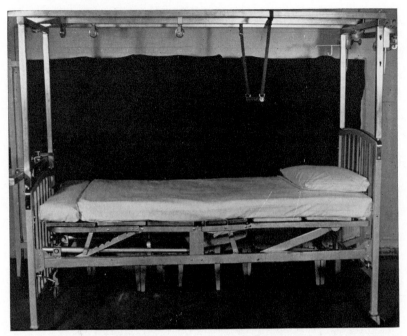

Fig. 76. Traction bed. The Balkan frame provides overhead bars for the attachment of pulleys.

of benzoin, and a razor with several spare blades. A lower shelf or a drawer might contain various types of pulleys, weights, carriers, ropes, footplates or spreaders, sandbags, shock blocks or pins for elevating the foot of the bed, hammocks for limb suspension, pelvic girdles, and chin halters.

Type of bed. The patient in traction must have a firm mattress that does not sag under his body. A bed that sags beneath the hips prevents the free play of the traction rope on the pulley and decreases the efficiency of the apparatus considerably. Furthermore, it may be the cause of a permanent flexion deformity at the hips of the patient who is in traction over a long period of time. The bed may be made firm by placing boards beneath the mattress. It is preferable that these boards extend lengthwise and that they be hinged at the backrest level.

It is desirable and, in most types of traction, necessary to have a bed with overhead bars. Some hospitals use wood-en Balkan frames which clamp to the regular bed, thus providing longitudinal bars and crossbars for the pulleys. However, traction beds that are equipped with the necessary bars and pulleys for the application of most types of traction may be purchased.

The trapeze (unless contraindicated) should not be omitted from the patient's bed. It facilitates nursing care and enables the patient to do many things for himself.

Shock blocks and bed lifter. As described previously, countertraction is usually obtained by the use of shock blocks. The bed lifter facilitates the placement of these blocks.

The hospital bed made in such a manner that the head may be lowered and the foot elevated makes it possible to obtain countertraction or shock position without using the blocks to elevate one end of the bed. This device facilitates treatment and saves nursing time.

Braun-Böhler inclined plane splint.

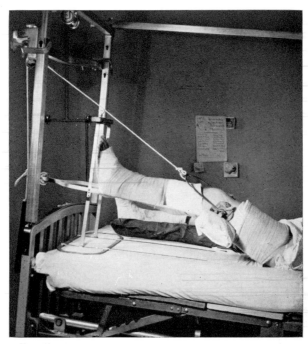

Fig. 77. The Braun-Böhler inclined plane splint may be used to support the limb following application of skeletal traction. Note that the splint supports the entire thigh and that the knee joint corresponds with the beginning of the inclined plane.

The inclined plane splint is frequently used for patients with fractures of the lower end of the femur, either in conjunction with skin or skeletal traction. Since this type of frame and traction rests on the bed, it does not maintain immobilization as automatically as a suspension apparatus. The physician should be consulted concerning the amount of motion permissible for the patient. As a general rule, it is permissible to turn the patient toward the splint for back care. In changing linen it is more convenient to use two folded sheets for the under part of the bed. One sheet rests under the splint, and the other reaches from the head of the bed to the level of the splint. It is thus possible to change the sheet under the patient frequently without disturbing the sheet under the splint. Two or three rolls of 5-inch muslin bandage may be used to cover the splint and to provide

support for the affected limb. The bandage is started around the base and wrapped smoothly and tightly over the inclined plane.

Splints. Half-ring or full-ring Thomas, Hodgen, Keller-Blake splints or the canvas hammock are used in applying balance or suspension traction. Suspension is frequently used with traction because it will permit the patient to move himself about in bed without disturbing the line of traction. Furthermore, suspension improves circulation and allows freer motion of the suspended part than would be possible if the patient had to lift the extremity against gravity.

TYPES OF TRACTION

Buck's extension, rubber surface traction, and Bryant traction may be described as straight or running traction which exerts a pull on the affected part but does not provide a balanced sup-

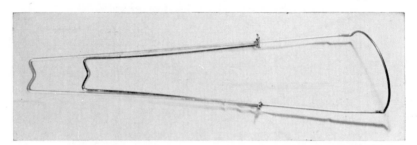

Fig. 78. The half-ring Thomas splint (Hodgen splint) with Pearson attachment.

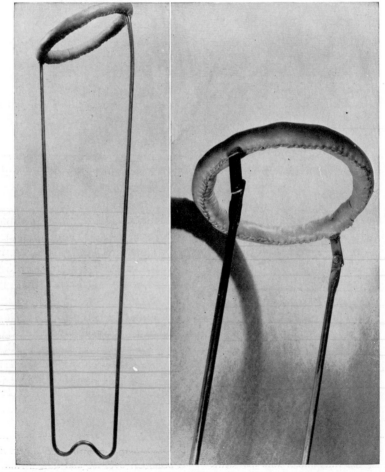

Fig. 79. Thomas splint for lower extremity and modified Thomas splint with hinge for upper extremity. (From Crenshaw, A. H., and Milford, L., editors: Campbell's operative orthopaedics, ed. 4, St. Louis, 1963, The C. V. Mosby Co.)

port by means of a hammock or splint.

With Russell traction, balanced traction, and Dunlop traction, the extremity has traction applied and is then supported by means of a hammock or splint held in place by balanced weights attached to an overhead bar.

Head traction, pelvic traction, and ankle traction are applied with some type of fitted apparatus, such as a corset, Sayre halter, or anklet.

Skill in the nursing care of the patient in traction is an attribute that comes with knowledge and experience. The patients in casts present their problems, but they are much simpler than the problems of the patient in traction. The patient in a cast may be moved as frequently as is necessary for the care of his back or for his comfort. He may lie on his back, abdomen, or side without endangering the immobilization of the diseased part. Patients in traction, on the other hand, usually have but one position to lie in, that is, the dorsal recumbent position. Good nursing care of these patients must include keeping the patient clean, comfortable, and free from pressure sores despite the handicap of his enforced and prolonged recumbency.

Buck's extension. Buck's extension (named after Gordon Buck, who described the apparatus in 1851) is probably used more than any other type of traction. In an emergency it can be applied with improvised equipment: two strips of 3-inch adhesive the length of the patient's limb, a block of wood to be used for a spreader below the foot, some type of pulley that can be purchased at any hardware or ten-cent store, and a weight that may be a window-sash weight or a canvas bag filled with salt or sand. A chair or sawhorse may be used to elevate the foot of the bed to provide countertraction. Hospitals usually have on hand more elaborate equipment for applying traction, but it is well for the nurse to understand how such traction can be applied and maintained satisfactorily with homemade equipment.

Some contraindications to the use of skin traction should be remembered and

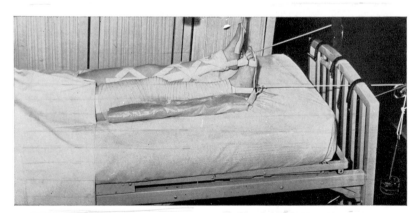

Fig. 80. Two types of adhesive traction for leg. Note pillow covered with plastic material under leg to eliminate friction and to free the heel of pressure. The left foot is supported by an adhesive strip to prevent drop foot. Aluminum footplate is used for right leg. Right leg traction is applied with a single strip and is held in place wth a spiral reverse muslin bandage. The left leg has three-tailed adhesive strips wound obliquely over leg and thigh. Note bracelet of stockinet and cotton over malleoli on left ankle. Also note strips crossed high above dorsum of foot to prevent circulatory impairment. Both extremities are maintained in a neutral position. External rotation is to be avoided.

observed. This type of traction cannot be applied to the patient with a severely injured extremity with open wounds or to the patient who is allergic to tape. Circulatory disturbances, dermatitis, or varicose veins may prohibit the application of traction to the skin. The patient with diabetes may present a problem if skin traction must be maintained for a long period of time. Traction applied to

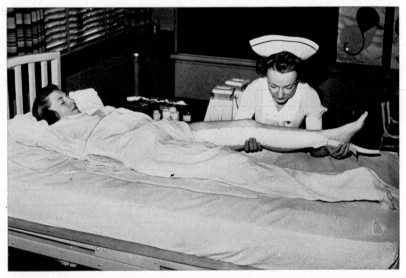

Fig. 81. Buck's extension (modified). Note notching of adhesive tape to fit leg contours.

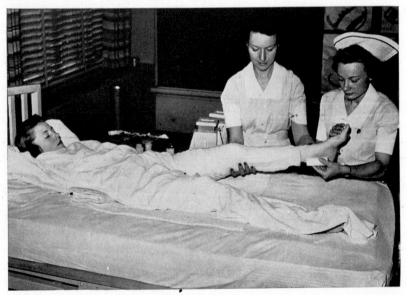

Fig. 82. Buck's extension is covered first with sheet wadding. Straps are retracted and sheet wadding is continued over malleoli as padding. Muslin bandage is applied over sheet wadding. When traction is being applied for fracture, tuberculosis, or other infections of joints, manual traction should be exerted during process of applying Buck's extension.

the skin with moleskin tape may slip if a large amount of weight is applied.

The area to which adhesive tape is to be applied is usually shaved. However, some physicians feel that shaving with a razor before applying tape is not advisable in that epithelium is invariably removed and infection may occur under the tape. Clippers are frequently used instead of the razor. When a razor is used, shaving must be done very carefully, and accidental denudation or cuts of the skin should be reported before the tape is applied.

There are a few landmarks on the leg that must be given special consideration when adhesive traction is applied. In almost all methods of applying traction strips of adhesive with tape webbing stapled or sewed to one end form the basis of the equipment. The adhesive tape extends from the malleoli to the thighs, and in many instances surgeons feel that these strips alone are sufficient for the pull. However, it is the custom in many clinics to use oblique strips of narrower adhesive tape to augment the lateral strips. These pass across the tibia and obliquely encircle the leg, crossing in the back of the calf and then above the knee. Although these strips add to the staying power of the traction as a whole, they present a distinct menace to the circulation of the foot if they are applied too snugly or if they are applied too near the dorsum of the foot. There is an inevitable amount of slipping of the adhesive tape when weights are applied, and oblique strips tend to be pulled down by the lateral strips and to cut into the flesh. An ischemia of the foot with resulting paralysis has been known to develop from the pressure on the dorsalis pedis artery which lies beneath.

Another landmark of which the nurse should be conscious is the upper 3 inches of the fibula, that is, the outer aspect of the calf just below the knee. It is here that the peroneal nerve lies close to the surface, and it can be easily compressed against the bone over which it passes. The result of this compression may be a peroneal paralysis. Such a paralysis is a serious thing, involving plantar flexion and inversion of the foot. This area should be well padded with felt or cotton before the tape is applied. The foot should be observed daily for the tendency to turn toward the midline of the body. Any complaint of pain or of a burning sensation under the tape should be reported to the physician immediately.

Although pressure upon the Achilles tendon will not cause paralysis, it must have special consideration. No tape should at any time pass directly over this tendon or very near above it. The tendon is exceedingly superficial and tends to become sore and denuded with great rapidity. An oblong piece of felt placed over this area before applying bandage or traction will eliminate danger to this area.

Oblique strips crossed on the tibia at any point are a threat to the underlying skin, and padding should always be applied at these points. Adhesive skin traction is not supposed to pull directly on bone. The pull is to be exerted on skin and subcutaneous tissues, and this fact should be borne in mind during application of the tape. Superficial bony points are to be guarded.

There are a few common errors in the use of apparatus that should be mentioned at this point. One of these is the use of a single pulley for more than one rope, a practice that limits greatly the efficiency of the pulley. Another is the use of a foot spreader so narrow that the adhesive tape connecting it to the leg contacts the bony points of the ankle, always vulnerable spots for pressure sores. A third error is the use of a foot spreader so wide that the adhesive strips constantly pull away from the skin of the leg, thus adding unnecessary discomfort to the patient.

Tincture of benzoin is frequently used for painting the skin before the application of the adhesive. This has a three-fold purpose: it serves as a disinfectant for the skin, it gives the tape greater properties of adherence, and it is said to allay itching beneath the tape. It is not always safe to apply it to the skin of an infant, because the adherence of the tape to the skin is so great that on removing it bleeding points are almost invariably encountered on the baby's skin.

In any case the skin should be dry and clean before the tape is applied, and in cold weather the tape may be laid over a radiator or hot-water bottle to increase its sticking power. Massaging the tape gently into the skin after its application will prevent much of the slipping that occurs when the weights are applied. Wrinkles or creases in the tape are to be avoided scrupulously in that they may be the cause of pressure areas on the underlying skin. Application of ether to dry skin wet with perspiration may aid in sticking the tape.

The adhesive should be applied with the knee in slight flexion to prevent hyperextension of the joint. The tape should cover a generous area of skin. The largest area of skin and subcutaneous tissue of the extremity is on the thigh, and the nurse should plan to utilize all of this, providing she does not receive contrary orders from the physician. One of the mistakes most commonly made by nurses and young doctors in applying traction is failure to extend the tape high enough on the thigh. A good rule is to extend the tape to the greater trochanter of the femur on the outside and 2 inches from the groin on the inside. Nurses should learn to know and use such landmarks as the femoral trochanter, which is the superficial bony knob on the external surface of the upper thigh 4 or 5 inches below the iliac crest. The tape should be measured from this point to a spot about ½ inch above the malleolus. The tape should never be applied directly to the malleolus but slightly above it. Beginning the application of the adhesive above the ankle is advisable, also, because space can be allowed for the tape to slip down, as it inevitably will do for the first 24 hours. If a moderately large amount of weight is used, a downward slipping of the tape for 1 or 2 inches may be expected in 24 hours. It is advisable to clip the tape obliquely every inch or so, beginning from the top. These nicks should be no more than ¼ inch in depth. They are to aid in fitting the adhesive tape more snugly and neatly to the contours of the leg.

The adhesive strips are then applied to the leg on its inner and outer aspects. English surgeons advise that the lateral adhesive strip be placed slightly back of the midline of the leg and the inner strip slightly in front of the midline. This tends to overcome outward rotation of the limb, so often a troublesome factor in traction work. However, under no circumstances should the strips be allowed to pass over the patella or over the popliteal space; this may happen if the tape is hastily or carelessly applied. The tape is massaged gently into the skin, and if circumstances permit, it is advisable to allow time to elapse between the application of the tape and attaching of the weights. Slipping will be much less likely to occur if this is done.

As has been stated, the use of these two straps alone is preferred by a number of surgeons. This is particularly true in children's hospitals, where the delicate quality of the child's skin is a consideration and where only small amounts of weight are necessary to obtain traction. In the adult services some type of transverse or spiral strip is frequently used to reinforce the longitudinal tape. For this type of traction a three-tailed adhesive strip may be used. It may consist of one wide piece of tape slit into three sections but undivided at its end or of three narrower strips stapled together at one end. The latter forms a neater dressing around the ankles. The center strip, slightly wider than the other two, is applied to the leg laterally and medially, as has been described. The other strips are wound around the leg obliquely, as shown in Fig. 80, with great care to avoid the pressure points mentioned.

A stockinet bracelet for padding the malleoli is an ingenious device used by some nurses. A 6-inch tube of stockinet, about 3 inches in width, is slipped over the foot to encircle the ankle region. Several layers of sheet wadding about 2 inches wide are wound loosely around the ankle over the stockinet, leaving the edges of the latter free to be folded over the sheet wadding and sewed together with a few basting threads. This provides an excellent padding that will neither slip nor fall off.

With the straight longitudinal adhesive strips unsupported by the transverse sections, a securely applied bandage is needed to maintain the position of the tape. In many clinics sheet wadding is applied over the adhesive in a simple spiral bandage, followed by a muslin or Ace bandage put on in an ascending spiral reverse. In these cases the sheet wadding is brought under the tape webbing at the ankle and provides effective protection of the bony points. It is a point of pride in many hospitals for nurses to be able to apply a beautiful and efficient spiral reverse bandage to the leg. Some orthopedists feel that the upper ends of the tape should be visible at all times in order that slipping may be detected without removing the outer bandage. It may be mentioned here that a figure-of-eight over the knee, which ordinarily would be used in applying a spiral reverse bandage to the leg, does not prove as satisfactory as a straight spiral or spiral reverse at this point. The reason is that the alternate periods of mild flexion and extension allowed some patients in traction usually displace the figure-of-eight bandage somewhat. Temptation to apply the bandage very snugly to improve its appearance must be firmly resisted. Circulation in the foot should be inspected after the bandage has been in place for several minutes. Signs of mild cyanosis will be present if the bandage has been applied too tightly.

When the three-tailed strip is used, a layer of gauze bandage is often applied over the tape for 24 hours or so. The surgeons who employ this type of traction usually request that it not be covered in order that the condition of the skin around the tape may be inspected daily. From the standpoint of the nurse this is most satisfactory, for unless bandages are removed daily it is altogether too easy for pressure areas to form under traction straps with none but the mildest complaints on the part of the patient. Needless to say, every complaint from the patient in traction deserves prompt attention. With these patients, as well as with those in casts, the nose is of definite assistance in detecting the musty odor that may result from pus forming under the bandage.

Once tape and bandage are securely applied, a footplate with buckles or a wooden spreader (if no plate is available) is attached to the sole of the foot. The spreader must be wide enough to keep the adhesive and tape webbing spread out somewhat from the malleoli. A small hook on the bottom of a footplate makes it possible to attach the rope. The spreader has a hole in its center large enough for the rope to pass through. A square knot on the surface of the spreader that faces the foot secures the rope, and the other end of the rope passes over a pulley secured at the foot of the bed. The weights attached to a carrier are suspended from this and must be high enough from the floor so that the patient's slipping down in bed will not cause them to come in contact with it. Canvas bags are sometimes used around traction weights to minimize noise and to prevent accidents from loosened knots. Weights must not be attached so high that if the patient alters his position in bed the knot will rest against the pulley. Rope should be of good quality, neither frayed nor pieced together. When a large amount of weight is applied to an extremity, nylon rope should be used. The added strength prevents sudden breaking of the rope and release of the traction.

All knots should be secure. The patient's comfort demands that no sudden release of knots occur to jar the leg in traction. All nurses should know how to tie a square knot and should make use

of it in their orthopedic nursing. Narrow strips of adhesive tape may be used to make such knots additionally secure.

The amount of weight to be used is dependent upon the doctor's order. As a beginning, 8 pounds is often used for the adult patient, and weight is added gradually until a maximum of 15 to 20 pounds is reached. For fractures large amounts may be applied at once. A large amount of weight should indicate to the nurse that she must be very solicitous in her observations of that patient's traction so that injury to the skin does not occur at any point. Children may have from 1 to 6 pounds of traction at the beginning, according to age and weight.

Orders regarding patients in traction are sometimes confusing to student nurses. For patients with scoliosis, for instance, it is occasionally the practice of surgeons to order a small amount of weight at the beginning with a substantial increase each day until a total of 30 or 40 pounds may be exerted on the head and pelvis. In patients with fractures the reverse may be true. A large amount of weight is frequently used during the first 24 to 48 hours, followed by a decrease in the amount after reduc-

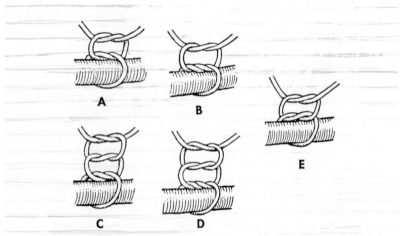

Fig. 83. Knots: **A**, square knot; **B**, surgeon's knot; **C**, square knot reenforced; **D**, surgeon's knot reenforced; **E**, granny knot. (From Mobley, H. E.: Synopsis of operative surgery, ed. 2, St. Louis, 1947, The C. V. Mosby Co.)

tion is obtained. For patients with scoliosis permission is frequently given to remove weights for short intervals during the day, but for those with fractures this would not be permitted. The maximum amount of weight for reduction of the fracture is put on immediately, and once reduction has been obtained, only such weight as is needed to maintain the bone ends in good position is used. However, this remaining amount of weight is important and should not be disturbed without specific order from the surgeon.

A word should be said about the danger of tape constriction in patients with fresh fractures to which traction has been applied. Traction for patients with fresh fractures should always be applied by the physician, but the nurse must realize that in trauma of this nature swelling inevitably occurs and an alarming degree of constriction may occur within the first 3 or 4 days. This must be watched for and reported to the surgeon immediately before any permanent damage is done to the extremity.

Rubber surface traction. Rubber surface traction requires the same equipment listed for Buck's extension, plus four long strips of soft porous sponge rubber. Three-inch adhesive strips are used for the skin traction without spiral reenforcements, and the sponge rubber strips are cut to the exact size of the adhesive tape. The adhesive side of the tape is applied to the sponge rubber and is rubbed well until it adheres securely. The rubber surface is then applied directly to the skin, as described for Buck's extension, and is secured to the leg by means of one or two 3-inch cotton elastic bandages. There is relatively little slipping when the weights are attached because of the suction of the rubber on the skin. The advantage of this type of traction is that the apparatus may be removed for physical therapy treatments and for hydrotherapy. Furthermore, it

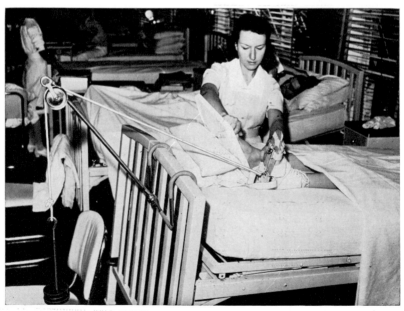

Fig. 84. Ankle traction with canvas boot and aluminum footplate. This type of traction is intended to be only temporary. Prolonged use results in pain and constriction over dorsum of foot and Achilles tendon.

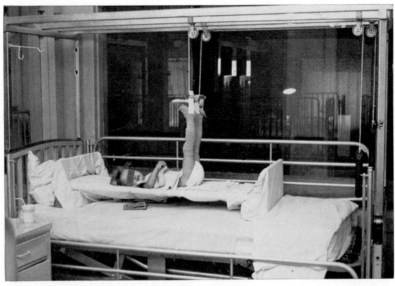

Fig. 85. Bryant traction for use in fracture of the shaft of the femur in young children. The frame is used to restrain child. Small blankets or divided linen must be used to keep the child warm.

can be used on skin that needs more watching than would be possible if adhesive tape were applied.

There are dangers, however, that the nurse must not ignore. To prevent slipping, the elastic bandage must be wrapped securely. This in turn may cause swelling and constriction of circulation, which is a real hazard with the older patient who has poor circulation.

Ankle traction. Ankle traction may sometimes be ordered as a temporary measure. It is obtained with a boot made of leather or canvas that is laced onto the foot and has straps extending below for rope and weight attachment. The shoe must be thoroughly padded over the dorsum of the foot as well as over the heel cord. Otherwise skin denuding and circulatory impairment will occur after a few hours in such traction. It is not the most satisfactory type of traction, although frequently its use is a necessity. Applying considerable weight to such a meager portion of the extremity is painful and dangerous. The nurse

should release the laces over the dorsum of the foot frequently and rub the area with alcohol. Ridged blue areas across the top of the foot inevitably occur after a few hours in this type of traction. Deep fissures have been known to form at this area within 24 hours.

Bryant traction. Both the Bryant traction and the Putti splint have their foundation in bilateral Buck's extension on the child's leg. Bryant traction is used in the treatment of a femoral shaft fracture in a child under 6 years of age. For this type of traction two overhead bars passing longitudinally over the crib will be necessary. One or two pulleys are attached to each bar. The legs are suspended from the bars at right angles to the body. When the weights have been applied, the child's buttocks must just clear the bed. Some form of restraint will be necessary to maintain this position, either a specially designed jacket or a Bradford frame with a harness restraint to keep the child in position.

When caring for this patient, the nurse

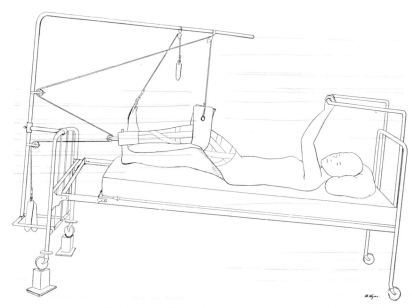

Fig. 86. Russell traction. Balanced traction adaptable to many types of thigh and hip fractures allowing relatively free motion of the patient in bed. Countertraction is obtained by elevation of the foot of the bed. The overhead trapeze adds greatly to the patient's independence.

will observe whether or not the child has normal motion in the ankle joints. Application of tape and bandage over the head of the fibula on the lateral aspect of the leg can cause peroneal nerve damage. The position of the bandage must be checked to see that it does not slip in such a manner as to cause increased pressure over the dorsum of the foot or about the heel cord.

Russell traction. Russell traction is in fairly general use in the treatment of fractures of the femur. When it has been properly applied and is in good mechanical working efficiency, it will restore muscle balance and make reduction of the fracture easier to maintain. Furthermore, it is a comfortable device for the patient, not the least of its merits.

The equipment required is not elaborate (Fig. 86). A single section of the common Balkan frame can be attached to the bed, with the overhead bar directly above the injured limb. Four pulleys are used. These pulleys are arranged

so that one is on the overhead bar at a level directly above the tubercle of the tibia of the fractured leg. A second is attached to the footplate or spreader. Two pulleys are attached to a crossbar at the foot of the bed and are placed at about the level of the mattress. A canvas hammock is often used for the knee sling, but a folded towel can be improvised to serve the same purpose.

Adhesive strips form the basis of the traction. In the original method these strips were applied only to the knee. Russell believed that it was best to extend the tape only from the ankle to the knee because he wanted the pull exerted at the point of insertion of the large muscles of the thigh into the tibia and fibula —namely, the hamstring and quadriceps muscles. However, many modifications to this original method have been devised by American surgeons during the past few years.

When the adhesive strips have been applied, the hammock is slipped under

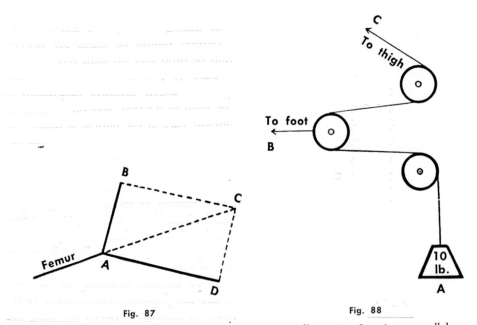

Fig. 87

Fig. 88

Figs. 87 and 88. Drawings to illustrate working of Russell traction. Imaginary parallelogram. Point **A** is the knee; **AB**, the rope suspending knee; **AD**, the line of the adhesive traction on lower leg; **AC** is the resultant or sum of the pulls **AB** and **AD**, which, if the traction is correctly applied, should be in direct line with the long axis of the femur. (From Calderwood, Carmelita: Russell traction, Am. J. Nursing 43:464-469, 1943.)

the knee and a rope is attached to it. This rope passes to the overhead pulley and then to the uppermost of the two pulleys on the crossbar at the foot of the bed. It is then passed over the pulley on the foot spreader and back to the remaining pulley on the end of the bed. Weight is then attached. The amount usually ordered for an adult is 8 or 10 pounds.

We are told that the pull of traction is twice that of suspension. Remembering Newton's third law of dynamics— "To every action there is an equal and opposite reaction"—and considering the 10-pound weight in the light of an action or effort, this pull can be readily understood by studying the diagram in Fig. 89. In order to balance A (the 10-pound weight) the person pulling on C would have to exert 10 pounds of effort. It can easily be seen then that the amount of

force being exerted on point B would be 20 pounds. If point B represents the patient's foot, the 20-pound pull on the foot is apparent.

The parallelogram of forces acting on the fractured femur about which surgeons speak is, of course, an imaginary parallelogram. It can be constructed by using the skin traction as one side of a quadrilateral and the rope suspending the knee as the other. Inasmuch as we know that the suspension is equal to about half of the traction, we make the vertical side of the quadrilateral only half of the horizontal length, thereby representing relative magnitude. With these two lines we can, of course, finish the construction of the quadrilateral or parallelogram. If the traction is in good mechanical efficiency, a diagonal passed through this parallelogram will pull in the direction of the long axis of the fe-

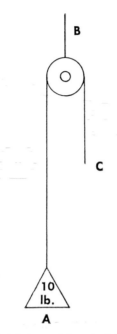

Fig. 89. Sketch to explain principle of weights in Russell traction. In order to balance **A** (the 10-pound weight) the person pulling on **C** would have to exert 10 pounds of effort. It can easily be seen then that the amount of force being exerted on point **B** would be 20 pounds. If point **B** represents the patient's foot, the 20-pound pull on the foot is apparent.

mur. This diagonal represents the resultant pull—that is, the combination of pulls of the suspension and traction, which are unified in the direction of the long axis of the femur.

Important nursing points are as follows: The angle between the bed and the hip should be approximately 20 degrees. The heel of the foot in traction should just clear the bed. Firm pillows should support the thigh and the calf along their entire length, leaving the heel free of the bed. The popliteal space must be watched for ridging and skin denudation. Back rest is usually permitted, and no difficulties are encountered in giving nursing care, because the fractured leg is not at the mercy of gravity and will not be altered in posi-

tion during any type of nursing care. Provision should be made for prevention of drop foot on both feet.

Care of patient in Russell traction. Russel traction includes suspension of the limb in traction, and for that reason nursing care of the patient is much simplified. The patient is usually allowed to sit up, to turn, and to move at will, because the line of traction is not disturbed by these movements. Care of the back, making of the bed, and giving of the bedpan are much simplified. Other nursing features that are important in caring for the patient in Russell traction are as follows:

1. To prevent wrinkling of the sling under the popliteal space a piece of felt may be inserted between the sling and the patient's skin. This will assist in eliminating pressure areas that sometimes form at this spot.

2. Whatever position the patient assumes, the angle of flexion of the hip in traction should be as near 20 degrees as possible at all times. (This is the angle between the thigh and the bed, not between the thigh and the abdomen.)

3. The heel should clear the bed. The ideal position for the heels of the patient in Russell traction is that of a person standing with his heels 4 inches apart. Abduction is to be avoided.

4. Two pillows are usually used under the traction: one of them is under the thigh to maintain the desired angle and the other is under the calf down to and including the Achilles tendon.

Care of patient in a Thomas splint. When a Thomas splint or any type of ring splint or suspension apparatus is used in conjunction with skin or skeletal traction, the patient is usually allowed more latitude in moving about in bed. If the leg rests on the bed, as it does in Buck's extension, any movement the patient makes with his body will alter in some degree the position of the traction. When suspension is used, however, the slack occasioned by the patient's movement is taken up at once by the suspension apparatus and the line of traction remains unchanged. Suspension allows freedom of the body as a whole while efficient traction on the limb is maintained.

We are told by Dr. McCrae Aitken—historian for Hugh Owen Thomas, who invented the Thomas splint—that Thomas invented the hip splint for a certain Sara McTurk in the year 1867. He had long disliked any type of traction apparatus that rested on the bed, because he noted the sagging of the limb that occurred when a bedpan was placed beneath the patient. The invention of the Thomas splint was an attempt to allow the patient to be moved for using the bedpan and for other nursing requirements without changing the position of the limb in traction.

Since the patient may be moved more safely, the problem of the sacral decubitus is not as troublesome as it is in patients with other kinds of traction. Furthermore, the splint is usually suspended or hung, and pressure on the heel of the leg in traction can easily be avoided. There are other nursing problems to consider, however, because of the pressure of the ring into the adductor and ischial area.

The ring of the Thomas bed splint is usually covered with smooth, moisture-resistant basil leather. It is usually considered advisable not to pad these rings with cotton or gauze.

When the daily bath is given, both the area of skin that is contacted by the ring and the leather ring itself must have special care. The patient may be turned toward the leg in the splint. The skin beneath the ring must be pushed backward and forward until all parts of it have been washed, rubbed with alcohol, and powdered. This is done by gently pulling the skin from under the splint above and below. The whole process contributes greatly to the patient's comfort and helps to preserve the integrity of the skin. Care should be taken not to apply the powder either to the skin or to the leather ring until they are well dried or the powder will cake.

The ring should be polished with saddle soap frequently and, if necessary, after each time the patient voids. A brisk rub is given to the leather, and this is followed by a rubbing with a soft dry cloth. The leather will take on a high polish that is moisture resistant. When the ring is thoroughly dry, it may be powdered sparingly. Alcohol should not be used on the leather—because it tends to harden it and make it uncomfortable for the skin. A soft, pliable, waterproof surface is the goal to be attained.

The tendency for pressure sores to form in the adductors and ischial region can be overcome by elevating the foot of the bed from 12 to 18 inches. The patient will thus pull away from the splint somewhat. In some cases this may be considered undesirable. The surgeon should always be consulted before this is done.

A half-ring Thomas splint (Fig. 78) is frequently used in balance traction. The splint is placed with the half ring on the anterior aspect of the thigh. With this arrangement the patient does not sit on the ring, there is less irritation in the groin area, and the difficulty and discomfort in using the bedpan are considerably lessened. The ring is not covered with padding and leather; consequently there is not the nursing problem of keeping it dry and clean.

Position of extremity in balance traction. The position of the extremity in traction is determined by the doctor, but it is well for the nurse to know that the limb is usually held in a neutral posi-

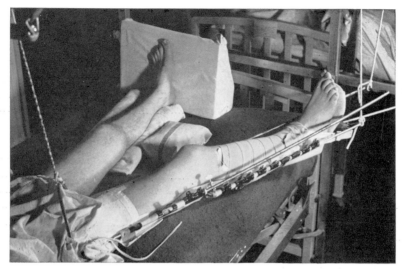

Fig. 90. Balance traction applied following cup arthroplasty. Note position of the extremities and use of sandbags to maintain this position.

tion (toes and kneecap pointing toward the ceiling) or in a position of slight internal rotation. The amount of abduction may vary with the patient. However, the nurse must recognize that when only one leg is in traction the position the patient assumes may greatly alter the amount of abduction being maintained. If the patient lies diagonally in bed, abduction is lost. Fig. 90 illustrates the use of a sandbag to remind the patient of the position he should maintain.

The patient's knee should correspond with the fastening of the Pearson attachment to the splint. Generally speaking, it is desirable to have the Pearson attachment (the part that supports the leg from the knee down) horizontal with the mattress and just high enough to swing clear of the bed. The position of the ring should be observed frequently. It needs to rest in the groin but should not cause undue pressure or irritation.

Pelvic traction. The pelvic girdle customarily used to apply pelvic traction is made of canvas, darted to fit the shape of the body. It is more comfortable if it is lined with flannel, which may be quilted in several thicknesses. This girdle is not to be made to fit the waistline except in its upper border. It is a pelvic girdle and is to pull from the bony crests of the ilia, so that its lower border will be considerably wider than the upper. It should fit snugly over the crests of the ilium and the pelvis, much as a girdle or garter belt does. On either side are tape-webbing straps, usually two or three, joined together to form one strip at about the level of the midthigh. If possible this strip should contain a steel ring for securing the rope for traction. The girdle is customarily fastened in front with tape-webbing straps and buckles.

Because it is exerting traction on bone, the crests of the ilia must have constant care and frequently, for the thin patient, padding over the crests will be necessary. Weight in pelvic traction is usually increased gradually, and although it may be started with as little as 5 pounds on each side of the pelvis it is usually increased considerably. The hazards of this amount of pull to thinly padded bony prominences are readily understood.

At the foot of the bed two pulleys about 2 feet apart are necessary. Ropes attached to the girdle extend through these and are attached to weight carriers and weights. It is the prerogative of the surgeon to order the number of weights, but when this is left to the nurse's judgment it is better to begin with too little than too much. Discouragement on the part of the patient during the first few hours may make further treatment difficult. Weights are not lessened or removed without the permission of the doctor who has given the order to apply them. Orders may occasionally be given to remove some of the weights at night to enable the patient to rest more comfortably. This type of traction may be applied to the patient with scoliosis to relieve pain and to gain some correction, or it may be applied to the patient with back pain to relieve muscle spasm.

The greatest complaint a patient in traction will have during his first 24 hours will probably have to do with pain in the lower part of the back, in the lumbar region. The thoughtful nurse will place some type of hard narrow pillow beneath this area, never one of the feather variety. If such a pillow is not available, a folded sheet will give considerable relief. The patient may remove the pad as necessary for comfort. This pain in the lower portion of the back is the result of a spasm of the extensor muscles of the back that occurs in conjunction with the pull upon the flexor muscles of the thigh.

At all times during the period that the patient is in traction the feet must be given protection. Some kind of foot support must be placed at the foot of the bed in such a fashion that the ropes are not contacted. Simple foot exercises carried out during morning and evening care will maintain the tone of the muscles. Dorsiflexion combined with toe flexion (not toe extension, which is the patient's usual tendency while dorsiflexing) is considered an adequate exercise for maintaining tone in muscles to be used for walking. When lying prone, the patient's feet must be supported or allowed to lie over the edge of the mattress.

Another point of discomfort to the patient newly in traction is a feeling of strain under the knee. A very small pad, such as might be made by a folded towel, placed under the head of the tibia will relax this joint satisfactorily and contribute much to the patient's comfort.

Frequently, the physician will request that the patient with acute back pain be placed in a semi-Fowler position in conjunction with pelvic traction.

Traction used in the treatment of fractures of the pelvis is discussed on pp. 411-413.

Head traction. It is preferable that head traction be secured with a well-made halter. (Sayre halter) ordered specifically for the patient who is to use it. Orthopedic and surgical supply houses have these available, or they can be custom-made of canvas or leather under prescription by a qualified brace maker.

In addition to the halter a spreader is needed. It should be wide enough to prevent pressure on the side of the head. The jaws and ears will become irritated if the spreader is too narrow. These two items plus the rope, weights, and pulley attachment are needed for the application of head traction with a Sayre halter.

Too much emphasis cannot be placed on the necessity for conscientious care of the chin during the period of traction. Alcohol rubs are almost always permissible, except for patients with acute inflammation, and should be given at stated intervals during the day. Cold

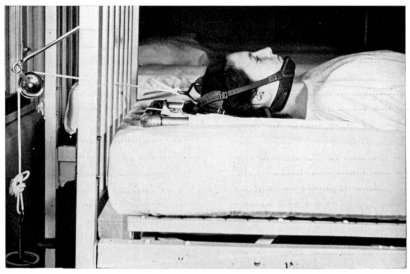

Fig. 91. Sayre chin strap for exerting traction on head.

cream massage, followed by alcohol to toughen the skin, provides an excellent skin treatment if the skin is in good condition at the beginning. Under no circumstances should massage or oils be applied in the presence of acne in that inflammation is likely to follow. This is especially true in hot weather. Soft material such as silk, sheet wadding, or silence cloth, inserted into the chin cup and changed frequently, gives the patient considerable comfort. Should the skin condition prohibit the use of the chin itself for traction, occipital traction can be substituted. In these cases the back of the head must be inspected closely each day for signs of irritation or pressure. The use of frequent shampoos for any type of head traction is indicated to improve the circulation of the scalp and to lessen the danger of decubitus ulcers.

Head traction may be applied to relieve muscle spasm and pain caused by an injured cervical disk or other injury. The patient suffering with cervical arthritis may receive relief when this kind of traction is applied. Head traction is

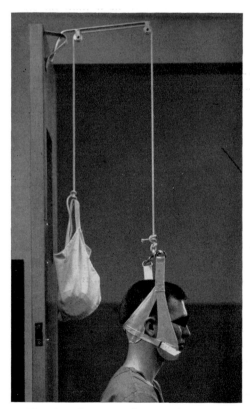

Fig. 92. Head traction that may be prescribed to be used intermittently in the home for the relief of cervical pain due to arthritis.

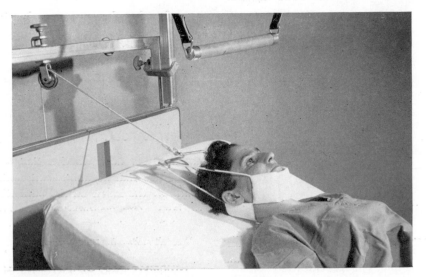

Fig. 93. A disposable head halter used to apply traction to the cervical region.

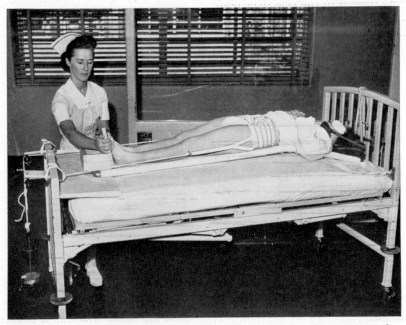

Fig. 94. Patient on Whitman frame with pelvic girdle and Sayre chin strap in place. Note boards to prevent frame from cutting into mattress. Foot support is always necessary, but some orthopedists feel that anything more than a pillow for this will disturb efficiency of traction.

used to relieve pain caused by the presence of a cervical rib or a scoliotic condition. Frequently, some type of head traction is applied following surgical correction of torticollis. The traction helps to maintain a position of overcorrection. Head traction with a Sayre halter may be applied to provide temporary immobilization and support when fracture of the cervical vertebrae has occurred.

Intermittent head traction is sometimes used in the home for short daily periods for patients with dorsum rotundum, cervical arthritis, and other conditions requiring hyperextension of the spine.

If a Sayre halter is being used indefinitely to maintain traction when cervical fracture or dislocation is present, difficulty may be encountered in giving adequate care to the chin and occiput. Traction must necessarily be constant, and, if considerable weight is being used, some danger to the skin over bony prominences may be expected. With the permission of the surgeon, the chin strap may sometimes be removed. One nurse exerts direct manual traction on the head. The grip is more comfortable to the patient if the nurse's palms are placed against his cheeks with her fingers flexed under his chin. The thumbs are not used during the process, and care should be taken not to encircle the patient's neck with the hands at any time during the process. A second nurse bathes and gently massages the skin and subcutaneous tissues of the lower jaw and chin.

Care should be taken to provide a spreader for head traction that is wide enough so that no unpleasant contact is made by the halter on the patient's ears or jaws. The occipital region requires special attention because pressure sores often develop in that area.

NURSING CARE OF PATIENTS IN SKELETAL TRACTION

Skeletal traction applied to an extremity. Various types of surgical apparatus for applying direct traction to bone have been used in the past fifty

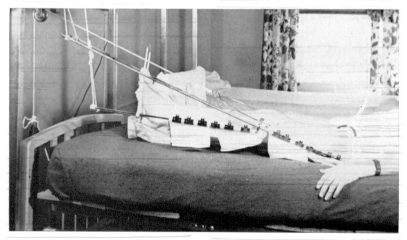

Fig. 95. Skeletal traction applied to the distal end of the femur. The limb is supported by means of a half-ring Thomas splint with Pearson attachment. The clips placed on the lateral aspect of the splint hold the canvas strips taut. The limb is in a neutral position and from the knee down is supported by the Pearson attachment. The position of the foot support can be adjusted to the patient's needs. Note U-shaped clamp attached to the Kirschner wire.

years. Nails, horseshoe clamps, stirrups, and ice-tong calipers have been used, but for the most part these have been supplanted by the Steinmann rustless steel pin and the Kirschner piano wire of chromic steel. The latter is perhaps the most commonly used type of skeletal traction and is preferred to the Steinmann pin because it is smaller in diameter and the disturbance to the bone occasioned by its use is almost negligible. Skeletal traction may be applied to the lower extremity through the proximal or distal end of the tibia, through the heel, and through the distal end of the femur. It may also be used in the upper extremity and in the skull.

The wire or pin may be inserted in the operating room or, if necessary, on the ward. The anesthetic used may be general or local. It is a surgical procedure and requires the most scrupulous aseptic technique in its performance. Usually, the area where the pin will be inserted is prepared surgically in advance of the procedure.

The wounds made by the introduction of the wire may be dressed with sterile gauze sponges secured by adhesive tape or small, quartersize circular sponges sealed with collodion. Whatever the type of dressing preferred by the doctor, the important thing is that it is not disturbed after it is applied unless evidences of gross infection become evident. Daily inspection of the wound is not necessary, and infections have been traced to overzealous dressing and cleansing of these wounds. Care should be taken not to allow the dressings to become contaminated by the patient's hands or through accidental spilling of fluids on the dressings.

It is usually wise to have a Thomas splint and Pearson attachment prepared and sent to the operating room with the patient. If the wire or pin is to be inserted on the ward, the splint should

be ready to be put on the patient's leg before the skin area is surgically cleansed.

Equipment to attach the weight to the U-shaped clamp that will be attached to the nail or wire should be ready on the ward when the patient returns from the operating room if the procedure is carried out there. Much discomfort can be eliminated if the weights are attached before the patient becomes conscious or before the local anesthetic has completely worn off.

Corks are usually applied over the sharp ends of the wire or pin to protect the nurses and patient from injury. All handling of the U-clamp, the rope, and the attached weights must be exceedingly careful to avoid causing pain and discomfort to the patient.

Skeletal traction is frequently used in fractures of the lower third of the femur, when it is essential that the fracture be treated with the knee in flexion. The Thomas splint with a Pearson attachment is generally used with this type of fracture. The splint and attachment are prepared with wide canvas strips or slings to support the thigh and lower leg. These strips should be fastened securely with large paper clips or safety pins on the lateral aspect of the splint to make tightening them more convenient. An overhead frame with pulleys is necessary for suspending the Thomas splint. The Thomas splint will usually be elevated at a 45-degree angle with the bed. The Pearson attachment is fastened to the Thomas splint at the knee joint. The knee is flexed to 45 degrees, and the lower leg lies in the Pearson attachment, which is horizontal with the mattress. Buck's extension is sometimes applied to the leg below the knee.

Equipment for preventing drop foot consists of an adhesive strip fastened along the sole of the foot and attached by rope to an overhead pulley. (Care must be taken not to exert pressure on the toes as contracture of the toe extensors will be likely to occur.) Also, commercial foot supports that clamp to the Pearson attachment are available.

Ropes are attached to the U-shaped traction clamp that holds the pin. This rope passes to a pulley at the end of the bed, where the weights are attached. The pull is in line with the Thomas splint and with the long axis of the femur.

The patient is allowed to move about rather freely in bed. He may sit up, or he may turn to his side as much as the traction will permit. The nurse must handle the apparatus with gentleness, however, for jarring movements are particularly dreaded by the patient. The rules applying to efficient skin traction also apply in skeletal traction, and nurses should be alert in their observations to see that the apparatus is mechanically correct and in good working order at all times.

When the wire or pin is to be removed, the skin is prepared as carefully as it was for the original procedure. Sometimes the surgeon will ask that the area surrounding the wire be saturated with alcohol solution for 24 hours before the removal.

The traction clamp and weights are removed from the limb, and the wire end on the outer aspect of the leg is sterilized with iodine, alcohol, and ether. The skin is then pushed inward, and the wire is cut beneath the surface of the skin. The wire is pulled through from the opposite side. Small sterile dressings are applied to the pin areas until healing takes place.

Skeletal traction applied to the head. Nursing care of the patient with skeletal traction applied to the head is included in the care of the patient with fracture of the cervical spine.

Bathing patients in traction. Patients in traction, like most other orthopedic patients, are bathed over the anterior surface of the body as the first step of their morning care. During the bath the toes are carefully cleaned and the sole of the foot is massaged with alcohol or oil. At this time the area around the traction tapes or bandage should be inspected. Particular attention is given to the back of the heel and the Achilles tendon, which so often become sore when adhesive tape and bandage have been applied too snugly. The dorsum of the foot is inspected for signs of ridging or cyanosis. If the protective bandage over the adhesive straps has become loosened either at the ankle or the groin, it should be reenforced or reapplied.

Nurses caring for patients in traction should make the observations listed below each time they give nursing care. To be effective traction requires constant vigilance, and nurses working on orthopedic wards should train themselves to take in many details of the apparatus at a glance.

1. Is the circulation in the extremity adequate? (Pallor, cyanosis, numbness, coldness, or swelling should be reported.)

2. Is the condition of the skin around the tape satisfactory? (Look particularly for signs of irritation, pimples, and purulent discharge. Use the nose as well as the eyes for the latter.)

3. Is the patient comfortable and warm? (Traction should never be a source of undue discomfort for the patient. If ropes interfere with the normal placement of bed linen, small blankets may have to be used and adapted to the individual patient's needs.)

4. Is the patient's bed position good, or does he use faulty body mechanics to thwart the purpose of the traction? Is the foot in traction protected against drop foot? Is provision made for maintaining the limb in a neutral position

and for preventing external rotation? Is there any inversion or eversion of the foot in traction? Is the opposite extremity in good alignment and protected against the pressure of the bedclothes? (It is particularly important to observe any tendency to lie with the foot in an inverted position. If this occurs, the padding over the area around the head of the fibula should be inspected. If this padding has slipped, it may mean that pressure is being exerted on the peroneal nerve, which lies close to the surface in this area. The peroneal nerve innervates the evertors of the foot, and injury to it may cause a partial or complete paralysis of the evertor muscles, making it impossible for the patient to turn his foot outward.)

5. Is the popliteal space free from pressure? (When the Russell traction is applied, a felt pad should be placed in the hammock to prevent wrinkling and undue pressure in any one area.)

6. Check the skin areas about the Achilles tendon and the malleoli carefully. These are likely spots for skin irritation.

7. Is the tape slipping at any point? Are the covering bandages adequate and secure?

8. Is the pulley working mechanically? (Watch for a stiff, unmoving pulley or a pulley with a shallow groove that allows the rope to slip off easily.)

9. Is the footplate or spreader wide enough to prevent irritation of the malleoli but not so wide that the tapes tend to pull from the limb?

10. Does the footplate or spreader contact the end of the bed when the patient slips down in bed?

11. Are the weights at a good level above the floor and also a considerable distance below the pulley? Are the knots secure?

12. Is countertraction provided?

13. Is there any impingement on the ropes either from the bedclothes or other apparatus? (Ropes should contact nothing but the pulley.)

14. Does the bed sag under the patient's buttocks? Are the heels digging into the mattress? (This causes friction, which lessens the traction. Also, the heel is a likely spot for decubitus ulcers. A small pad or folded sheet placed beneath the calf of the leg will help eliminate this problem. It prevents excessive weight on the heel and does not cause marked flexion of the knee.)

Without explicit permission weights are never removed at any time during the nursing care given these patients. This is an axiom of such serious import that it can scarcely be emphasized too strongly. The damage that can be done in fractures of the extremity by this kind of thoughtlessness may on some occasions be almost immeasurable. This is equally true in patients with tuberculous and septic joints.

When the patient has been bathed on the anterior surface of his body, the undersheet should be changed from the unaffected side. If the patient is a child, one nurse will be enough to assist with back care. If the patient is heavy, the procedure should not be attempted without two assistants. Both assistants stand on the opposite side of the bed from the nurse who is bathing the patient. One assistant supports the entire limb in traction, maintaining good alignment. The other places one hand across the patient's buttocks and the other under the shoulder girdle. For this procedure the nurse or attendant must use good body mechanics to protect herself against strain and fatigue. She should flex her hips and knees sufficiently to keep her back straight. She should stand in the foot forward position as close to the bed and the patient as possible, and she should tense her corset muscles for the activity before she begins to lift.

In washing the patient's back close attention should be paid to the sacral area, which is an extremely vulnerable spot that must have constant care to prevent breakdown of the skin. It should be emphasized that nurses giving care to such patients should take the trouble to inspect this area. The fact that the area is below the eye level often makes the nurse content to wash and rub the part without sufficient inspection. As sensitive as one's fingers are, they miss change of color, the purplish redness of the skin in the early stages of pressure before skin breakdown has occurred. Further damage may be prevented at this time, and it is important to detect the oncoming trouble before it progresses further. If signs of pressure are present, the area should be massaged gently and covered with a thin coating of talcum. A rubber ring may be provided, or squares of sponge rubber may be used. If squares of unclipped sheepskin are available, they may be placed under the sacral area. Most important of all, especially for the patient who cannot be turned, is frequent massaging of the part. This can be done, of course, without raising the patient each time. The nurse may slip her hand under the area and give an acceptable massage several times a day without changing the patient's position. Even moving the skin back and forth for a short period may prevent undue pressure on any point for a dangerous period and will be valuable.

The undersheet and drawsheet are usually changed from the side that is not in traction. If the patient is a child it is sometimes more convenient to change bed linen from the bottom or from the top of the bed. Many variations of bedmaking and bathgiving procedures are necessary in caring for the patient in traction, and no one way can ever be set down dogmatically as the best for all patients.

An overhead bar, or trapeze, is almost indispensable for the adult patient in traction. With this device he can support himself for back care and thus spare the nurse much unnecessary lifting. For patients with fracture or septic and tuberculous joints a second nurse or attendant should be on hand to steady the limb and keep it in proper alignment while the patient is receiving back care.

Prevention and treatment of pressure sores. The problem of preventing pressure sores on patients in traction is an extremely serious matter. Traction seems to predispose patients to this condition, first, because in many instances alteration of position is not allowed, and, second, because a great number of patients in traction are elderly. It is very common for the older person in traction to have a continual 30- to 45-degree back elevation as a safeguard against pulmonary congestion. This, of course, places a considerable portion of the body weight on the sacral area, and pressure sores tend to occur at that point with great frequency. In addition, the elderly patient often has dry tender skin, and the protective fat pads are gone from over bony surfaces. Often their nutrition is inadequate, particularly regarding protein and vitamin C, both of which are exceedingly important elements for promoting tissue health.

It is important that nurses recognize these hazards before trouble begins to occur. They should consult the doctor in regard to proper diet and obtain his assistance and advice in meeting the problem. He will often be able to help them in planning for change of position. Usually, some latitude will be allowed the elderly patient who must be in traction over a considerable period.

A great deal of the problem of pressure sore prevention is the responsibility of the nurse. She must recognize that trauma of any nature that endangers tissue integrity is a great factor in the production of skin abrasion, and the trauma need be no more than that caused by a few crumbs in the bed. Trauma can occur to the skin from wrinkles in the undersheet, the rubber sheet, or the drawsheet; it can occur from grit in talcum powder. A wet bed is a well-recognized cause of skin abrasion, and the necessity for keeping the bed dry and smooth can hardly be overemphasized. Patients who lift themselves on their elbows many times during the day may develop pressure sores at these areas. Another vulnerable site is the heel of the unaffected foot because the patient has a tendency to push himself up in bed with this foot.

Pressure areas go through certain rather well-defined stages. The first stage of redness will usually be accompanied by the patient's complaint of a hot burning pain at the site involved. After a day or so the initial reddened area may cause the patient little pain because of the paralysis of the sensory nerve endings in the skin. The redness in the area may take on a purplish cast which will not disappear upon blanching. The skin may break, because of an almost undetectable vesicle formation. Unless this progression is checked, ulceration may follow, and the denuded area may become the source of secondary infection by an endemic staphylococcus. Culture of these sores and appropriate antibiotics may be indicated in selected cases. Tissue necrosis may cause deep craterlike holes in the skin and underlying soft tissues that may reach down to the bone.

Fundamental to all treatment for this condition is removal of pressure. Frequently, permission may be given to turn the patient to his side for short periods to relieve pressure on the sacral area. If this is done, the nurse should be careful to keep the legs in good alignment. The top leg should be supported with pillows to prevent sagging.

A brisk rubbing to restore circulation to the threatened area can be given, but it should not be vigorous enough to endanger the skin. Alcohol may be used to toughen the skin, but it is advisable to use oil on the area once during the week to prevent excessive drying. Sponge-rubber squares or squares of unclipped sheepskin are often effective in preventing the progress of pressure areas if they are used during the early stages.

Small pressure pads placed around such points as the heel and the malleoli should not be circular but semilunar in shape. Too often the circular pad with its doughnutlike hole cuts off what little circulation is left to the part. A half moon that only partially closes the area accomplishes relief from pressure without the accompanying circulatory loss. Sponge rubber, cut into varying sizes and shapes, makes excellent pressure pads for heels, elbows and other bony prominences.

Some physicians prescribe drying powders such as boric or zinc. Tincture of benzoin is sometimes beneficial in the early stages of denudation.

Treatment for the advanced pressure sore with its craterlike hole is a more difficult problem.

If a culture taken from a decubitus ulcer grows a staphylococcus organism, the patient should be isolated and precautions taken to protect other patients and personnel. Gloves and mask should be worn when dressings are changed. The physician may request that the ulcer be cleansed several times daily, depending on the amount of drainage. Because of its infection-inhibiting properties, pHisoHex solution may be the prescribed cleansing agent. Daily irrigation with sterile saline solution, Dakin's solution, or solutions containing antibiotics are commonly used. Elase ointment, because of its action on necrotic tissue, may be placed on the ulcer. Packs of gauze impregnated with penicillin ointment or other antibiotics are frequently used. A and D Ointment, granulated sugar, and many other drugs may be prescribed and used with varying degrees of success. The physician

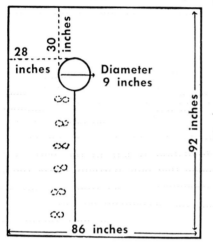

Fig. 96. Diagram of fracture or traction sheet. (From Wilde, Delphine: Some fracture nursing problems, Am. J. Nursing 39:964-967, 1939.)

frequently requests that dressings be omitted for certain periods of the day to permit drying of the area. Sunlight or treatment by the bactericidal lamp has been helpful in many cases. Dressings should be held in place with a minimum amount of tape, because adhesive itself can be a frequent cause of skin breakdown. With some patients it is advisable to use cellophane tape or Blenderm surgical tape. These tapes are usually less irritating to the skin.

Surgical closure of a decubitus ulcer may be necessary to facilitate rehabilitation. Pressure sores treated conservatively heal slowly and, in some instances, healing is superficial. The area breaks down when activity is started, revealing a larger underlying ulcer. It is necessary, therefore, to precede surgical closure of a pressure sore with several weeks of preparation. The patient must understand the importance of assuming positions that eliminate pressure on the involved area, and thus provide for a more adequate blood supply. Frequent cleansing and irrigation of the area are

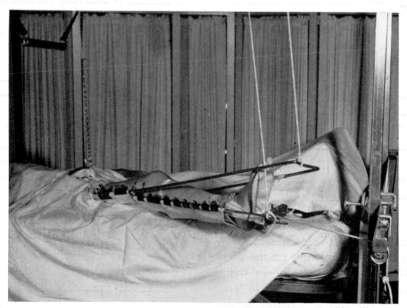

Fig. 97. Traction sheet. A small blanket may be used to keep the extremity warm.

prescribed to lessen infection and to promote growth of healthy tissue.

Bedmaking. In making the top of the bed the efficiency of the traction and the warmth of the patient are the important considerations. The appearance of the bed is always secondary. If divided linen is available, making the bed is a relatively simple matter. This linen may be made from standard sheets from any hospital linen room. A sheet measuring 86 by 92 inches may be slit 28 inches from the left side up to a distance of 62 inches. The raw edges may be neatly bound or hemmed with cotton tape ties attached at 2-inch intervals. This will provide a very simple sheet for a patient whose left leg is in traction. A more comfortably fitting sheet may have a hole 9 inches in diameter at the 56-inch level. This hole in the linen will fit neatly around the patient's thigh. For a patient in bilateral traction a double split should be made at the proper distance. Blankets may be made in the same fashion, and another divided sheet will serve nicely for a bed covering. If spreads are desired, the tape ties may be neatly covered by securing them beneath the spread at a distance of 4 inches from the divided section on one side and at the edge of the divided section on the other side. This 4-inch flap will then serve as a cover for the ties, making a neat bed possible for these patients. Large flannel socks may be slipped over the toes to keep them warm in cold weather, and cradles can be used to suspend blankets if necessary. If a small watt electric bulb is used, the patient's warmth need not be so much a matter of concern to nurses during the winter nights, but care must be taken to protect the bulb in some kind of wire cage. When divided linen is not available, there are several satisfactory ways to make the bed of a patient in traction. A sheet may be pre-pared by folding it in half with a small blanket in between. This may be used for the upper unit of the patient's bed, covering his chest and abdomen. The lower part may be made with a similar sheet and blanket passing over the normal leg and under the leg in traction, which may be protected by a flannel sock and a small lightweight woolen blanket. The nurse's well-worn ingenuity comes into play each time she cares for such a patient, and no set rule can be laid down except that the comfort of the patient and the efficiency of the traction come before the appearance of the bed in orthopedic wards. Undersheets and drawsheets must be snug and tight, but the upper part of the bed may be made according to the individual case.

Traction and bedpans. Because a great majority of patients in traction lie in a bed that has the foot elevated for countertraction, some difficulty in the use of the bedpan may be encountered. There are certain small tapering pans on the market that can be slipped under the patient without disturbing the traction or altering the position of the hips. These fit snugly against the flesh of the buttocks and prevent backward seepage. Female urinals are convenient and eliminate lifting. However, for enemas, when it is necessary to use a large pan, a rubber-covered pillow placed lengthwise along the back will prevent fluid from running backward into the bed. When there is no trapeze with which the patient can help himself onto the pan, nurses are cautioned to protect their own backs carefully for the effort. Bending the knees and hips and contracting the muscles of the buttocks and abdomen will enable the nurse to assist the patient more satisfactorily and with less danger to her own back.

Activity to prevent atrophy and stiffness of uninvolved extremities. It is always important that the parts of the body not in traction be kept in the best condition possible. No unnecessary stiffness or atrophy should be allowed to occur because of the immobilization of the injured part. Frequently, exercises for the uninvolved portions of the body are ordered by the physician and may include flexion and extension of the hip and knee of the good leg; dorsiflexion and inversion of the ankle; static exercises to strengthen the quadriceps, gluteal, and abdominal muscles; exercises to develop the extensors of the elbows and wrists to facilitate future crutch walking; and breathing exercises. The patient with only lower extremity involvement is also encouraged to use his upper arms and shoulders freely, particularly in positions of outward rotation and abduction. Activities such as combing his hair, fastening his gown at the back of the neck, or lying with his arms out at the sides with elbows flexed and palms upward are beneficial and prevent shoulder restriction that often results from long bed rest. Equipment must, of course, be supplied to encourage the patient to lie in good physiologic positions: a footboard or box, rolls for under the knee, and a firm pad for under the lumbar region; the latter is indispensable for the comfort of the patient who has traction applied with the legs in full extension.

Diversional therapy. It is also extremely important that the patient be given something to do. A patient in traction is confined so closely to his bed for such long periods that restlessness and depression occur rather easily. If an occupational therapist is available, she will be able to suggest many crafts suitable for this type of patient. Otherwise the nurse should provide some type of activity attractive to the patient, so that he will have the satisfaction of creating something with his hands while he is bedfast. Wherever possible, schooling should not be interrupted.

Patients in traction may be moved without too much difficulty to recreational courts or porches to provide variation in their daily program. If swinging weights are attached to the bed, moving should not be done by one person. Someone should be responsible for holding the weights during the moving process so that they do not swing or become dislodged from the pulley. Shock blocks will have to be removed and replaced during this moving. For this reason beds which may be raised or lowered or beds with pins for elevating the foot of the bed, if available, are to be preferred. These beds can be moved safely without being lowered.

There is a type of self-contained traction on the market, which dispenses with pulleys, weights, and ropes. The moving of beds is much simplified with this type of traction, and other nursing procedures may be carried out with much less interference with traction efficiency.

Crutch walking

The orthopedic patient usually has ample time to anticipate the moment when he will be able to move about on crutches. It is a goal that he sets for himself and looks forward to with great eagerness because once again he will be able to get around and do things for himself. This is the feature that usually

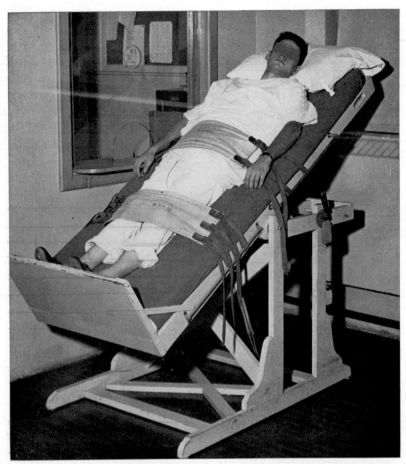

Fig. 98. The tilt table is used to help the patient adjust to the standing position. Several times daily he is placed on the table, and gradually the vertical position is attained. This activity has psychologic as well as physiologic values.

appeals most to him. Sometimes this same eager patient is considerably disappointed when he begins to use those crutches. He is weak; progress is slow; and many limitations of which he was previously unaware become apparent.

The nurse needs patience and foresight in her management of this situation. Many institutions have physical therapy departments to teach patients to walk on crutches. This is ideal for the patient. He receives careful instruction and guidance from a physical therapist skilled in this procedure. In the smaller hospitals, however, no such assistance is available to the nurse, and she must assume the responsibility for this part of her patient's treatment.

MEASURING FOR CRUTCHES

The nurse must first of all have some knowledge of crutches. The most common and satisfactory way to measure the patient for a crutch the correct length is to have him lie on his back with arms straight at the side. When the patient lies with the arms elevated over the head, measurement is often inadequate; contracture of the muscles in the axillae are essential for correct measurement. The tape measure extends from the axilla to a point 6 to 8 inches out from the patient's heel. He should be measured in the shoes he will wear to learn to walk. When it is inconvenient to have the patient lie down, measurements can be made by subtracting 16 inches from the patient's total height.

Crutches that are more than 2 or 3 inches too long should not be cut off to fit the patient without some provision being made for altering the handbar, which will otherwise be too low. The position of the handbar should allow practically complete extension of the elbow. The wrists are to be held in hyperextension. The palms of the hands should bear the weight.

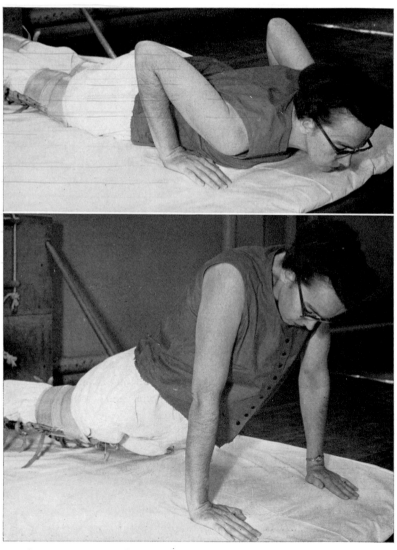

Fig. 99. Push-up exercises are done prior to walking on crutches. This activity is of special value in strengthening the triceps muscle (elbow extensor).

Crutch tips should be of good quality and should be inspected from time to time for wear. A worn crutch tip is a menace and must be recognized as such, for slipping is likely to result. Slipping may be undesirable for a normal person, but for the handicapped person it may spell disaster.

Padding over the axillary bar is not necessary, but frequently it is used because the patient thinks it is more comfortable. Some authorities believe that such pads encourage the patient to lean on the crutches, thus bearing too much weight on the axillae. Since crutch paralysis is not an infrequent complication from too much pressure on the axillae, under which the radial nerves lie, it is well to discourage this attitude from the beginning.

PREPARATORY EXERCISES FOR WALKING ON CRUTCHES

In hospitals or clinics where intensive treatment of disabled persons is carried out, attention is first directed toward developing and strengthening the muscles of the shoulders, chest, arms, and back. The patient is made to recognize the fact that he must have strong upper extremities and back muscles to support his weight when he becomes ambulatory. It is important that these things be accomplished before he begins to walk. An overhead trapeze is extremely valuable in encouraging the patient to use his arms and shoulders to lift his weight from the bed. He should begin standing exercises as soon as his general condition permits him to do so. Prolonged lying in bed can lead only to loss of muscle tone and incipient deformities that will make standing and walking all the more difficult when they are finally undertaken.

During the time the patient is carrying out active and active-resistive exercises to strengthen the upper extremities,

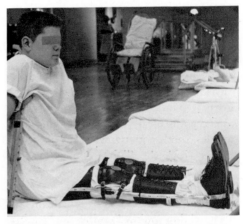

Fig. 100. Short crutches may be used in preparation for walking on crutches. Using the crutches to lift the body weight off the bed or mat is valuable in strengthening the shoulder depressors, elbow extensors, wrist dorsiflexors, and finger flexors.

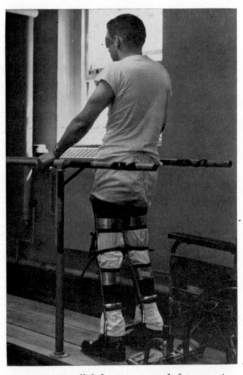

Fig. 101. Parallel bars are used for exercises in balancing, standing, and walking. They provide added security and safety for the disabled person.

the weak legs are carried through the full range of joint motion several times during the day to prevent muscle contractures and to minimize joint stiffness.

In preparing the patient to use crutches push-up exercises from the prone position are useful in strengthening the triceps muscles. Sawed-off crutches that may be used in a sitting position in bed will help the patient to become accustomed to the sensation of having crutches under the arms and will also give him the feeling of bearing his body weight on his hands. He can be taught how to hold his shoulder girdle as he practices with these sawed-off crutches, so that he will avoid hunching and will keep the shoulders at a normal or slightly depressed level. He can learn to shift his weight on the crutches while he is still sitting in bed. These sideways shifts will enable the patient to transfer himself to the wheelchair when he is ready for that experience. Exercises may also include the use of weights. With weight lifting the finger flexor muscles, the wrist dorsiflexor muscles and the triceps muscles are strengthened.

GOOD CRUTCH-WALKING POSTURE

The standing position is not attempted until the patient has mastered the bed exercises and has learned to transfer himself without help into a stabilized wheelchair. Standing with crutches may take a considerable time to master, for it is vitally important that the patient learn to balance himself on the crutches before he undertakes any further activity. Two hospital beds, placed with foot ends together and stabilized with wooden blocks, may be used as parallel bars for exercises in balancing, standing, and walking.

Nurses will not usually be required to teach the severely handicapped patient to walk on crutches. However, they must know what constitutes safe and

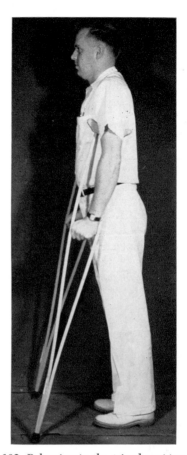

Fig. 102. Balancing in the tripod position.

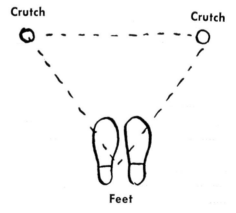

Fig. 103. Diagram showing proper standing position with crutches. The two crutches and feet make a triangle. (From Nelson, Doris: Crutch walking, Am. J. Nursing 39:1088-1093, 1939.)

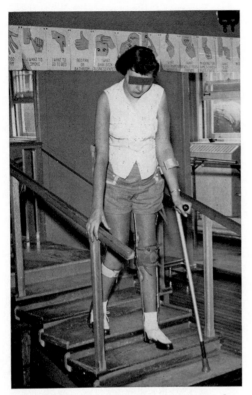

Fig. 104. Aluminum forearm crutch (Canadian type).

efficient crutch walking for this type of patient if they are to supervise such activities on the wards or in the home. They should be able to recognize the patient's maximum degree of good crutch-walking posture and to encourage it at all times. The desirable stance is one in which the head is held straight and high, with the pelvis over the feet if that is possible with the muscular power the patient possesses. The crutches are placed about 4 inches in front and about 4 inches at the sides of the feet, which makes a large standing base. As in all crutch walking, the patient should extend his elbows and carry his weight largely on his hands. He must not hunch his shoulders, and very little weight should be taken by the axillae at any time. However, the crutches will

lean somewhat against the rib cage and are grasped there by the adductor muscles of the arm and chest.

If involvement is such that this position is impossible—that is, when the patient has little or no use of the muscles of the hip joint, the back, or abdomen—he is usually taught to balance himself in the tripod position. In this position the weight is forward from the ankles, with the hips forward and the crutches ahead and out at each side. It is important to keep the pelvis as far in advance as possible with patients who have severe muscular involvement. They have litle muscle power in the front of the body to support them if the pelvis is held too far behind the feet, and so they must depend on anterior hip joint ligaments to stop them from going too far forward.

The patient must, of course, always be assured of his own safety. Usually, one attendant will stand behind him and one in front, but care is taken not to touch the patient unless it is absolutely necessary for his safety.

Attention to details of good posture is essential when the patient begins to walk. If he starts badly, he is likely to continue in the same attitude. Rounded shoulders, stooping back, slumping, flexion at knees or hips, outward rotation of hips, and eversion of the feet are postural defects particularly common to the patient walking on crutches. Fatigue, overdetermination to make progress, and muscular weakness from prolonged bed rest may account for some of this. Discouragement also may play its part. If the patient is allowed to see himself in a mirror, there is sometimes amazing automatic improvement in posture.

Sitting with back and feet well supported either on the bed or in a chair should precede actual walking by several days for the patient who has been bedfast for a long time. This is followed by standing at the side of the bed in good position, hips and knees extended, back straight, chest forward, and head up. Contracting the abdominal and gluteal muscles will assist with later easy natural locomotion and good posture. As the patient stands at the bedside he can be helped to shift his weight from one foot to the other without slumping, provided his disability permits. Alternate knee flexion and extension and deep-breathing exercises may be used to prepare the patient for walking. This is the slow approach, and the patient may be impatient to start actual locomotion. The situation and reasons for the delay must be carefully pointed out to him. Getting a patient out of bed and allowing him to walk on crutches in the space of one day usually ends in tears and discouragement.

The patient should learn from the first day the proper way to balance on crutches, as a safety measure and to give him a feeling of security. The starting position is a tripod formed by the patient's body and the two crutches. The patient stands with his feet slightly apart, and the crutches are placed forward and out from the body in such fashion that a line drawn between them would form the base of a triangle whose apex would be the patient's feet. All the factors of good standing posture must be observed. In teaching the patient to walk on crutches our aim is ultimately to enable him to walk without the crutches. Faulty unnatural habits developed during this period will inhibit ultimate return to a normal gait. Hips will tend to sag backward, the chin will be low on the chest, and the eyes will be directed toward the floor. These defects should be corrected before the patient actually begins to walk.

The patient is taught to extend and stiffen his elbow and to place the weight of his body on the wrists and the palms.

He is taught to avoid bearing any weight at the axillary level, because the radial nerve passes under this area superficially and pressure on it may cause paralysis of the extensor muscles of the hand and arm. It is, however, usually considered permissible to allow the patient with considerable arm and trunk involvement to lean on the axillary

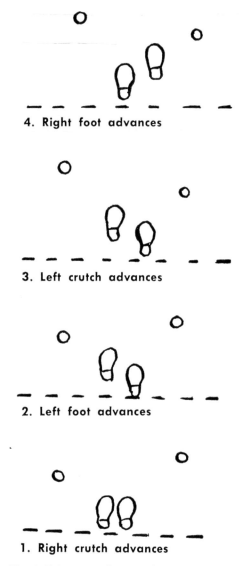

4. Right foot advances

3. Left crutch advances

2. Left foot advances

1. Right crutch advances

Fig. 105. Diagram showing the four motions of a four-point gait. (From Nelson, Doris: Crutch walking, Am. J. Nursing **39:**1088-1093, 1939.

bar for brief periods in order to rest the hands. The patient should be aware of the danger involved in using this position too frequently.

Persons beginning to walk on crutches have a tendency to try to lift a crutch when bearing weight upon it. Nurses should be alert to this tendency and explain the fallacy to the patient. The habit of taking a longer step with the weaker leg is a common mistake also made by beginners. Patients should be instructed to attempt rather short steps of equal length with both legs.

The Canadian crutch, without axillary rest, is preferred in some clinics. The advantage in the use of these crutches is that there is more tendency on the part of the patient to make better anatomic use of the hips and pelvis in locomotion. In other words, the patient tends to depend on himself and his own muscles more than on the crutches, which are really not much more than

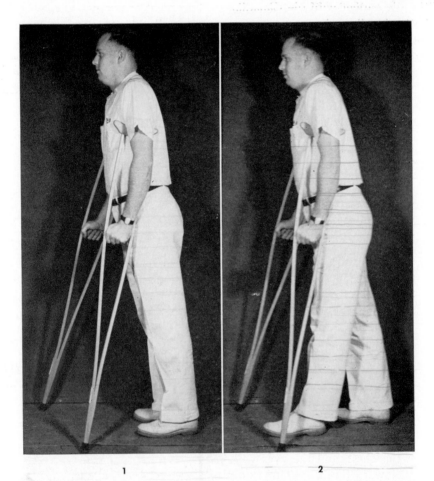

Fig. 106. Four-point crutch walking. **1,** Right crutch. **2,** Left foot. **3,** Left crutch. **4,** Right foot. Parts **2** and **4** of this group also illustrate the two-point crutch-walking gait: opposite foot and crutch are advanced simultaneously, i.e., right crutch and left foot are advanced together followed by left crutch and right foot. With the four-point and two-point crutch-walking gaits, weight is taken on each extremity. It is frequently used by the patient with poliomyelitis, arthritis, or cerebral palsy.

canes. Absence of the axillary bar is considered to be advantageous also in that likelihood of crutch paralysis is decreased greatly.

These crutches are particularly useful for the patient who is likely to need them only for a short period, but the longer crutch with the axillary bar gives more adequate support. It is usually considered advisable to use the standard type of crutch for patients who have involvement in the trunk, hips, and arms. In fitting the patient with the Canadian crutch the handbar should be in such a position that the shoulder girdle can be relaxed comfortably when the hand is dorsiflexed on the bar with the elbow in almost complete extension.

TYPES OF CRUTCH WALKING AND THEIR USE

The type of disability that the patient has determines the type of crutch walking he should do. Where help is available through a hospital physical therapist, it should be solicited in making the choice. In general, the following will apply to the most common types of orthopedic patients:

1. When the patient may partially bear weight on each limb, teach the four-point or two-point crutch gait. This is applicable to patients with poliomyelitis, arthritis, cerebral palsy, etc.

2. When the patient must bear little or no weight on one extremity, teach the method of advancing both crutches

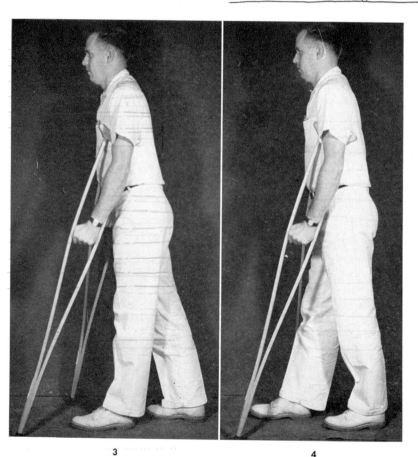

3 4

Fig. 106—cont'd. For legend see opposite page.

and the affected limb at the same time, the three-point crutch gait.

3. Swinging through crutches is sometimes permissible when paralysis of hips and legs is complete. This is the type so frequently seen on the street. It does not simulate normal walking in any way and leads to atrophy of legs and hips.

Modifications are recognized to be essential. For instance, although swinging between crutches is not recommended as a permanent practice for patients with poliomyelitis, it may frequently be necessary when speed in walking is essential. Also, the use of one crutch or cane is an advanced procedure for the preceding method. The crutch is used on the normal side, because it is put forward at the same time as the disabled limb, thereby taking the weight off that foot.

Four-point crutch gait. The four-point gait can be performed to a count of 1-2-3-4. The patient puts one crutch forward, then the opposite foot, the other crutch, and the opposite foot. This is hard for a normal person to do, although it approximates normal walking motions of arms and legs. However, with a little practice the patient becomes automatic in its use.

Two-point crutch gait. The two-point

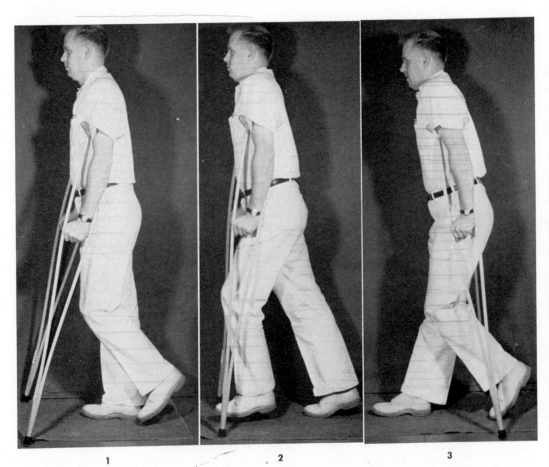

1   2   3

Fig. 107. Three-point crutch-walking gait is used when there is involvement of one extremity. It may be used when no weight bearing has been ordered or when partial weight bearing is permitted. The affected extremity advances with the crutches, and the patient's weight is taken on the hands as the normal extremity comes forward.

gait is the same as the four-point gait, except faster. With this gait the patient advances the opposite crutch and limb simultaneously—left crutch and right limb, right crutch and left limb.

Three-point crutch gait. Walking on crutches is usually an ordeal for the patient who has been inactive over a period of time. Everything possible should be done to make the experience safe and comfortable. The patient will need instruction and constant encouragement if he is to learn to use crutches without undue fatigue. When no weight bearing has been ordered or when partial weight bearing is permitted on the affected extremity, the three-point gait is usually considered preferable. The patient may be taught the mechanics of this gait by means of a diagram before he is out of bed. The affected limb and both crutches are advanced at the same time. Then, with the body weight balanced on the two crutches and the weak leg, the normal leg is advanced. The patient should be instructed to take steps of equal length; otherwise he will tend to take a long step when using the crutches and a very short one when advancing the normal extremity.

When the physician wishes the patient to begin bearing weight on the

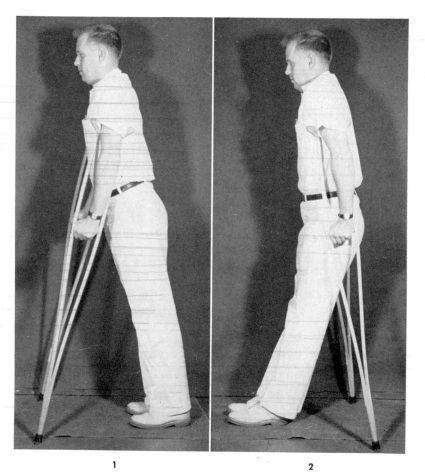

1   2

Fig. 108. The swing-through crutch gait is used when both lower extremities are paralyzed. The limbs are braced and swung forward together.

affected leg, it should be begun gradually. As the patient advances in the ability to manipulate himself on crutches, one crutch may be discarded. The single crutch should be used on the normal side because its purpose is to carry the weight of the body when the normal leg is advancing forward.

Swing-through crutch gait. The swing-through gait is frequently used by the patient with poliomyelitis with paralyzed lower extremities. The limbs are braced and swung forward together. This is a rapid gait but does not simulate normal walking.

Tripod crutch gait. The tripod gait is often taught to patients with severe involvement of the lower extremities. The right crutch is advanced first, then the left crutch, and the body is then dragged

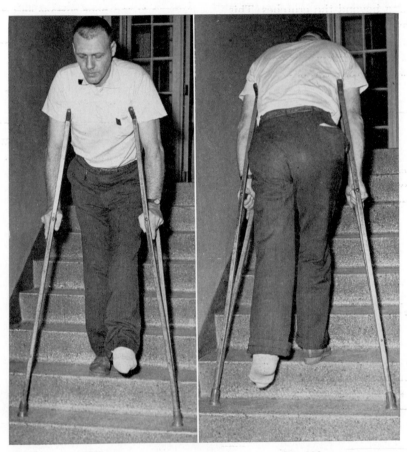

Fig. 109   Fig. 110

Fig. 109. Down the stairs with crutches. The crutch walker who is accustomed to the three-point gait will place his crutches on the lower step, take his weight on his hands, and bring the normal extremity down to the lower step with the crutches. Then with the body weight on the normal extremity the crutches are placed on the next step and the procedure is repeated. **Fig. 110.** Up the stairs with crutches. When going up steps, the body weight is taken on the hands and crutches and the normal extremity is advanced to the upper step. The body weight is then taken on the normal extremity, and the crutches and involved limb follow. A safe rule to remember when teaching the three-point crutch gait is that the involved limb always goes with the crutches.

up to the crutches. If the upper extremities and shoulders are strong, the patient can use the swinging crutch gait. For this gait the crutches are placed together in front of the body. The patient then bears down on the crutches and lifts his body so that it is brought up to the crutches. The next step in advance of this method is the swing-through gait, when both crutches are placed ahead and the body is lifted and swung beyond the crutches. This is more involved than the first swing gait because the body is swung through the crutches and therefore comes to the floor ahead of the crutches.

HAZARDS OF WALKING ON CRUTCHES

Everything possible should be done to ensure the patient's safety, for a fall is extremely hazardous after a long period of inactivity. Even a mild mishap may lead to a fracture. When the pa-

tient begins to walk, there should be one worker in front and one behind him. He should not be encouraged to lean on his assistants, but he should feel confidence in their presence at all times. No wet spots, loose rugs, or other obstacles to safe walking should be near the patient. Crutch tips must be intact and should be replaced when there is any sign of thinness in the rubber. Suction crutch tips, as the name implies, adhere to the floor surface and decrease the possibility of slipping.

Common errors for which the nurse should be alert are: walking with the knee and hip flexed, the foot everted, and the hip in outward rotation; a tendency to walk with the weight on the ball of the foot and with the heel elevated; and a slouching posture, with the eyes fixed on the floor, the chin on the chest, and the shoulders and back rounded.

Nursing care of the orthopedic surgical patient

Nurses will remember from their surgical nursing experience that hemorrhage, wound infection, and pain are the three great obstacles to success in surgery. In orthopedic surgery, impairment to circulation caused by mechanical obstruction must be added. Nurses should be alert for symptoms that indicate the presence of any of these conditions.

GENERAL CONSIDERATIONS

A great number of reconstructive operations on bones are performed on people past middle age. Steindler states

that when the constitutional background of the patient is abnormal, it will have a definite primary influence upon the surgical risk. It is for this reason that laboratory tests are done on a large scale. In addition to the routine laboratory tests done on all surgical patients, such as blood count, hemoglobin estimation, bleeding and clotting time, and urinalysis, the orthopedic surgeon often requests determinations of serum calcium, phosphorus, and phosphatase, as well as of the blood sedimentation rate. All these things are especially necessary in older persons in whom the surgeon suspects metabolic changes in the bones. Renal function tests are sometimes ordered, because certain anesthetics offer a definite threat to the patient with kidney damage. Surgery adds a heavy burden to the kidneys by diminishing body fluid through perspiration, lack of ability to take fluids properly over a period of some hours or days, vomiting, and hemorrhage. Nurses should be able to read laboratory sheets with some degree of facility and intelligence in order to understand more satisfactorily their patients' condition. Understanding preoperatively the risk facing the individual patient will enable the nurse to assist in his recovery more confidently. A high sedimentation rate is not a good prognostic sign. Excessively high or low blood pressure may lower the patient's vital capacity. Specific gravity of less than normal in the urine adds to the gravity of the outcome. Blood urea nitrogen of over 35 mg. per 100 ml. of blood indicates a considerable degree of kidney damage. It is a well-known fact that postoperative mortality in patients with nephritis complicated by hypertension is high. Any patient who has been confined to bed over an extended period is not considered a good surgical risk.

Dehydration, present or threatened, is an outstanding danger that may be recognized preoperatively. An increase in fluid intake is of greater value before operation than afterward. A daily intake of at least 3000 ml. containing a high percentage of glucose is advisable, and a diet predominating in carbohydrates is advised by some authorities for 48 hours preceding orthopedic surgery.

Delayed coagulation time demands special treatment. Frequently, an intravenous injection of 10 ml. of 5% sterile calcium chloride solution is given for 2 days preceding operation. Transfusion is of greater value if it is given before operation than afterward. Men-

struation is not considered a definite contraindication to orthopedic surgery, although some surgeons will postpone the surgery because coagulation time is somewhat lengthened during this period. It should always be reported to the doctor before the patient is sent to the operating room.

The mental condition of the patient demands respect. This is particularly true with the spastic child. Severe excitability is known to bring about acidosis. When possible, the patient with cerebral palsy should be allowed to obtain some mental equilibrium before surgery is performed. Some surgeons will scoff at preoperative psychic depression. Others feel quite definitely that such depression adds to the gravity of a postoperative prognosis, particularly when premonition of death exists. Such mental states should be reported to the doctor by the nurse as accurately as is a definite physical symptom.

Excessive obesity causes the surgeon concern because of the impairment in respiration that sometimes accompanies it. Wound infection and fat embolism are possibilities to be feared, especially in these patients. A marked degree of weight loss is not considered a good indication, because a loss of glycogen reserve is likely to exist. After operation persistence of nausea and vomiting will increase the gravity of such a patient's condition extremely, in that acidosis may occur very quickly.

Inhalation anesthesia is usually preferred by orthopedists, largely because it is a controllable anesthesia; that is, it can be discontinued at once if the patient's condition seems to warrant it. Spinal anesthesia is sometimes used in older persons or in those with hypertension. Danger signals in this type of anesthesia are rapid fall of blood pressure and diminution of the respiratory rate. The surgeon will usually order ephedrine in these cases.

PREOPERATIVE PREPARATION OF PATIENT

Preoperatively, a general physical examination will be performed by the physician. His preoperative instructions will usually consist of orders for increased fluid and carbohydrate intake, cathartics, enemas, and preoperative sedation. Antibiotics may be administered to patients who have had osteomyelitis or some septic bone condition in former years. Children are predisposed to acidosis after operation, and in their case, sugar in the form of stick candy is given the night before surgery. Although breakfast is omitted for all surgical patients receiving general anesthesia, some orthopedists order the juice of one orange to be given 2 or 3 hours before surgery to all young children. The use of strong cathartics is not recommended by most surgeons. Enemas may or may not be given. If they are ordered, they are usually given the night before the operation, the morning of the operation, or both, depending on the surgeon's wishes. Barbiturates may be given the night before surgery to ensure proper rest. These are especially advisable for the nervous patient and are frequently given the morning of operation also, particularly when rectal, spinal, or local anesthesia is to be used. The usual preoperative medication of morphine or a derivative combined with atropine or scopolamine is used, except in very young or elderly patients.

Attention to the physical and mechanical data should not shut from the nurse's mind the psychologic treatment that must accompany much of the preparation of any patient for surgery. Most orthopedic conditions are not acute. The patient has perhaps anticipated this operation for some time. Probably, if he is an adult, he has debated the advisability of having the procedure performed over a long period of time. The emotions he feels are a mixture of hope and doubt

—hope perhaps that he will regain the use of a long paralyzed limb and fear that the surgery and long convalescence may be of no avail. It is a great moment in his life, and the nurse should recognize this. She should realize that the difference between the operative procedure for the orthopedic patient and that done for the ordinary surgical patient lies in the hope he has that some lost function of his body will be restored to him. This hope often overrides the natural fear. While she is preparing the operative site, the nurse has an opportunity to establish rapport with the patient and to listen to his story so that she may gain some knowledge of his social background. Also, it is a good time to explain to the patient his own part in his recovery and the necessity for patience and cooperation to ensure a successful outcome.

PREPARATION OF OPERATIVE SITE

Because the consequences of infection in bone surgery are so grave and may lead to crippling through stiffness of the joints or chronically infected bone, the preparation of the operative site must be carefully and conscientiously executed. The exact procedure used will vary from clinic to clinic. Recently, however, there has been a tendency to omit the long 48- or 72-hour sterile orthopedic preparation. The orthopedic patient may be given a preparation similar to that given the general surgical patient.

The antiseptic solutions used vary in different clinics. The method of preparation, however, is much the same. It is now well recognized that mild soap and water are probably the best agents available, not only for removing dirt and grease from the skin but also for eliminating bacteria safely and effectively. Some surgeons feel that no other antiseptic is necessary for cleansing the skin.

After the preliminary cleansing of the skin shaving is the next step in the op-

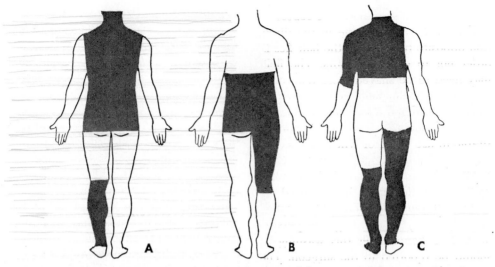

Fig. 111. A, Drawing illustrating sites commonly prepared for surgery of the spine with autogenous graft from left tibia. B, Site prepared for bone operation on hip. C, Sites prepared for operations on shoulder, ankle, and knee.

erative preparation. The area to be shaved is usually designated by the doctor in his preoperative orders, but the nurse should know what constitutes the area of preparation for all types of orthopedic surgery. Surgery performed on the toes will usually require a surgical preparation to the knee; surgery on the ankle, to the midthigh. In spinal surgery the area will depend on the site of injury or disease. If the operation is to be performed in the high cervical area, the shaving will no doubt include the back of the neck and occiput and will continue to the buttocks. Preparations for operations on lower spinal fusions will include the backs of the buttocks and the upper parts of the thighs and will extend upward to the shoulders. If a graft is to be taken, the leg will be prepared from ankle to midthigh or groin. Knee operations usually indicate preparation of the leg from the toes to the groin. For operations on the hips the preparation usually extends to well below the knee and to the lower border of the ribs, the umbilicus being the limit anteriorly and the spine posteriorly. The pubic area is always included. The nurse must remember that a preparation for operation on one joint should include preparation of the joint above. This is not always a rule, but it provides a generous enough area that little dissatisfaction will be found.

Nurses should develop a deep respect for the importance of the skin, recognizing the fact that the intact skin serves as a mechanical barrier to keep bacteria out of the body. Indeed, some investigators feel that a clean, healthy, and intact skin may actually have a self-disinfecting power. Nothing that is done during the sterile preparation should lessen in any way the defensive powers of the skin.

The shaving must be most carefully done. The blade should be new and of good quality. It is not a procedure to be hurried. Two things can happen with a hurried shave: denuding of the skin area or omitting a small field of fine hair. Hair is not easy to disinfect and may be a source of infection. A denuded area is a grave threat and may mean postoperative infection. Most surgeons will refuse to operate in the face of it. Abrasions of the skin of any sort should be reported.

Shaving is usually done in the direction opposite from which the hair lies in order not to omit fine hairs. The field may need to be shaved more than once to ensure a clean field. A wet shave is usually considered more satisfactory, but in case of emergency, when it is not desirable to use water or when the electric razor is used, a dry shave may be given.

After the area is shaved the extremity for operation must have special attention. It must be thoroughly washed and absolutely clean. If grime persists on feet or hands after this washing, it should be reported to the surgeon. The toenails or fingernails must be clipped and thoroughly cleaned. Frequently, it is necessary to soak the foot or hand in warm sudsy water for 30 minutes prior to scrubbing.

After these preliminary but important details have been attended to, the procedure that follows will vary somewhat according to the wishes of the surgeon. In general, however, the area that has been shaved is well scrubbed with mild soap and water for 3 to 5 minutes. A brush is used for this scrubbing unless the skin is sensitive and tender, and then sponges may be used. The nurse must recognize that this mechanical cleansing of the skin prior to the preparation in the operating room is of the utmost importance and must be done conscientiously.

A tray or cart for these preparations should be on every orthopedic service. It should contain an extension light, a razor with fresh blades, unsterile towels for protecting the bed from moisture, bottles containing mild liquid soap, the antiseptic preferred by the doctor, ether or benzine, and water. A small cup or basin to contain water for the shave, a paper sack, cotton balls or sponges, gloves if they are used, and adhesive tape will complete the tray.

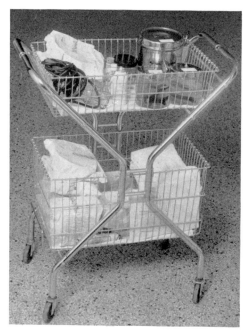

Fig. 112. Equipment necessary for cleansing and preparing the skin for a surgical procedure can be taken to the bedside in this lightweight cart.

BLOOD TRANSFUSIONS

The transfusion of blood has become a common procedure and is done frequently on a busy hospital service. Yet the transfusion of blood carries a death risk as great as that from an uncomplicated appendectomy. The observations made by the nurse during this procedure are a vital part of the patient's care. The alert well-informed nurse can prevent some dangerous reactions, and her prompt recognition and treatment of others can be life-saving.

When the blood is delivered to the patient area, prior to the time that it is to be given, it should be placed in a refrigerator and kept at a temperature above freezing until it is to be transfused. Blood should not be permitted to stand at room temperature for several hours.

Before the transfusion is started both

the physician and the nurse should compare the patient's name and registration number on the label of the blood container with that on the patient's identification wrist band. In addition to the patient's name the type of blood and the Rh factor appearing on the bottle label should be checked against the accompanying slip. Dangerous reactions and deaths have occurred because blood has been given to a patient for whom it was not intended.

During the entire transfusion the recipient should be watched carefully. It is essential that the drop indicator on the transfusion set be checked frequently and adjustments in the rate of flow be made when necessary. The soft tissues around the needle should be checked for swelling. A hematoma caused by blood going into the subcutaneous tissues can be very painful and may result in serious slough of tissue. The complaints of a patient receiving blood must not go unheeded. Any complaint of respiratory difficulty, such as pain or tightness in the chest, fast breathing, wheezing, coughing, pain in the abdomen or lumbar region, or the appearance of chills or hives, is an indication for the nurse to stop the transfusion and to notify the attending physician. The appearance of respiratory difficulties may necessitate the prompt application of tourniquets on all four extremities, the upper arms and the thighs. The purpose of the tourniquets is to prevent pulmonary edema by pooling the blood in the extremities away from the heart. The tourniquets should be pulled tight enough to hold back venous blood but not tight enough to occlude arterial pulses. The tourniquets should be released one at a time for 2 minutes, then replaced and another one released. No tourniquet should be in place more than 10 minutes without a respite.

Do not permit the tubing to empty completely before discontinuing the transfusion. Near the end of the transfusion watch the apparatus carefully so that the blood flow may be stopped when there is still 20 ml. or so in the container or tubing. If the transfusion has been discontinued because of a reaction, place the used equipment containing the residual blood in the refrigerator. The labels and unused blood should be available for posttransfusion tests in the investigation of transfusion reactions.

After a transfusion take the patient's temperature at 2-hour, 4-hour, and 6-hour intervals. An elevation in the temperature should be reported to the physician.

A 24-hour collection of urine should be made for all patients receiving transfusions. Note the volume and color of each specimen as it is collected. Oliguria is the output of a dangerously small amount of urine, usually less than 600 ml. in a 24-hour period. If a single specimen, collected over a known period of time, has a volume of less than 25 ml. per hour, or if a red color is present in a urine specimen after transfusion (probable hemoglobinuria), save the specimen and notify the physician.

Immediate transfusion reactions

Transient fevers. These are often initiated by a chill. The fever may occur during or soon after transfusion. The cause may be the presence of polysaccharides called pyrogens in the blood mixture. These pyrogens are produced by the growth of nonpathogenic bacteria in the fluids or equipment used in the transfusion. These substances are not destroyed by sterilization. A second cause may be the presence of small amounts of heated plasma protein left in reused equipment. A third cause may be the onset of a hemolytic reaction in which the donor's or recipient's erythrocytes are destroyed. Early hemolysis may be excluded by drawing a fresh specimen of the patient's blood, centrifuging it, and demonstrating the lack of pink coloration in the plasma or serum.

Urticaria. Hives occur in about 1% of the patients receiving blood transfusions. During or soon after giving the blood patches of hives or angioneurotic edema appear on the skin. This can be promptly dealt with by an intramuscular injection of 0.3 ml. of a 1:1000 solution of epinephrine. The transfusion can then be continued.

Hemolysis. Destruction of the red blood cells may occur from (1) damage to the donor's blood by improper storage, overheating, or freezing of the blood, or the mixing of the blood with distilled water, glucose solutions, or solutions other than isotonic sodium chloride, (2) the transfusion of blood containing red blood cells that are destroyed by the recipient's antibodies, or (3) the administration of blood whose plasma contains strong antibodies against the recipient's blood cells. Some of these incompatibilities cannot be detected by the usual laboratory tests. However, some may occur from errors in blood grouping or crossmatching, errors in labeling blood containers, or errors in reading the labels by the nurse or physician. Hemolytic reactions often start with a chill and fever, accompanied by pain or a constrictive sensation in the chest and pain in the lumbar regions or thighs. These symptoms should indicate the immediate discontinuance of the transfusion, notification of the physician, examination of a fresh urine specimen for hemoglobinuria, and the collection of a fresh blood specimen from the patient for examination of plasma hemoglobin. Between 6 and 24 hours after transfusion hemolysis has occurred the patient may develop painless jaundice that lasts a day or two. Two dangerous complications may result from hemolysis. A state of immediate shock may occur in which the patient has few symptoms except lethargy, and low blood pressure. Death may occur in a few hours. More insidiously, the kidneys may be damaged so that the urinary output is less than 600 ml. in a 24-hour period. Complete cessation of urinary excretion is called transfusion anuria; when some urine, but an insufficient amount, is produced, it is termed oliguria. The prognosis is the same for both; normal urinary excretion may resume any time up to 3 or 4 weeks, or death may occur from renal failure.

Circulatory overload. This occurs when the increase in blood volume from transfusion causes acute cardiac failure and pulmonary edema. The patient suddenly becomes extremely short of breath, with wheezing respirations and cyanosis of the lips. When these signs occur, the transfusion should be discontinued at once and tourniquets (as described previously) placed on all four extremities. Preparation should also be made for a phlebotomy, which the physician may wish to perform.

Air embolism. This condition occurs rarely but it is possible whenever a leak is present in certain parts of the transfusion apparatus, or when all the blood has run out and air follows it into the vein. The patient has pain in the chest with severe dyspnea and cyanosis. The nurse can hear thumping in the heart at a distance. Prompt action may be life-saving. If this occurs, the transfusion should be discontinued and the physician notified. The patient should be placed on his left side so that the air bubbles float upward in the right ventricle away from the outlet to the lungs, and oxygen should be administered.

Delayed transfusion reactions

These need not concern the nurse directly but are mentioned for general information.

Transmission of disease. In the United

States infectious hepatitis (serum type), or homologous serum jaundice, is the most common disease transmitted by transfusion. The donor is a carrier of the causative virus but usually has no clinical signs or symptoms of the disease; thus there is no method of excluding him from giving blood. The incubation period in the recipient is roughly from 60 to 120 days. The patient may become jaundiced with signs of severe liver damage, and there is considerable mortality. In some parts of the world transfusion malaria is a serious problem. With ordinary storage of blood the malarial parasites outlive the erythrocytes. The only method of preventing the disease is to reject all donors who have had untreated malaria within 5 years. Transfusion syphilis is usually not possible to contract from blood that has been refrigerated for more than 2 days, because the causative treponemas are readily killed at low temperatures. Syphilis may be transmitted by transfusion of fresh blood when the donor has a chancre and enough time has not elapsed to confirm the diagnosis of syphilis by a positive Wassermann reaction. The disease differs from that acquired by physical contact in that when the blood of a syphilitic person is given to another person, the recipient will also acquire the disease but without the chancre. The incubation period of syphilis acquired in this manner is from 1 to 4 months.

Isosensitization of the recipient. If a patient does not possess a particular blood antigen, he or she may be sensitized when cells containing this antigen are received in transfusion. Antibodies gradually develop in the recipient over weeks and months, so that a succeeding transfusion with the same antigen results in destruction of the red blood cells. Women who are Rh negative may also be sensitized from a fetus that received Rh positive antigens from the father's genes. In this case the mother's antibodies may hemolyze the red blood cells of her infant to produce a disease called erythroblastosis fetalis. The red blood cells of a woman sensitized in this fashion will also hemolyze blood containing the antigen when it is received in transfusion.

POSTOPERATIVE NURSING CARE

A recovery room where intensive nursing care can be provided for the postoperative patient is almost a must in the modern hospital. Here the recovery room nurse can give her undivided attention to the postanesthetic patient. Constant observation for signs of shock and hemorrhage or for an obstructed airway is a vital part of her concern. The administration of blood or intravenous fluids started in the operating room usually continues in the immediate postoperative period. Emergency equipment and drugs are readily available and the timely use of suction and oxygen have greatly reduced postoperative hazards. Encouraging and helping the patient to cough and to breathe deeply at frequent intervals are almost routine postoperative orders. Use of a breathing tube to build up carbon dioxide is helpful when deep breathing and coughing are vital to the patient's welfare. In addition to a recovery room many hospitals provide postoperative units or intensive care units, where the patient who has had major surgery may receive care for several days. By grouping these patients together in small units superior and constant nursing care can be provided. Many postoperative complications can be prevented when good nursing care is provided the first few days after surgery.

In orthopedics it is absolutely essential for all patients other than those receiving surgery of the foot or hand and arm to have a firm bed. This frequently

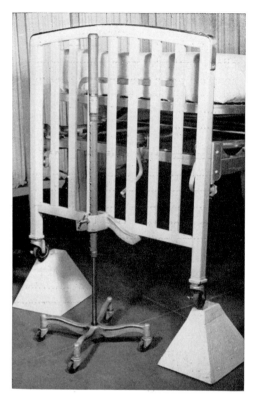

Fig. 113. A hydraulic bed lifter and shock blocks. This apparatus is used frequently on a busy orthopedic service for the elevation of beds to maintain countertraction or to secure shock position.

necessitates the placement of boards under the mattress. Preferably these boards are placed lengthwise, but when long boards are not available, the shorter ones may be placed across the bed. A sagging bed has no place in orthopedic nursing. Almost every type of postoperative patient will need one or more rubber-covered pillows. However, the use of large numbers of pillows never assures the safety or comfort of the patient in a cast. Care in the arrangement of pillows will frequently eliminate the need for a number of them. Body alignment should approximate the body alignment desirable for all bed patients. The chest should be the part of the body farthest forward. All nurses know

that this is true, because it applies to good posture in any position, but frequently they forget to apply it to the patient in the hip spica cast. The extremities should be supported along their entire length, not merely at one or two points such as the knee and heel. Pillows placed under the head should support the shoulders as well. If the head is to be elevated, one pillow should support the back from the lumbar spine to the shoulders and two pillows are arranged crosswise to support both shoulders and the head. A common error is to elevate head and chest without providing for this support under the back, and the result is that an actual bending of the body occurs just above the body section of the hip spica cast. This causes the edges of the cast to press against the soft portion of the abdomen and frequently results in a feeling of fullness and pressure in the abdomen that is mistaken for distention. It will usually be found that once a pillow has been placed lengthwise under the cast to the sacrum this troublesome feature can be eliminated.

Pillows should be arranged so that the leg portion of the spica cast is supported along its full length and no strain is imposed on the groin section, which is always vulnerable to cracking. Some surgeons prefer that sandbags be used to support the cast from the bed in order to prevent excessive weight from falling on it. Sandbags may be placed under the hip, knee, and foot on the cast side so that the weight of the body falls on the unaffected side.

Leg casts usually require three pillows for elevation or an overhead frame with one crossbar and a hammock that may be suspended from the frame. This will eliminate the use of pillows and ensure constant elevation of the limb. If no cast is to be put on the body, a lumbar pad consisting of a long narrow hair pillow or a folded sheet will do much to pre-vent postoperative backache—still a threat even after anesthesia.

When skeletal traction is being used, it is well to have the equipment for es-tablishing traction at hand for imme-diate application. This will consist of pulleys for the foot of the bed, rope, footplate, and weights. An overhead frame or Braun-Böhler splint may be necessary. With all patients who are to have hip spica casts it is advisable to have the overhead frame ready with a trapeze for helping the patient to lift himself. For reconstructive operations on the hip a Thomas or Hodgen splint with a Pearson attachment or some mod-ification of these will probably have been ordered by the doctor. The splint must be properly prepared with the Pearson attachment in place. Small tow-els, or preferably strips of bandage 6 inches wide, and at least 2 dozen safety pins are needed for preparing the Thomas splint. If desired, canvas strips and metal clips may be used in place of the towels and safety pins. Buck's extension equipment should be acces-sible if the nurse is not sure that it will be applied in the operating room.

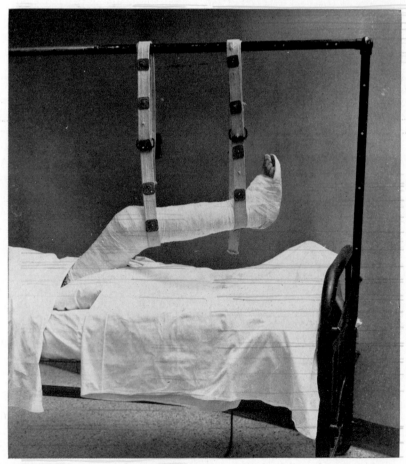

Fig. 114. Method of suspending long leg cast in elevated position. (From Speed, J. S., and Knight, R. A.: Campbell's operative orthopaedics, ed. 3, St. Louis, 1956, The C. V. Mosby Co.)

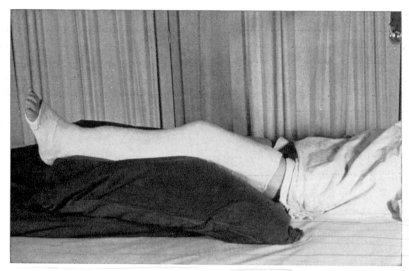

Fig. 115. Placement of pillows to support long leg cast. Note that the support is continued along the entire limb in order to eliminate strain on any muscle group. The patient's foot extends beyond the edge of the top pillow, thus preventing pressure or weight on the heel. With some patients it will be necessary to place a sandbag or trochanter roll along the lateral aspect of the thigh to prevent external rotation of the extremity.

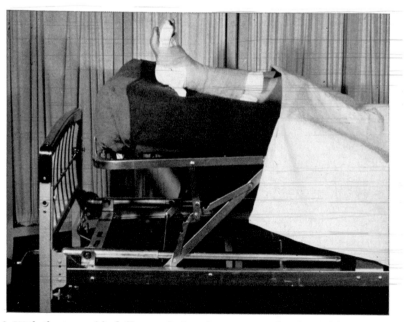

Fig. 116. With the type of bed illustrated, short leg casts may be elevated by raising the knee roll and the lower portion of the springs.

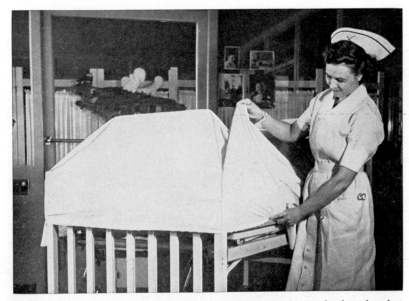

Fig. 117. Method of making the end of an orthopedic bed when a footboard is being used or the patient is wearing a long leg cast. The top linen may be placed over the end of the bed, thus avoiding pressure on the toes. Pinning this linen with safety pins at the corners will secure the linen at the end of the bed neatly. Merely tucking the ends in does not provide a permanent position for the upper covers.

After any type of orthopedic operation it is important that the nurse know the limitations of activity for her patient. This is essential for intelligent care, and it is as unwise to restrict the patient unnecessarily over a long period as it is to allow him more activity than the doctor wishes. Every orthopedic nurse should ascertain the limits within which she may work with her patient. When and how often may he be turned? Will he be allowed to lie on his side with proper support, or is the prone position more advisable? May he have his backrest elevated at intervals? It is also advisable for the nurse to inspect the cast early. Are all the toes visible? Is the cast cut out enough around the buttocks for good care? (It is almost never necessary for the cast to come down over the gluteal crease, and if it is left in this fashion it is usually the result of oversight.)

It will be said many times in the course of this book that close observa-

tion of circulation in extremities in plaster is one of the nurse's chief responsibilities. To quote directly from Lovett and Jones, "Every plaster cast where there is any definite slowing of the return of blood in the fingers or toes or any considerable swelling of fingers or toes should be immediately bivalved, the lid removed, and all constricting soft bandages cut through. The latter point is more important."*

It must be remembered, too, that apparatus or casts applied for the remedy of acute conditions, such as fractures, osteomyelitis, or septic joints, may be followed, or rather are likely to be followed, by constriction and circulatory embarrassment as late as 3 or 4 days afterward. The cardinal symptoms the orthopedic nurse should watch for are

---

*Jones, R., and Lovett, R. W.: Orthopedic surgery, Baltimore, 1929, Williams & Wilkins Co.

(1) pain, (2) color—cyanosis, anemia, or blanching, (3) swelling, (4) depressed local temperature, (5) diminished sensation, (6) loss of motion, and (7) sudden elevation of temperature that cannot be accounted for.

ORTHOPEDIC SURGICAL DRESSINGS

Dressing of orthopedic surgical wounds should be done by the most scrupulous technique. Patients with infected wounds should be segregated from those with clean ones, preferably in a different ward or room. Clean wounds are always dressed before infected ones, and there should be a separate dressing tray or cart for use on infected wounds. Greater control of environment is, of course, possible if a special room is set aside for dressings. Wartime experiments showed conclusively that many hazards exist in wound dressings that were not formerly recognized as being important. For example, if clean and infected bone cases are housed in the same open ward, the bedclothing may be a source of contamination. Bedclothes contain great quantities of lint and dust, and if they are exposed to purulent discharges from wounds and dressings these particles may be loaded with bacteria. The gradual spread of certain strains of bacteria through an entire ward by this method was demonstrated forcefully during World War II.

For this reason some orthopedists make it a rule not to dress wounds until at least an hour after all the beds have been made, in order that dust and lint may have a chance to settle. Sweeping or dusting is never done during dressing periods. Even turning a patient in bed may be hazardous in that it will release quantities of lint and dust. Blankets and soiled linen should be carefully handled and never shaken in the ward as the beds are made. They should not be thrown on chairs or on the floor where dust and lint may be deposited. It is preferable to have containers for soiled linen in the ward, and place the linen in them immediately as it is removed from the bed. In some institutions nobody is admitted to the ward during the dressing period and windows and doors are kept closed. Doctors, nurses, and the patient wear masks while the dressing is being done.

Bandage scissors are sometimes a source of infection in surgical dressings. It is inexcusable to cut the outer dressings of both infected and clean wounds without disinfecting the scissors. In removing dressings it is wise to cut the bandage and remove it in one piece. Unwrapping soiled bandages may fill the surrounding air with bacteria-loaded lint that may infect other wounds. It is considered safer not to touch anything with the hands until the outer bandage is applied unless the hands have been washed in the meantime. All saturated dressings should be reenforced immediately after they are observed, and when the wound is a clean one, the reenforcement must be sterile to avoid contamination by capillary action. This means, of course, that the dressing should be applied with a sterile forceps. The practice of placing sterile dressings on a wound by hand is uniformly condemned by surgeons.

POSTOPERATIVE COMPLICATIONS

Nurses caring for patients who have had bone surgery should be familiar with the symptoms of fat embolism. This condition will usually occur within the first 24 hours but can be distinguished from symptoms of shock by the fact that it usually does not occur until 12 hours after surgery. When the pulmonary vessels are involved, symptoms are rapid breathing, increased pulse rate, and pallor followed by cyanosis. Some war surgeons have noted that the condition is often accompanied by petechiae over the chest and shoulders. If the fat embolus is in the brain, it will manifest itself in delirium, pupillary changes, twitching of the muscles, and coma. The condition is severe and frequently fatal. The patient must be kept absolutely quiet. If he is in a cast no attempt should be made to remove it in trying to save his life. Intravenous therapy, heart stimulants, and artificial respiration may be ordered.

Thrombophlebitis may occur as the result of immobilization or enforced bed rest. The causes of this condition are a general slowing of the blood flow, collapse or compression of the veins, and endothelial damage. Complaints of pain in the calf of the leg, swelling, or heat and redness of the extremity should be reported immediately to the attending surgeon. Rest, avoidance of sudden movements, and elevation of the extremity are usually ordered as treatment. When an anticoagulant (heparin) is prescribed, frequent determinations of clotting times are required. When Dicumarol is substituted for the heparin, measurements of prothrombin time daily or at other suitable periods of time are indicated. To prevent dislodgment of a clot the surgeon may desire to interrupt the involved vein or veins.

Pulmonary embolism is another grave complication that sometimes follows surgery. It comes on much later than fat embolism, usually in from 10 to 20 days, although it may occur much later. If the embolus is large, death may occur instantly. If there is a partial block, the patient will complain of sudden severe chest pain.

Gradual stretching of nerves may bring about epileptiform convulsions. These are not as grave as the convulsions that accompany fat embolism and occur later, usually from 2 to 6 days after operation. The dyspnea is slight,

the pulse does not become increased, the respiratory rate is approximately normal, and recovery may be expected after 2 to 4 days. Treatment is removal of plaster and sedation.

The presence of backache after operation as a result of the complete relaxation of the muscles of the back during anesthesia is so commonly known that it seems hardly necessary to mention it. It is almost axiomatic that the lumbar spine be supported with a firm pad during anesthesia and after return to bed to prevent this disturbing postoperative complication.

Urine retention may occur in patients who have had orthopedic surgery. It is frequently necessary to catheterize adult patients who have had operations on the back or hip. This may continue to be a problem for several days postoperatively, and the utmost care must be taken to prevent cystitis or kidney infection.

It is not uncommon for the adult patient who has had a major orthopedic operation to have abdominal distention. Rectal tubes, enemas, and neostigmine methylsulfate may be ordered to relieve discomfort. In some instances relief is not obtained until Wangensteen suction has been started.

The alert orthopedic nurse will provide measures to prevent postoperative pneumonia. This applies to any surgical patient but is of special importance for older persons. They must be encouraged to cough up mucus and to do deep-breathing exercises. Their position must be changed frequently, and as much activity as possible should be permitted.

The risk of operative intervention on spinal deformities of great extent (severe scoliosis or kyphosis) is increased by the effect these deformities have upon the rib cage, the lungs, and heart. The large vessels of the thorax, too, may be affected. Patients with severe scoliosis should be observed postoperatively for dyspnea, cyanosis, and edema of the lower extremities.

PREVENTION OF WOUND INFECTION

In surgery of bones and joints the greatest possible care is exercised to prevent infection. The outcome of most orthopedic operations depends largely on bone union, and bone will not unite in the presence of infection. Furthermore, the presence of postoperative infection of bones and joints often leads to lifelong crippling. For these reasons techniques used by nurses in preoperative skin preparation and in postoperative dressings should be as nearly faultless as possible.

The prevention of wound infection will depend to a large extent on attention to the following details:

1. Careful skin preparation preoperatively
2. Meticulous operating room techniques
3. Observation of wound site to keep dressings and cast intact and free from contamination
4. Careful dressing cart technique—masks, use of forceps rather than fingers, segregated space for dressings, etc.
5. A clean ward for clean patients where no patients with infected bone conditions are housed simultaneously
6. Careful removal of any foreign bodies or dead tissue from wounds, since such foreign objects will increase the susceptibility to infection five-hundredfold

Postoperative drainage from clean surgical wounds should be reported by the nurse as soon as it is observed. Staining of the cast either by serum or by purulent drainage must be watched for. Immediate reenforcement of saturated dressings with a sterile pad so that capillary action will not bring about further contamination is important.

Children who have been walking barefoot are often predisposed to tetanus infection. When dirt is grimed into the soles of the feet before surgery, it is sometimes difficult to attain the surgical cleanliness desired. The physician should be informed of this circumstance. Occasionally, prophylactic antitoxin may be given to these patients before surgery is performed.

EARLY AMBULATION AFTER ORTHOPEDIC SURGERY

Although bed rest is being whittled down to very short periods in patients with surgical conditions that are not of the skeleton, a certain amount of recumbency is still indispensable for many orthopedic patients. Even in orthopedic wards the tendency is to promote as early ambulation as is compatible with the healing time of bone.

New sets of skills are necessary for the nurse who wishes to help her patient toward an early and uncomplicated convalescence; there is nothing helter-skelter about the procedure. It requires wisdom, understanding, and knowledge of new techniques. It is not merely a matter of saying "arise and walk." Equipment for preparing the patient for ambulation is seen in most hospitals today. One sees trapezes on many beds and portable overhead frames of lead piping on wheels, that make it possible for patients to exercise arms and shoulders for using crutches. Sawed-off crutches are often provided the badly affected patient for learning to manage crutches while he is still in bed. Footboards are used for support and for maintaining the standing reflex. Pulleys and ropes for resistive exercises are not uncommon. Printed lists of simple instructions for bed-conditioning exercises prescribed by the physician are seen.

Present-day nurses know that standing is preferred to sitting for the patient's first out-of-bed periods, and they understand the relationship of the cough and the elimination of mucus to his welfare. Standing is almost always preferred to sitting in early rising after surgery. There are certain dangers that attend the patient who is allowed out of bed early only to sit for many hours in a chair. For patients who must sit it is important to see that the seat is not too long, because a long seat causes pressure on the popliteal vessels, with the inevitable danger of thrombosis. A backward tilt to the seat is preferable because it serves to keep the hips from slipping forward toward the edge of the chair—a posture that encourages sag-

ging shoulders and rounded back. The elderly thin patient must not sit with his legs crossed because of the danger of peroneal palsy from pressure on the very superficial peroneal nerve on the outer aspect of the knee.

Wheelchair restraints should provide a good sitting position for the patient. Hips should be maintained in contact with the back of the chair, and shoulders should be persuaded to an upright position so that stooping forward does not occur as the patient operates the chair.

No restraint is foolproof, and all of them need constant adjusting.

The procedure for getting a patient out of bed by having him turn to his side, flex his hips and knees as though sitting, and then swiveling him gently to the sitting position is entirely accep-

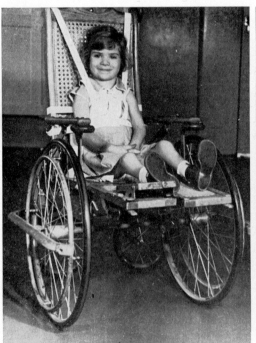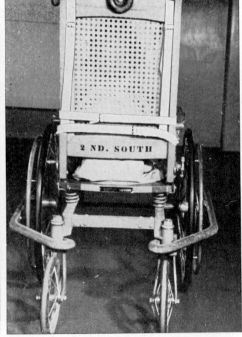

Fig. 118. Wheelchair restraint, front view and rear view. To prevent accidents small children and elderly patients need safety belts of one kind or another whenever they are placed in a wheelchair. Webbing straps and buckles may be attached directly to the chair and thus provide added safety for the patient who is forgetful or not cognizant of the danger of falling from the chair.

table in orthopedic nursing. Unfortunately most orthopedic patients are encumbered with apparatus that makes getting up a much more complicated procedure. Nevertheless, adaptations may be made to fit the needs of each patient without too much difficulty if sufficient help is available.

STUDY QUESTIONS

1. You have been assigned the care of a patient who has been placed in a hip spica cast:
   (a) What preparation will you make prior to the patient's return from the plaster room?
   (b) Describe the placement of pillows to support the wet cast.
   (c) What observations will you make pertaining to circulation of the extremity enclosed in the plaster?
   (d) Describe the procedure you will use for turning this patient onto his abdomen.
   (e) When placing the patient on a bedpan, what nursing measures will you use to protect the cast and to ensure comfort for the patient?
   (f) When the cast is dry, how will you finish its edges?
   (g) If the cast becomes soiled, how will you clean it?
2. Construct a brief nursing-care plan for the patient newly removed from a hip spica cast.
3. Bleeding noted by staining of the cast after

surgery can be checked for progress by what simple method?
4. Describe a desirable setup for providing clean orthopedic dressings in an open ward.
5. Discuss early ambulation in the treatment of orthopedic patients.
6. Discuss reasons for applying traction.
7. Describe several methods of securing traction.
8. Distinguish between skin and skeletal traction. List several types of skin traction.
9. What is meant by a Balkan frame?
10. When is Bryant traction used?
11. Distinguish between Buck's extension and Russell traction.
12. List observations you would make when caring for the patient in traction pertaining to the following: position of extremity, position of patient in bed, countertraction, weights, and the footplate.
13. What are some of the areas that frequently become denuded after the application of Buck's extension?
14. Why is it important that no pressure be exerted on the head of the fibula in applying traction?

REFERENCES

American Academy of Orthopaedic Surgeons: Orthopaedic appliances atlas, vol. I, Ann Arbor, Mich., 1952, J. W. Edwards.

Arey, M. S.: Walking with crutches, Nursing World **126**:36-39, 1952.

Bird, B.: Psychological aspects of preoperative and postoperative care, Am. J. Nursing **55**:685-687, 1955.

Bleck, E. E., Duckworth, N., and Hunter, N.: Atlas of plaster cast techniques, Chicago, 1956, The Year Book Publishers, Inc.

Bruck, H.: The drying of plaster casts, Am. J. Nursing **46**:400-402, 1946.

Calderwood, C.: The patient comes out of his cast, Am. J. Nursing **44**:202-205, 1944.

Calderwood, C.: Russell traction, Am. J. Nursing **43**:464-469, 1943.

Crenshaw, A. H., and Milford, L., editors: Campbell's operative orthopaedics, ed. 4, St. Louis, 1963, The C. V. Mosby Co.

Crutchfield, W. G.: Skeletal traction in treatment of injuries to the cervical spine, J.A.M.A. **155**:29, 1954.

Dalton, A.: Using a Stryker frame, Am. J. Nursing **64**:100-101, 1964.

Davis, L.: Christopher's textbook of surgery, Philadelphia, 1956, W. B. Saunders Co.

Deaver, G., and Brown, M. E.: The challenge of crutches, crutch management, Arch. Phys. Med. **26**:397-403, 1945.

Eastwood, D. W., and Mabrey, J. K.: Suction and maintenance of an airway, Am. J. Nursing **53**:552-553, 1953.

Jager, B. V.: Untoward reactions to antibiotics, Am. J. Nursing **54**:966-968, 1954.

Knocke, L.: Crutch walking, Am. J. Nursing **61**:70-73, 1961.

Latham, H. C.: Thrombophlebitis, Am. J. Nursing **63**:122-126, 1963.

Nicholson, J. T., Robert, M., and Heath, R. D.: Bryant traction—a provocative cause of circulatory complications, J.A.M.A. **157**:415-418, 1955.

Olmsted, L.: Crutch walking, Am. J. Nursing **45**:28-35, 1945.

Schmeisser, G.: A clinical manual of orthopedic traction techniques, Philadelphia, 1963, W. B. Saunders Co.

Scuderi, C.: Atlas of orthopedic traction procedures, St. Louis, 1954, The C. V. Mosby Co.

Shands, A. R., Raney, R. B., and Brashear, H. R.: Handbook of orthopaedic surgery, ed. 6, St. Louis, 1963, The C. V. Mosby Co.

Skinner, G.: Head traction and the Stryker frame, Am. J. Nursing **52**:694-697, 1952.

Stanton, J. R.: Venous thrombosis and pulmonary embolism, Am. J. Nursing **55**:709-711, 1955.

Steindler, A.: Orthopedic operations: indications, techniques, and end results, Springfield, Ill., 1950, Charles C Thomas, Publisher.

Wilde, D.: The patient in a spica—abed and afoot, Am. J. Nursing, **50**:429-432, 1951.

Wilde, D.: Traction and suspension, Am. J. Nursing, **53**:1465-1468, 1953.

Chapter 3

Congenital deformities, including nursing care

Deformities that are present at birth are considered congenital. They may follow hereditary patterns or be the result of embryologic defects.

It is estimated that 2% of newborn infants have congenital malformations. It is now known that only 25% of the cases are of genetic origin, whereas 75% are the result of external factors influencing an originally healthy ovum. The importance of these external factors became evident when it was found that women who develop rubella in the fifth week of pregnancy might give birth to a child with cataracts. Rubella contracted in the ninth week of pregnancy may lead to lesions of the inner ear, and if the virus is contracted between the fifth and tenth weeks of pregnancy, the child might be born with cardiac deformities. A new sedative, Thalidomide, given to pregnant women resulted in many children being born with multiple congenital deformities, especially phocomelia. These malformations do not depend merely on the nature of the causative agent but more on the stage of pregnancy at which it acts on the embryo and on the vulnerability of certain cells in the embryo. Poisons or parasites, such as toxoplasmosis, can produce ocular and/or nervous lesions. Roentgen rays or irradiation from radioactive substances can cause anencephalia, exencephalia, hydrocephalus, and ocular anomalies. Irradiation given late in pregnancy may cause spina bifida, velum palatinum, fissures, and all types of limb malformations. Avitaminosis, particularly of A, E, B_2, or pantothenic acid deficiency, can cause malformations, whether they are caused by a lack of supply, a lack of absorption, or the presence of substances that impede their normal utilization. Many of the progesterones (4-Pregnene-3, 20-dione) can lead to virilization in female fetuses. They may cause total or partial fusion of the labia majora, hypertrophy of the clitoris, or opening of the ureter into the vagina. Over four hundred drugs are known that have teratogenic effects in animals, but only a few of these drugs can cause malformations in humans. It is important when treating a pregnant woman to prescribe only those drugs that are imperative to her well-being, such as insulin, cortisone, and isoniazid.

The types and variations of deformities are almost limitless. Many deformities, however, are not disabling. Those encountered frequently will be described in this chapter.

CONGENITAL DISLOCATION OF THE HIP

The term congenital dislocation of the hip implies that the head of the femur is outside the confines of the acetabulum at birth. Actually, there are degrees of dislocation, from incomplete to complete, and these are identified by definite terms.

Subluxation, or predislocation, is an incomplete dislocation. This is more common than dislocation and is more difficult to detect. If they remain untreated, however, many subluxations eventually result in complete dislocations, and for this reason they assume importance in early recognition.

The exact cause is unknown, but the defect is primarily improper acetabular development. This does not cause symptoms, but when certain signs are present the condition should be suspected and verified by a roentgenogram of the hips. Limited abduction of the hip in the flexed position and/or a click sign when the hip is being abducted are the most useful objective findings. Treatment consisting of a Frejka pillow splint should be instituted immediately.

Congenital dislocation refers to those cases in which there is an actual complete dislocation. This can occur during intrauterine life or result from an untreated subluxation sometime after birth. In either case it demands early recognition and treatment to obtain a satisfactory result.

The signs of congenital dislocation vary with the age of the child. Walking is often delayed, and the mother may have noted an extra gluteal fold on the affected side. Occasionally it is brought to attention by a shortness of the leg, an unusually broad perineum (especially in bilateral cases), or an unusual trochanter prominence. Should the dislocation be unrecognized until walking begins, the most obvious sign will be a waddling limp. On examination it is usually apparent that the affected leg is shorter, the range of hip motion is freer than normal, there is lack of stability

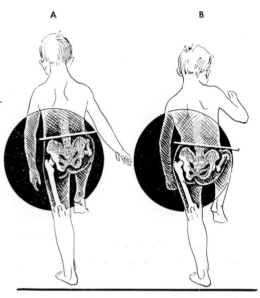

Fig. 119. A, Negative Trendelenburg sign. When the body weight is placed on the normal limb (stable hip) and the opposite limb is elevated, the pelvis rises on the side of the lifted limb. B, Positive Trendelenburg sign. When the body weight is placed on the unstable hip (as in congenital dislocated hip) and the opposite limb is elevated, the pelvis drops on the side of the lifted limb.

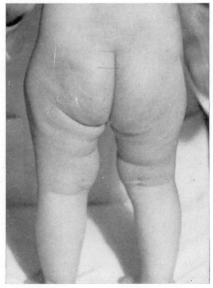

Fig. 120. Congenital dislocation of the left hip. Note prominent trochanter on the affected side and asymmetry of gluteal folds.

on the push test, and the trochanter is higher than normal. In standing the child will demonstrate a positive Trendelenburg test. A positive Trendelenburg test is indicative of an unstable hip joint. When the body weight is put on the normal or stable hip and the affected limb is elevated, the pelvis on the side of the dislocated hip rises (this is true with normal hip joints). However, when the body weight is taken on the dislocated hip and the normal limb is elevated, the pelvis drops on the side of the normal limb. To compensate for the pelvic drop the body shifts to the opposite side to maintain balance.

Treatment must be started immediately after the diagnosis is made. The aim is to reduce the dislocation to a normal position. This is ordinarily accomplished by a closed manipulation performed while the patient is under anesthesia. The reduction must then be maintained for sufficient time to allow the acetabulum to develop to a point that will maintain reduction. This may require months, during which time the

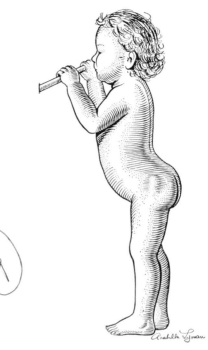

Fig. 122. Bilateral congenital dislocation of the hip in older child. Note prominence in the gluteal region and swayback. The swayback position compensates for the backward displacement of the hips.

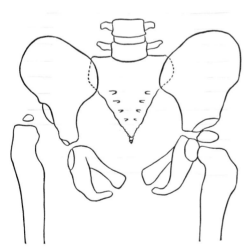

Fig. 121. Copy of roentgenogram of congenital dislocation of right hip. There is upward and backward displacement of the head of the femur and thickening at the base of the acetabulum (prenatal).

hip will be immobilized in a plaster spica cast. The surgeon in charge will vary the position to obtain proper placement of the femoral head within the acetabulum. Various splints are available as substitutes for plaster casts and have the advantage of being removable. These are more applicable in the later stages of treatment.

Operative reduction is necessary when closed manipulation has failed to correct the dislocation. The aftertreatment is similar to closed reduction both in time and in the type of fixation apparatus.

Late results. When treatment is begun early (within the first 18 months of life), the outcome will be excellent. A few patients treated early and many treated late will show degenerative

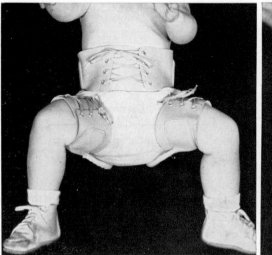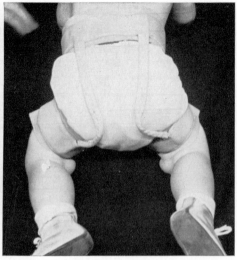

Fig. 123. Anterior and posterior views of the splint used in treatment of congenital dislocated hip.

changes of the hip by the time middle age has been reached. These degenerative changes cause painful disability sufficient to require further treatment. For the details of treatment at this stage as well as for unreduced dislocations found in adults see Chapter 11.

Treatment and nursing care. The nurse's function in detecting and reporting congenital anomalies is an important one. Whether she is a hospital nurse working with infants in the obstetric nursery, a public health nurse giving bedside instruction to a new mother, a nurse in the pediatric ward, or a school nurse, she will have many opportunities to detect abnormalities. To do this intelligently she must, of course, have a clear understanding of what is normal in the structure, function, and development of the child. In addition to this she needs to know the symptoms of the common orthopedic conditions that are found at birth. Although most congenital deformities cannot be prevented, nurses should recognize the fact that certain birth injuries can sometimes be prevented by good medical supervision and care during the period of pregnancy and delivery. They should use their influence to see that all mothers are given good obstetric care.

The nurse giving a bath to the newborn infant may become aware of deviations as she bathes him and watches his activities while he is unclothed. Abnormal conditions—such as limitation of joint motion, excessively free joint motion, limpness or a disinclination to move a part, a tendency to lie in one position constantly, alteration of body contours, or asymmetric folds in the skin—may rightly arouse her suspicions that something is wrong.

All congenital anomalies, however, are not detected at this early stage. The child may have reached school age before an abnormality is noted; sometimes the condition will be manifested only when the child is tired, and then a slight limp or alteration in gait will be detected.

The importance of early recognition, of course, is that it makes early treatment possible. Early treatment is para-

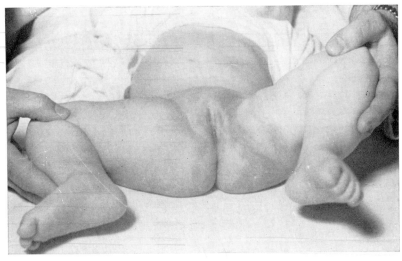

Fig. 124. Limitation of left hip abduction in an infant with congenital left hip dislocation.

mount in the management of these patients. Delay may make any attempted treatment only palliative. The nurse needs to realize this factor in order to help the family accept the necessity for securing immediate medical treatment when the abnormality is recognized. She should be cognizant, however, of the tremendous emotional components in this kind of condition and appreciate the feelings of the family. She will often meet parents who are afflicted by shame, pride, despair, or bewilderment, and she must be prepared to combat these reactions with sympathetic understanding and informed common sense.

"The key that opens the door of diagnosis is suspicion," says Osgood.* The nurse does not voice her suspicions aloud, but uses her utmost influence to see that the child she suspects of having an abnormality is given the benefit of medical examination without delay.

It is hardly possible to overestimate the importance of early recognition of congenital dislocation of the hip. The

results of the treatment are always best if it can be started early, if possible during the first 3 months of life. The possibilities of a perfect result, diminish rapidly as the child grows older.

The importance of observing the newborn infant for signs of the condition cannot be overemphasized. When bathing the infant, the nurse may note an extra fold in the buttock or thigh, or perhaps a widening of the perineum. In flexing the baby's hips and knees with his feet flat on the table she may observe that one knee is lower than the other. She may detect that all motion in the suspicious hip seems abnormally free except for limited abduction. When the physician's attention has been called to these observations, the nurse may see him fix the baby's pelvis with his hand and grasp the lower end of the femur to determine if piston motion, or telescoping, is present. Roentgenograms of the hip on which these signs are noted will assist the physician in making his diagnosis if an established dislocation is present.

If the anomaly of the hip is not de-

---

*Osgood, R. B.: Compression fractures of the spine, J.A.M.A. **89**:1563-1568, 1927.

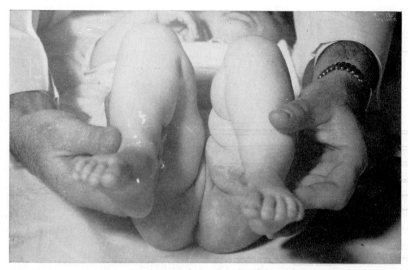

Fig. 125. Apparent shortening of the left thigh as the result of left hip dislocation. The left knee appears lower. Two extra skin folds are present in the left thigh.

tected in infancy or early childhood, other symptoms become apparent after weight bearing is established. Nurses should be familiar with these symptoms.

The child will walk with a lurching or a waddling gait because of the instability of the femur on the affected side. In addition to this, the buttocks may seem abnormally broad and there will be lumbar lordosis accompanied by a protuberant abdomen. By 10 or 11 years of age the lordosis has usually become very marked and unsightly, and scoliosis may have developed if the dislocation is unilateral. There will be shortening of the limb and often an adduction deformity of the leg. When this stage is reached, great difficulties stand in the way of treatment but much can be done to ensure the child a fairly stable hip and to reduce the possibility of arthritis and allied conditions in later life.

Treatment of congenital dislocation of the hip will vary somewhat according to the age at which the child is seen and the kind of dislocation present. The closed reduction is probably still the preferred method if the child is seen within the first few years of life. It will usually involve the use of a spica cast, and the nursing care the child receives after this may do much to determine the success or failure of the treatment. Open reductions are sometimes necessary to supplement the closed reduction. Palliative operations, such as shelving operations and the various types of osteotomies, may be necessary if both closed and open reductions fail. If the condition is diagnosed during what is called the predislocation stage of the postnatal type, an abduction splint may sometimes be used.

Nursing care with the Frejka pillow splint. The student nurse working on an orthopedic service will seldom have the opportunity to care for a small patient wearing a pillow splint. However, during her experience in the orthopedic outpatient department she will undoubtedly observe its application and may be asked to instruct the mother in the use of the splint. With this apparatus the child can be cared for in the home. The splint consists of a square pillow (stuffed with kapok), which is held in place by a romperlike garment. The romper is made with a pocket to hold the pillow and with straps that are placed over the baby's shoulders and pinned securely. The pillow part of the

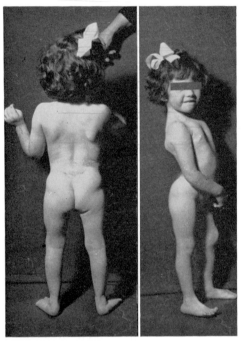

Fig. 126. Bilateral dislocated hips in older child. Note marked lumbar lordosis, protruding abdomen, wide perineum, and prominent trochanters.

garment that is placed between the baby's legs is wide enough to maintain the thighs in a position of abduction, flexion, and external rotation. The splint is applied over the regular diaper. To protect it from becoming wet or soiled the child must wear plastic panties, or a Pliofilm apron between the diaper and the pillow.

The mother needs to know why it is important for her baby to wear this splint. Then she must understand how to apply it correctly. Because the pillow splint must be applied each time the baby's diaper is changed, the desired position of the hip joint may not be maintained if the mother is not cautious. The splint is worn for several months or until roentgenograms show a normal hip. During this time the child will need to be checked at frequent intervals by the orthopedist.

Nursing care in the closed reduction method. The closed or bloodless reduction method, used by Lorenz a half century ago and somewhat modified during the past twenty-five years by Putti, Ridlon, and others, is probably the preferred method of reduction for children under 5 years of age. This reduction is performed when the patient is under anesthesia. The child is usually

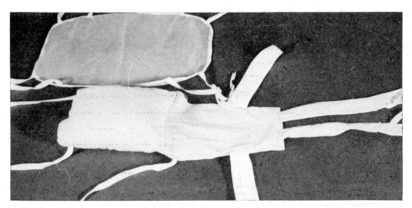

Fig. 127. The Frejka pillow splint ready for application. The pillow has been placed in the pocket part of the garment.

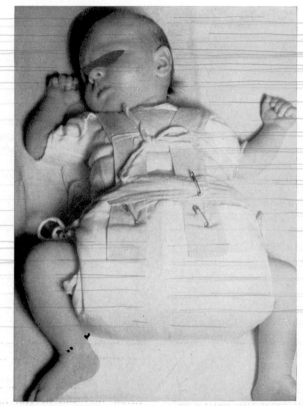

Fig. 128. Correct application of the Frejka pillow splint. The pillow maintains the thighs in flexion, abduction, and external rotation.

placed in a double hip spica cast after the manipulation. The cast is very carefully applied and well molded to maintain the reduction. It may be applied with the hip in a position of 90-degree flexion and 60- to 70-degree abduction, or it may be applied with the hip in a position of abduction and internal rotation. In either instance the double hip spica cast is used whether the dislocation is unilateral or bilateral. When the frog or Lorenz position is employed, it is usually followed in 3 to 4 months by a change to the Lange or functional position of inward rotation and abduction.

The care of a young child in a hip spica cast requires forethought and ingenuity to prevent soiling and soaking. Even 24 hours of neglect can ruin such a cast hopelessly. A half century ago, even though congenital dislocation of the hip was recognized early, the specialist often did nothing about the deformity until the child was at least 2 years of age. Most of the pioneer workers with this condition believed that it was not feasible to try to correct the dislocation by forcible correction in infancy. If the child was not diaper trained, the application of a spica cast seemed impracticable because of the danger of soiling. Reduction of congenital dislocation of the hip has long been associated with problems of nursing care.

There usually will be a stockinet lining to the cast in which the child is enclosed. Some surgeons place small towels over the abdomen and back before the stockinet lining is put on the

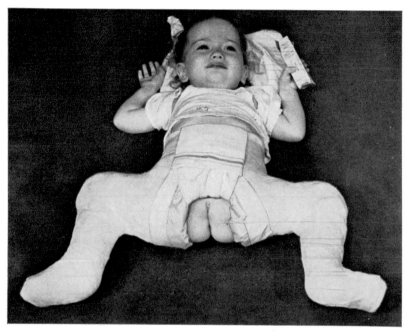

Fig. 129. Arrangement of towels for protecting inner surface of hip spica cast after reduction for congenital dislocation of the hip. (Courtesy Dr. Arthur Steindler, Iowa City, Iowa.)

patient. These towels may be changed frequently to help keep the baby's skin in good condition. The towel edges may be pinned together on the outside of the cast after the plaster is dry. In changing the towels a clean one is pinned to the soiled one; the latter is then gently pulled from under the cast at the same time the clean one is pulled into place. Even though these towels are not applied when the cast is put on, they may be used on the wards. A thin towel can be inserted beneath the cast with a tongue depressor or comb, but care must be taken to avoid pinching the baby's skin in the process.

Some plan of care must be devised to protect the cast from soiling and wetting. The small Bradford frame (suspended to the crib by iron hooks or placed on boxes) has served this purpose well. The Bradford frame is equipped with a two-piece canvas frame cover that leaves space beneath the buttocks for the bedpan. The edges of the frame cover should be protected by pieces of waterproof material at the buttocks area. A bedpan is kept underneath this opening at all times. As soon as the cast is dry, it should be waterproofed against soilage.

Sheets are commonly used to cover Bradford frames. Sometimes these are merely laid on the surface of the frame, but there is considerable danger of wrinkles unless it is possible to smooth the sheets several times during the day. Sheets fastened with safety pins prove satisfactory, but the time element in the use of many pins is something of a worry. Furthermore, the use of sheets for this purpose is uneconomic in that it frequently results in many tears in the linen. Frame covers with tapes sewed at the sides at 2-inch intervals and cut to fit large, medium, and small frames are particularly convenient for quick changing. It has been found that only three sizes are necessary, in that tapes make alteration possible. It is much easier to tie a cover over the canvas than to pin on a sheet.

A harness or jacket restraint will be necessary to secure a baby to the frame. For frame restraints a Y-shaped harness restraint with the arms of the Y going over the shoulders and the base of the Y attached to the foot of the frame is frequently used. Crosspieces at the level of the child's hips and abdomen fasten under the frame with buckles, and the arms and base of the Y are also fastened by buckles to the head and foot of the frame.

A jacket or vest restraint like the one illustrated in Fig. 130 provides fairly satisfactory immobilization for the child on a frame. There is some danger in using all types of jacket and harness restraints if the child slips down in bed. This must be borne in mind.

Restraints should never be placed too near the child's neck because with any alteration of his position they may cause respiratory embarrassment. Restraining pieces should not cross under the arms, because if the child slides down in bed the shoulder girdle may be elevated into a position of deformity. Poor habits of respiration are fostered if crosspieces are too tight over the chest. A crosspiece over the abdomen should not be tight enough to cause distress after eating.

Rubber-covered pillows may be used in place of the frame to support the small child in a hip spica cast. It is desirable that the child's head and shoul-

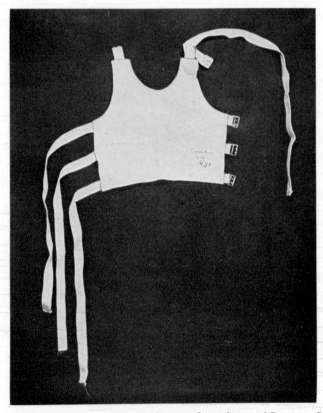

Fig. 130. Vest or jacket restraint for use with or without frame. (Courtesy State University of Iowa Hospitals.)

ders be elevated slightly to prevent urine from running back under the cast. The casts of small children should be protected with waterproof material shortly after they are applied.

Considerable difference of opinion exists concerning the use of diapers. In the past orthopedists have disapproved of them because they tend to become soaked across the groin area and soften the cast at the most important point, that is, at the hip level. Diapers may be omitted entirely if a frame is used. It has been found, however, that if the cast is protected with waterproof material (as described previously) it can be kept clean and dry without using a frame. One diaper is folded as a perineal pad and placed across the perineum before the outer diaper is applied. The perineal diaper covered with a strip of waterproof material will absorb much of the moisture and protect the cast from wetting. It will, of course, be necessary to change it frequently. When the mother is instructed to care for the baby and cast in this manner, the baby can be held and cuddled and thus given the affection and attention so important to the small child.

Convalescent treatment. The child is usually immobilized in a plaster cast for several months. When the roentgenographic findings are satisfactory, a regime of controlled functional treatment will be begun. Immobilization for too long a period is universally avoided because it has been found to result in cystic atrophy or epiphysitis of the hip. A period of physical therapy, consisting of radiant heat, massage, hydrotherapy, and exercise, followed by limited periods of walking, will usually be prescribed. This phase of the child's treatment is one in which he must be observed and examined frequently because redislocation may occur at this time. Nurses should understand that it is the general opinion of orthopedists at present that the main cause of redislocation is anteversion of the head of the femur. To maintain the femoral head in the acetabulum in a stable manner inward rotation of the leg is considered essential and outward rotation is usually avoided for a long time. One of the things that is accomplished by physical therapy is the strengthening of the inward rotators of the hip, that is, the gluteus medius, gluteus minimus, and the adductor magnus muscles. Functional treatment of congenital dislocation of the hip seeks

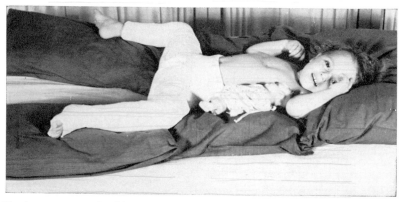

Fig. 131. Arrangement of rubber-covered pillows to support hip spica cast. Note space for the bedpan and the folded diaper across the perineum. Head of bed may be elevated slightly to help prevent wetting of the cast.

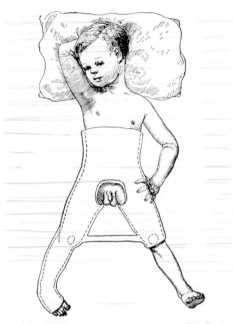

Fig. 132. Bilateral hip spica cast with affected right hip in abduction and internal rotation—sometimes called the Lange position. Commonly used to maintain correction after open reduction of congenital dislocation of the hip. (From Shands, A. R.: Handbook of orthopaedic surgery, ed. 4, St. Louis, 1952, The C. V. Mosby Co.)

to maintain abduction of the leg and to avoid outward rotation. Motion in all other directions is usually permitted.

Apparatus to assist in keeping the legs in this position is used in some localities. The device pictured in Fig. 133 consists of an iron bar with a plate at each end. The plates are attached to the patient's shoes. They are fastened in such a way that inward rotation, flexion, and extension of the hip are possible, but outward rotation is strictly limited at 75 degrees or under. There is a sliding mechanism on the bar that makes it possible to increase or diminish abduction. Usually, the legs will be kept at a 100- to 120-degree angle.

This bar is used from 2 to 6 months after the cast is removed. The

bar is removed only for the daily bath, at which time the legs must not be allowed to roll into outward rotation. Roentgenograms are usually taken every 2 months to check the progress of the joint and the building of the acetabulum. The bar may be removed as the child progresses, and walking may be permitted for short periods. Walking time is increased as the roentgenograms show progress in the development of the hip joint. Night splints may be used for several years after reduction

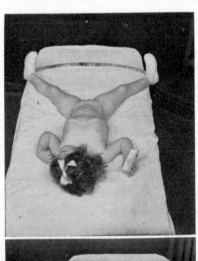

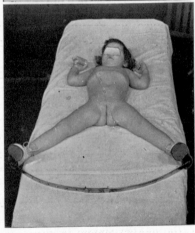

Fig. 133. Abduction bar for treatment of congenital dislocation of the hips. Bar is adjustable, but feet are locked against external rotation. Internal rotation is free. (Courtesy Dr. Arthur Steindler, Iowa City, Iowa.)

of the hip to offset the chance of recurrence or redislocation.

Instruction for home care. After the cast has been thoroughly dried and finished and the position of the hip has been checked by roentgenography, the child may be allowed to return home. The mother should be carefully instructed in the care of the patient and the cast. This instruction cannot be given hurriedly if the child is to have adequate care. A discussion of many details will enter into the instruction. Nurses should bear in mind that most mothers tend to be afraid of damaging the cast. It is essential that they realize that it is possible to give the child wholly adequate care in the cast if they will take the time to do so. Methods of keeping the cast clean and dry and of caring for the skin beneath the cast should be demonstrated. The necessity of using the fingers to clean under the cast must be particularly emphasized. Many times cast sores are overlooked near the edges of the cast, where they should be discovered without difficulty. Inexpensive substitutes for waterproofing the plaster should be suggested and methods of applying the diaper demonstrated. The mother must be instructed to observe signs that the child is growing too large for his cast, and she should be made aware of the danger of a weak or broken cast and the necessity for returning to the hospital or clinic at once for repairs when such is discovered.

The freedom the child is to be allowed should be discussed. Most surgeons permit the child to stand or even walk in the crib if he so desires. Sitting astraddle chairs or kiddy-cars is often permitted. If the child's feet are not in the cast, the mother should be instructed in methods of maintaining good position for them. With the surgeon's permission simple exercises can be taught to prevent atrophy and loss of function in the

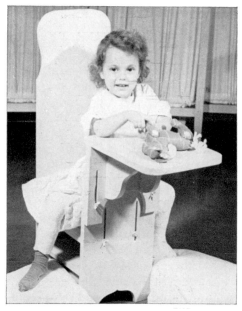

Fig. 134. Adjustable chair which may be used with child in hip spica cast after reduction for congenital dislocation of the hip.

feet. Usually, dorsiflexion and inversion exercises will be prescribed. Where it is at all possible, a public health nurse should be notified of the homecoming of a child after a hip reduction. She will be able to assist the mother during the first daily bath and will be able to clear up any details that have escaped the mother's memory.

Preparation for surgery. Skeletal traction may be used as a preparation to open reduction or other surgery on congenital dislocation of the hip. It has been found that this procedure will shorten the time necessary for reduction while the child is under anesthesia and will often eliminate the use of undue force in placing the head of the femur in the acetabulum. The purpose of traction is to bring the head of the femur down to the level of the acetabulum. Usually, the orthopedist will maintain this traction for 10 days to 2 weeks before the operation is performed.

With the patient under anesthesia, the

Kirschner wire or Steinmann pin is drilled through the condyles of the femur. It is advisable to have the caliper attachment, weights, ropes, and pulley at the bedside so that they can be applied and the traction setup completed before the child awakes. Application of the traction after waking usually causes the child considerable discomfort. The caliper, which is fastened to the nail or wire, should not be allowed to rest directly on the child's leg because it will cause bruising. A felt pad may be kept between the caliper and the lower leg. The line of traction should be in direct line with the femur. A small pillow covered with powdered oiled silk may be placed under the calf of the leg to keep the heel free of the bed, thereby preventing friction.

Nursing care after surgery. Open reduction of the hip may be attended by a certain degree of shock during the first 24 hours after surgery. Intravenous fluids will usually be given, and shock position may be required. The child should be kept warm and observed frequently for signs of hemorrhage. During the first day or two following surgery, nurses should avoid exposing the child in an effort to dry the cast. It has been found that too rapid evaporation of the moisture in the cast's surface sometimes cools the child's skin excessively and prolongs shock.

The child will usually be immobilized in a spica cast, and after recovery from the effects of surgery, nursing care will not vary greatly from that given to a child with a closed reduction.

The treatment of neglected or recurrent dislocation of the hip in older children will usually include surgery. Nursing care after the shelving operation or after osteotomy will be similar to that given to the child with open reduction of the hip.

After removal of a hip spica cast that has been worn for several months following surgery, patients seem vulnerable to fracture of the shaft of the femur as a result of bone atrophy that takes place during long periods of immobilization. Gentle handling of the extremity is essential, and extreme care should be exercised in getting the child up in a chair or on crutches. If the child is being discharged from the hospital the parents should be instructed to guard the child's activity carefully against possible jars and falls. Fracture of the femur has been known to occur from merely turning over in bed. The fracture may often be overlooked, inasmuch as the pain associated with it is attributed to the general discomfort resulting from the removal of the cast. Nurses should be alert for any complaint that might indicate a pathologic fracture. Any accident, however minor, should be reported to the physician at once.

CONGENITAL CLUBFOOT

Congenital deformities of the foot are of many kinds and are primarily hereditary in that they can frequently be traced through several generations. The typical clubfoot (Fig. 136) is composed of three main elements of deformity, i.e., equinus, varus, and forefoot adduction, and is known by the common term, talipes equinovarus, which was derived from the Latin.

Intrauterine positions of the foot can easily be mistaken for true clubfoot deformity, but examinations will reveal the difference. A true clubfoot, if examined, cannot be corrected to a neutral position in all elements of deformity, whereas an apparent positional deformity corrects itself quite readily. This is important to decide because treatment should begin immediately after a true clubfoot is known to exist, whereas no special treatment is necessary for a positional clubfoot. This also holds true for other foot

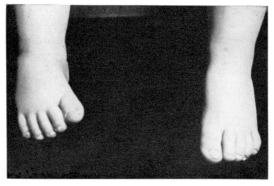

Fig. 135. Forefoot adduction of the right foot.

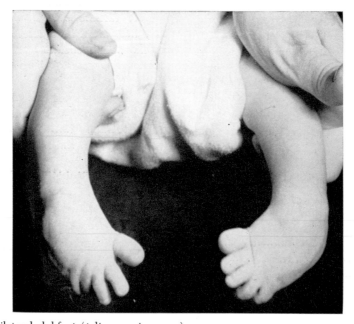

Fig. 136. Bilateral clubfoot (talipes equinovarus).

deformities, such as pes adductus and talipes calcaneovalgus.

A true clubfoot may be unilateral or bilateral and occurs not infrequently in association with other defects such as spina bifida and arthrogryposis. In any patient with clubfoot, therefore, other defects should be carefully looked for during examination.

Treatment of a clubfoot is quite successful in most instances. The principle of the treatment is to attain correction of all elements of deformity by manipulation and to maintain correction throughout the early growth years. This has been accomplished by various techniques, ranging from simple adhesive strapping to manipulation under anesthesia. Time and experience have taught us that excessive force can be harmful to the growing centers. The most common technique used is repeated manipulations and plaster casts. By this method the foot is stretched gently into

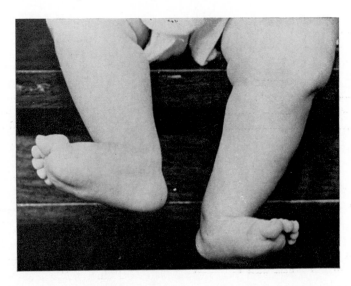

Fig. 137. Calcaneovalgus deformity of both feet. (From Kenney, William C., and Larson, Carroll B.: Orthopedics for the general practitioner, St. Louis, 1957, The C. V. Mosby Co.)

a corrected position and a cast is applied to hold the gain. This is repeated at intervals of a few days until correction is attained. Ten or more manipulations over a period of several months may be required. Weight bearing plus some type of retentive apparatus at night will usually maintain correction.

Many variations may be made in an effort to accommodate prolonged treatment to specific needs in each case. Frequently one element of deformity, namely equinus, will be more resistant to treatment and will require special effort even to the point of operative correction. In other instances muscular imbalance will prevent maintenance of correction so that operative transfer of tendons, such as shifting the tibialis anticus pull to a more lateral position, will be indicated.

In addition to the therapy outlined, it is important to follow these patients until growth is complete to be certain that recurrences of deformity do not occur.

Treatment and nursing care. In no congenital orthopedic condition is early recognition and treatment more important than in clubfoot. Although severe clubfoot conditions are not likely to be overlooked at delivery, a mild involvement is sometimes not noticed for periods of weeks or months. Delivery room nurses and those in the obstetric nursery should be especially observant of exaggerated attitudes in the baby's feet. It is not abnormal for an infant to lie with the feet slightly inverted, that is, turned inward with the soles of the feet toward the midline of the body. The normal infant can easily assume and maintain the opposite position if slight manipulation is used. A child with talipes equinovarus cannot maintain the everted position. Any indication, however mild, that the baby's ability to change the position of his feet is limited should be reported at once.

A few years ago considerable persuasion was sometimes necessary to convince parents that the baby with a clubfoot needed immediate attention. Much argument was put forth against taking the baby from its mother and breast feeding for such treatment. Public understanding is now more widespread, but the nurse will occasionally encounter parents who are extremely reluctant to begin treatment early. It will be necessary to help these parents to understand the necessity for early treatment. Clubfoot is a condition of which control has been definitely established; that is, the treatment is known, its results are almost certain, and the risk attending it is very minor. At present there is little excuse for the neglect that is still prevalent. The nurse who has an opportunity to listen to an orthopedic specialist talking to parents regarding these children will do well to observe his words. She will note, first and foremost, his insistence upon early treatment, but of equal importance will be his insistence on continued treatment. Too often these children are given prompt early treatment, and then, after they have been dismissed with an apparently satisfactory foot, the doctor's insistent demand that the child be seen at frequent intervals for several years afterward is ignored. The deformity, like most congenital deformities, tends to recur. The child is brought back to the clinic three or four years later with a badly deformed foot for which radical treatment is necessary. The watchword, therefore, is early treatment and prolonged observation by the specialist. One doctor made the comment that he taught a mother faithfully the care of her son with clubfoot to be carried out over a long period of years, and then when the patient was grown he instructed the wife in the same fashion. This is a manifest exaggeration, but the idea is clear.

Treatment and nursing care may be given in the form of the Kite method, manipulation and casting of the clubfoot, adhesive strapping of the clubfoot, manipulation without casting of the clubfoot, the Denis Browne splint, braces, and shoe corrections.

Kite method. Early treatment is always conservative. Up to a few years ago it varied a great deal in manner and apparatus, and to a certain degree this is still true. The method of Kite, who believes that as many as 90% of clubfeet can be treated by the conservative method until the child is about 8 years of age, is followed to a great extent. It is a method of gradual correction that systematically deals with the different aspects of talipes equinovarus deformity. It is done by cast with a series of wedging maneuvers that seek first to correct the adduction deformity of the forefoot, then the inversion deformity, and finally the equinus deformity. From the standpoint of the nurse the case may seem simple enough. She should remember, however, that each wedging is a threat to the patient's circulation. Often the circulation of the extremity is closely observed after the application of the original cast, but the wedging may escape notice. The doctor should forewarn the nurse, and night nurses especially should be solicitous about inspecting the child's foot after such wedgings. Considerable strain is placed on tendons, blood vessels, and ligaments after the equinus correction, which forces the plantar-flexed foot into a position of dorsiflexion. Undue pain or circulatory impairment should be reported at once.

Manipulation and casting of clubfoot. Sometimes, with the child under anesthesia, the feet are treated by a series of corrective casts applied after forcible manipulation is carried out. Frequent changes of the cast are required in this kind of treatment.

The very young baby in the plaster cast should always have close attention. The danger of circulatory impairment is so important that it should never be overlooked, but in the midst of a busy orthopedic ward, where spinal and hip

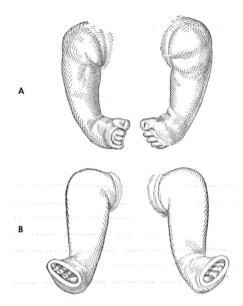

Fig. 138. Bilateral talipes equinovarus in the infant. **A**, Before correction. **B**, Undergoing correction in plaster casts. (From Shands, A. R., Raney, R. B., and Brashear, H. R.: Handbook of orthopaedic surgery, ed. 6, St. Louis, 1963, The C. V. Mosby Co.)

operations are so urgent in their demands upon nursing time, the baby with clubfoot is sometimes given less attention than he deserves. The foot should be inspected frequently. All the toes should be visible. This is frequently a point that must be called to the doctor's attention so that more of the cast can be cut out to reach the two smallest toes. The cast is usually applied in a position of flexion at the knee that will prevent its slipping downward, a complication that previously was common when the cast was applied only to the knee. In certain emergencies, when circulatory disturbance is manifest and severe and when no doctor is available, the nurse may be required to cut the cast. Bivalving the cast usually is preferred. Most doctors advise against cutting windows over the dorsum of the foot to relieve circulation, but in other clinics this is a routine measure to pre-

vent pressure over the dorsalis pedis artery. The bandages under the cast must also be released in case of severe circulatory embarrassment. The removed portion of plaster should be taped lightly over the opening to prevent window edema.

The parents are warned about the necessity for keeping close watch on circulation when they take the infant in the clubfoot cast away from the clinic. They are advised also to watch for signs that the child is outgrowing his cast and to report to the clinic any severe chafing of the skin. Some kind of waterproofing should be applied around the thigh edge of the cast. These edges must be carefully smoothed and taped to avoid chafing the soft skin of the thigh. Failure to waterproof this portion of the cast lessens its life considerably; a diapered child inevitably will wet the cast each time he voids. In an older child the parents must be warned that if the foot part of the cast gets soft and thin from wear, much of the correction so far attained may be lost. It is not unusual to have these children return to the clinic with the cast no thicker than a stocking and with about as much corrective force.

Adhesive strapping of clubfoot. Some surgeons use adhesive plaster strapping to obtain gradual correction of the clubfoot condition in infants. They believe that plaster of paris is outgrown quickly and therefore is impracticable, whereas the adhesive tape can be changed for alteration in the corrective process as the need arises. A simple method of applying adhesive tape for this purpose is given by Sever. A single narrow strip of adhesive tape about 1 inch in width is brought around the forepart of the foot from the inner to the outer aspect and is carried up the outside of the leg. The knee is kept flexed at a 90-degree angle as this is done, and the tape is brought over it and well up on the thigh. It is necessary to exert considerable traction on the tape to secure the foot in a position of overcorrection. The danger from tape, snugly applied to the baby's skin is, of course, apparent immediately. Adhesive plaster and the skin of young babies, as most nurses realize, do not have an affinity for each other. It is extremely urgent that the edges of the adhesive tape be carefully watched for signs of skin erosion and that the danger of circulatory impairment to the foot be foremost in the nurse's mind.

Manipulation without casting. Mild clubfoot deformity in the very young infant is sometimes treated by frequent manipulations without the use of a corrective cast. Manipulations are usually begun immediately after birth and are carried out every 4 hours, preferably before the baby is fed. Because the manipulation is accompanied by some discomfort for the baby, it is better to perform the treatment before rather than after the feeding; if done afterward, the baby soon learns to expect unpleasantness after the feeding and will cease to take his feeding well. These manipulations may be continued until the child is 2 years of age or until the surgeon feels satisfied that reduction is complete and unremittent. Frequently this treatment is employed to lead up to later treatment by cast or splint.

There are many variations in the manner of performing manipulations, and the nurse should have demonstrations given her by the surgeon for each individual patient upon whom she must carry out such treatment. Occasionally the surgeon may feel that a complete reduction should be sought in the first manipulation and will usually perform this himself. Complete reduction is considered to be accomplished when the foot has been forcibly brought into full calcaneovalgus position to such a de-

gree that the little toe touches the outer side of the leg. British authorities feel that this drastic early manipulation ultimately saves the child much discomfort.

The nurse must understand that, when she forces the clubfoot into the position of overcorrection by whatever method the surgeon prefers, she must grasp the foot below the tibial epiphysis. There is danger that the epiphysis may be displaced by too vigorous manipulation. This can be avoided by grasping the foot well below the malleoli with one hand while holding the ankle rigid and stable with the other hand.

The Denis Browne splint. The Denis Browne splint has proved a useful device for the treatment of clubfoot in young children. The splint works on the mechanical principle that it is possible to correct the position of one foot by means of the other. In this treatment the muscles of the leg and foot may be used and strengthened while the deformity is being corrected, thereby eliminating some of the atrophy and joint stiffness that often occur when casts are used for correction. Many modifications of the original splint have been made, but the general principle remains the same. The splint is composed of a flexible horizontal bar attached to a pair of footplates. A device under the plates allows for rotation of the footplate on the horizontal bar. The apparatus is constructed so that each footplate is manipulated by means of the other. Various methods of securing the splints to the feet are used. Bandages, tape, and plaster of paris have been tried. Adhesive tape is probably the most commonly used method in this country at present. Sponge rubber or felt is used to cover the footplates on the surface contacting the foot.

The technique of strapping the foot to the plate varies somewhat in differ-

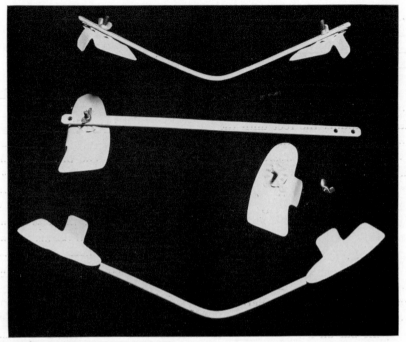

Fig. 139. Details of construction of Denis Browne splints. (Courtesy Dr. Arthur Steindler, Iowa City, Iowa.)

ent clinics, but certain basic principles must be observed to assure the success of the treatment.

1. The skin of the foot must be inspected carefully to see that it is clean and free from abrasions. For the original strapping it is prepared by washing and drying and may be painted with tincture of benzoin. For subsequent strapping, however, most surgeons prefer that the skin be left as it is, and washing or cleaning of the area with benzine or other solvents is not done.

2. There should be careful apposition of the foot to the footplate. The heel and sole must be firmly held to the plate; the sidepiece should contact the infant's ankle.

3. In applying the tape no wrinkles are allowed in the tape that might be the cause of pressure areas beneath.

4. There should be no open spaces between the strips of tape, or window edema may occur.

Some physicians feel that it is wise to begin the treatment by attaching the feet to the plate for a short time in the position of the deformity rather than to attempt immediate correction. The bar is bent in the shape of an inverted V and applied to the footplates in such a fashion that the position of the feet is not changed. Swelling and skin irritation may sometimes be reduced and pliability of the foot encouraged by this method.

During the period of correction, which may take from 6 to 8 weeks, strapping is changed frequently, usually every 5 or 6 days. The child is allowed to leave the hospital only when there is absolute assurance that the parents will return him promptly for change of strapping. Usually it is considered preferable to keep the child in the hospital during the first period of treatment, that is, until correction has been obtained.

After one or two strappings the connecting bar may be straightened to the horizontal position. The feet will follow the position of the bar and adduction and inversion of the feet will gradually be corrected until a neutral position is obtained; that is, the feet will point straight ahead. After that, effort is made to rotate and abduct the feet until they reach 90 degrees of outward rotation, which is the position of overcorrection essential in the treatment of clubfoot.

In order to secure a valgus position, some orthopedists prefer to angulate the bar into a true V shape at the time the foot has reached the neutral position.

As treatment proceeds, effort is made to stretch the calf muscles. This may be done by increasing the V angle of the bar when the foot is in 90 degrees of outward rotation. If the deformity is unilateral, the bar on the normal side is bent horizontally so that the normal foot is held in physiologic position at all times.

The more vigorous the baby's activity the greater will be the correction, for as the child flexes one leg and extends the other, the foot on the flexed side is forced into a valgus position, which, of course, is the corrected position for varus deformity. Furthermore, with the foot in the valgus position, flexion of the knee will cause the foot to go into dorsiflexion, thereby stretching the posterior calf muscles. This is necessary for correcting the equinus deformity. It can readily be seen that with this treatment the baby provides his own corrective manipulation by his normal activity. Five or six weeks of this activity may be sufficient to obtain correction, but maintenance of correction will require a far greater length of time. The splint may be used as described for 5 or 6 months, after which shoes may be attached to the plates. Usually the shoes will be attached in reverse, that is, the left shoe will be used for the right foot and the

right shoe for the left foot. This apparatus may need to be worn 6 months or longer. After the child reaches walking age, alterations are frequently applied to the walking shoe. An outside wedge or patch of leather, $\frac{3}{16}$ inch in thickness, may be placed on the sole. This alteration aids in overcoming any tendency the child may still have toward adduction or varus. The physician sometimes prefers that the child wear a shoe without a heel in order to continue stretching the Achilles tendon. The night splint is usually continued for a year or longer even after the child begins to walk.

Pediatricians have commented upon the increased likelihood of upper respiratory infections in children who are having clubfoot correction by the Denis Browne splint method as compared with those whose treatment is by cast. There seems to be some relationship to the fact that nurses tend to pick up babies in clubfoot casts more frequently and that babies in splints are often left in their cribs during the entire day, for bathing, dressing, and even feedings. Nurses are urged to see that these babies are taken from their beds frequently and either held or placed in chairs for at least part of the day. The well-being of the baby may depend a great deal upon this simple factor.

It cannot be overemphasized that the skin of babies upon whom adhesive tape is being used for any reason must be carefully watched for signs of swelling, excoriation, or blueness. Any abnormality of the skin around the tape should be reported to the physician immediately.

When the child is discharged from the hospital in the Denis Browne splint, some physicians instruct the parents to remove the plates from the bar once or twice daily. They feel that this will aid in preventing pressure areas. The parents are also instructed to check the position of the baby's heel at frequent intervals.

If the heel is found to be slipping up, the instructions usually are to remove the foot from the plate and to return the child to the clinic at once.

Parents are sometimes asked to place a crossbar above the baby's crib and to attach the bar of the splint to this for part of the time. It is felt that this will aid in eliminating the equinus position that results from constant resting on the bed. Instructions to parents should include advice to keep the baby in the sitting position at intervals during the day.

Braces and shoe corrections. When an overcorrected position of the clubfoot has been attained by the use of casts, the child is fitted with a splint designed to maintain the correction. This splint may be worn continuously at first and then discarded gradually as the leg and foot muscles become stronger. The Denis Browne splint may be used for this purpose. The footplates and abduction bar are fastened to the child's shoes. The position of the feet is controlled by the abduction bar and by the mechanism used in fastening the bar to the shoes.

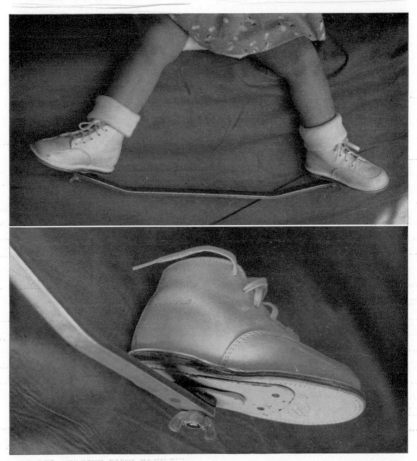

Fig. 140. After correction of clubfoot deformity, the modified Denis Browne splint may be prescribed to maintain correction. The splint is worn continuously at first and is gradually discarded as the child's activity increases and as muscles of the foot and leg become stronger. The desired position of the foot is controlled by positioning the abduction bar and by the screw mechanism that attaches the shoe to the bar.

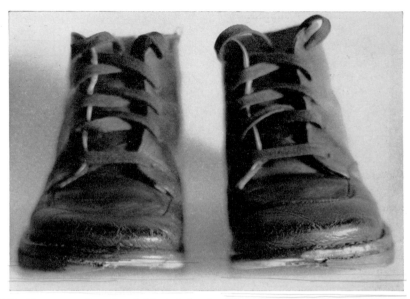

Fig. 141. Shoe corrections for clubfoot deformity. The elevation on the lateral aspect of the shoe sole helps prevent recurrence of the varus deformity. The importance of maintaining these shoe corrections cannot be overemphasized if recurrence of the deformity is to be prevented.

The feet are usually held in a position of abduction, eversion, and dorsiflexion.

Exercises may be prescribed by the physician and demonstrated to the parents at this time. Experience has shown that follow-up exercises are a most neglected feature of home care. Upon return visits to the clinic parents are questioned and frequently admit that they have omitted them for one reason or another. These exercises, however, are important. They are not difficult to perform, and parents should be urged to continue them faithfully for the welfare of the child. Failure to carry out such orders may mean that the parents have no clear conception of the importance of the exercises. A little time given to explanation will pay surprising dividends.

Shoe corrections may consist of an elevation to the outer border of the sole and heel. This will place the foot in a slightly everted position and aid in the maintenance of overcorrection. Here

again the parents must be warned that when shoe corrections are worn down the child should be brought to the clinic. It is disheartening to observe children returning to the clinic in run-over heels and worn-down shoe corrections after a long and costly series of treatments by the orthopedist. Doubtless, fuller instructions given to the parents by doctor and nurse would obviate much of this carelessness.

Treatment of the older child. The older child with recurrent or neglected clubfoot will usually require some type of operation. It is never possible to reconstruct the foot to perfect contour and function by surgery, but a good weight-bearing foot that will minimize the deformity can usually be obtained. In order to eliminate chances of disappointment after surgery, the parents and the patient should be given a realistic understanding of what the operation will accomplish. Only careful explanation of the expected result before the operation is performed will prevent disappointment.

Soft tissue procedures, such as tendon lengthenings, stripping of the plantar fascia, or capsulotomies, are performed for neglected clubfoot. Surgery on the bone may be required for maximal correction in some patients. These may be wedge resections, osteotomies, or astragalectomies.

On a busy orthopedic ward, where major surgery is being done daily, these patients may seem of only minor importance. The risk is not minor, however, and the danger of congestion and hemorrhage is great. They will usually be immobilized in a cast that extends to the thigh and will be kept elevated with pillows or a hammock.

The nurse should be alert for seepage of blood at the site of surgery and also at the thigh where the cast ends; frequently hemorrhage may be detected there. An overhead frame with a hammock to support the cast is the preferred apparatus to support the leg. Pillows may be used but are not so stable, and many pillows are necessary to obtain a comfortable degree of elevation. The patient is usually much more comfortable with the limb in the hammock, and it does not interfere with nursing care because he can be moved from side to side as long as elevation is maintained. This is usually about 48 hours but may be longer if congestion or pain is excessive. The nurse must heed complaints of the patient and interpret them intelligently. She must know where the line of incision is so that she may be alert for any odor. Knowledge of the line of incision is necessary also in order to detect pain at other points at which pain should not be present. A complaint of pain at the heel, the patella, or the dorsum of the foot is not an expected aftermath of such surgery and should be reported at

once. When the surgeon has given an order to have the cast cut over any of these points, the cutting should be done at once, not at the end of the day when it is easier to secure an orderly. Too often casts may be marked for cutting in the morning or early afternoon, but the actual process may be delayed for hours if the nurse is not faithful (and persistent) in her attempts to get a cast cutter to the bedside.

Dressing cart technique should be rigidly aseptic when the cast is cut and the first dressing done. Frequently, spreading of the incision may occur if stitches are removed too soon. The surgeon will usually ask for some type of sterile adhesive strap for approximating the wound edges.

The three principal causes of failure in the treatment of clubfoot are (1) delay in beginning treatment, (2) imperfect nerve supply to muscles, as in conditions such as spina bifida, and (3) failure to obtain and maintain complete overcorrection of the deformity. Nurses will easily recognize their part in helping to eliminate at least two of these causes of failure—the delay in beginning treatment and the failure to continue medical supervision after correction has been obtained. Parents should be guided to the realization that follow-up treatment in clubfoot is as important as the active correction. They must have a clear understanding of their responsibility in this matter.

WRYNECK (TORTICOLLIS)

Signs and symptoms. At birth or shortly after, the child with wryneck may have a tendency to hold the head to one side. On palpation of the neck a mass may be felt in the sternocleidomastoideus muscle. There is limitation of motion in attempts to move the head away from the affected side.

Cause. The cause of wryneck is con-

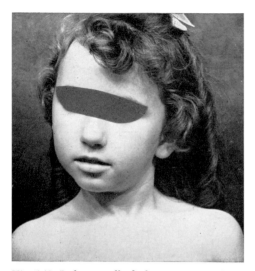

Fig. 142. Left torticollis before correction. Note asymmetry of the face, rotation of the head to the right, and tilt of the head toward the affected side.

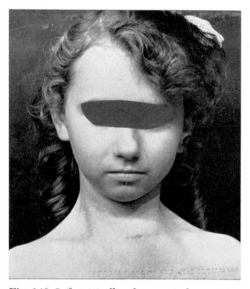

Fig. 143. Left torticollis after surgical correction

sidered to be an engorgement of the muscle as a result of overstretching during the passage through the birth canal. Some observers hold to the theory that the affected muscle was inherently weak before birth.

Anatomy. After tearing occurs in the muscle, there is hemorrhage and extravasation of blood into the fibers. During the healing process this undergoes organization and development of scar tissue. The scar so completely involves the muscle fibers that elasticity is lost and contraction occurs. As the child grows older, this also leads to the development of a facial asymmetry.

Treatment and nursing care. In most cases of congenital wryneck discovered shortly after birth, correction and cure can be assured within a month or two by the daily use of heat, massage, and carefully regulated stretching of the affected muscle.

In cases that have gone untreated or unrecognized, fibrosis takes place in the muscle and permanent deformity develops. Operative treatment is necessary. This consists in the resection of the tendon of the muscle from both the sternal and the clavicular attachments. Usually, about ¾ inch of the tendon is removed.

There are various methods recommended for maintaining correction after operation, but probably the safest is the application of a plaster of paris cast that covers the chest, neck, and head in an overcorrected position. This requires that the chin be brought high above the shoulder of the affected side.

The cast should be left on for approximately 6 weeks. After its removal a Thomas collar may be worn, and massage and stretching may be continued for several weeks.

Early recognition and treatment are essential. It is now generally recognized that much facial and postural deformity can be prevented if conservative treatment is begun early. The deformity may be so mild at birth that it is unobserved; or, being observed, the opinion may be held that with function the child will outgrow it. As time goes on, however, the ligaments on the affected side be-

Sternocleidomastoideus muscle

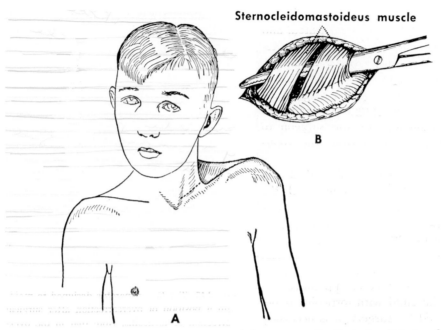

B

A

Fig. 144. Operation for torticollis. **A**, Line of skin incision. **B**, Clavicular and sternal attachments of sternocleidomastoideus muscle withdrawn from wound and divided. (From Crenshaw, A. H., and Milford, L., editors: Campbell's operative orthopaedics, ed. 4, St. Louis, 1963, The C. V. Mosby Co.)

come so shortened and twisted that facial deformity becomes pronounced. Very early in the child's life an elongated swelling may be noted in the lower half of the sternocleidomastoideus muscle. It is quite tender at this time, and the child will cry if it is touched or if the neck is stretched. This swelling and tenderness eventually disappears, and the mother usually decides that there is nothing further to fear. Later, however, it can be observed that muscle tenseness exists. A band of fibrous connective tissue develops that, by contraction, pulls the head into the characteristic attitude—the ear on that side seems to be pulled downward toward the clavicle, and the face itself is turned in the opposite direction. When this condition is left without treatment, a slowly developing atrophy of the side of the face near the affected muscle will occur and become very apparent as the

child grows older. This, of course, is followed by tissue changes. The soft tissues on the deformed side will become adaptively shortened and be followed by certain definite bony deformities in accordance with Wolff's law.*

The nurse caring for a young baby should be alert to detect any signs of limitation of movement in the head or neck. Frequently, when the stage of tumor and tenderness is missed, the deformity may escape notice because there are no marked symptoms except this limitation.

In mild cases after the stage of tumor

---

*Wolff's Law: Every change in the form and the function of bones, or in their function alone, is followed by certain definite changes in their internal architecture, and equally definite changes in their external conformation, in accordance with mathematical laws. Julius Wolff, 1868. Briefly, the law may be remembered as form follows function.

and tenderness has passed manipulation and exercises are usually instituted, and often these alone will suffice to overcome the deformity. These manipulations should be prescribed and demonstrated to the nurse by the surgeon for each patient, and progress should be checked frequently by the surgeon to ensure proper results from the treatment.

Surgery is usually indicated if the manipulative treatment fails or if the child is not seen until he is 2 years or more of age. In severe cases surgery is sometimes performed on the young infant, in which case one of the foremost nursing problems is to care for the baby properly in the traction apparatus.

When the child with torticollis is being prepared for surgery, it is necessary to shave above the hairline on the affected side. Specific instructions should be obtained from the surgeon as to the extent of the area he wishes to have shaved. When a young girl undergoes a tenotomy of the sternocleidomastoideus tendon, it is possible to part her hair low on the affected side, comb it to the opposite side, and braid it tightly. Postoperatively, the patient is especially happy to have this long hair to comb over the shaved area.

Casts are not always applied immediately after surgery. Postoperative nausea and the possibility of respiratory embarrassment make it safer to apply the cast the following day. Some type of retentive apparatus may be used in the interval. Head traction is difficult to apply and can be dangerous if it is inefficiently done, particularly in such a young child. A flannel sling for the chin may be devised to exert head traction, but it must be inspected frequently lest it slip and impair the child's breathing or smother him by slipping upward. The amount of weight used will be ordered by the doctor, but it is usually very little. Sand-

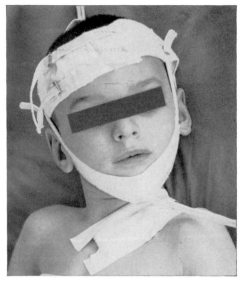

Fig. 145. Traction apparatus designed to maintain a position of overcorrection after surgical correction of torticollis. Note that in the overcorrected position the chin points toward the incision and the back of the head is pulled upward.

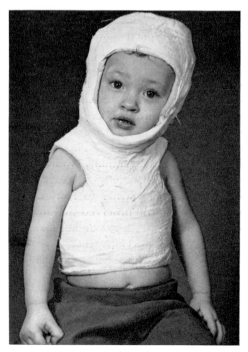

Fig. 146. Right torticollis. The position of overcorrection is maintained 4 to 6 weeks postoperatively.

bags may be used to control the position of the head.

The ordinary Sayre chin strap may be used, augmented by sandbags to maintain a position of overcorrection. In this type a long sandbag is placed low, forcing the chin toward the side on which the incision has been made. The second sandbag is placed on the opposite side, exerting pressure on the forehead and ear. The sandbags must be closely watched because they tend to slip.

Traction of this nature may be worn for a week or two, after which a brace is often applied. This brace is usually one that comes well down over the spine and may be a Taylor body brace with some type of corrective chin apparatus.

If the cast is applied in surgery before the patient becomes conscious, considerable care must be exercised to prevent aspiration of vomitus. Suction apparatus must be available. The area around the chin and mouth needs to be protected with pieces of waterproofing that may be tucked in until the cast is dry enough to finish the edges. A towel should also be tucked in around the face to further eliminate soiling.

After the cast is dry the scalp section of the cast will usually be cut out to permit care of the head, and constant attention to this area will be necessary to prevent itching and irritation from plaster crumbs. At feeding time it will be necessary to protect the cast with a towel or napkin to prevent food from falling inside the cast. The ears must be inspected frequently to see that no plaster crumbs or pieces of food are lodged in them. Scalp and ears become sore easily when this type of cast is worn. These patients are soon ambulatory and are often left to care for themselves, but it must be remembered that careful supervision will be necessary daily to detect signs of skin irritation, pressure areas, or cracking and softening of the cast.

The cast may be kept on from 6 weeks to several months, according to the severity of the condition. After it is removed, physical therapy will be ordered, consisting of massage, manipulation, and gymnastic exercises. These treatments may need to be continued over a considerable period, particularly in the older child. The parents should understand that torticollis cannot be completely corrected by surgery alone. A long period of follow-up care under the constant supervision of the physician will be necessary. If the child is dismissed soon after the cast is applied, the mother will need careful instruction in the details of caring for the patient and his cast.

CONGENITAL ELEVATION OF THE SCAPULA (SPRENGEL DEFORMITY)

Symptoms and signs. Deformity is apparent in the upper part of the back of patients with congenital elevation of the

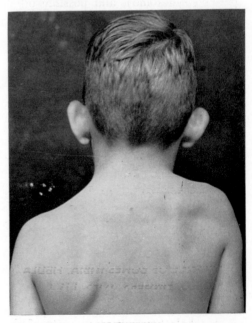

Fig. 147. Sprengel deformity.

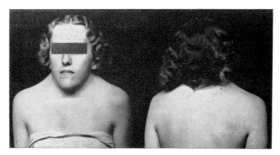

Fig. 148. Klippel-Feil syndrome. (From Kenney, William C., and Larson, Carroll B.: Orthopedics for the general practioner, St. Louis, 1957, The C. V. Mosby Co.)

scapula. One or both shoulder blades are high. There is usually some limitation of the movement in the shoulder joints.

Anatomy. It is the opinion of most authorities that the term congenital elevation is a misnomer. The scapulae are normally high during the period of development, but descend and rotate before birth. It is therefore a failure of descent of the scapulae. The deformity may be associated with other congenital deformities, such as abnormalities in the shape of the vertebrae, webneck (Klippel-Feil syndrome), and possibly other deformities.

Treatment. The treatment of choice for congenital elevation of the scapulae is that recommended by Schrock. This consists in the complete subperiosteal and submuscular release of the scapulae, followed by rotation of the bone within this compartment to its normal position. Immobilization for a period of a few weeks follows, allowing reattachment of the periosteum. The scapulae are now in their normal position. In properly selected cases in younger children this treatment gives complete correction of the deformity.

ABSENCE OF BONES (TIBIA, FIBULA, RADIUS, FINGERS, TOES, ETC.)

Clinical picture. A child may be born with whole extremities or parts of the extremities missing, or with various bones missing. Extremities or digits may be partly missing, and there may be constricting bands or circular creases.

Causes. Absence of bones seems to be caused by the arrest of development during the early stages of embryonic growth. Constrictions and retarded development in the extremities in many instances are thought to be caused by amnionic bands or scars or intrauterine constrictions.

Anatomy. The deformity that develops from the absence of a bone is always characterized by loss of the propping or strutting effect of this bone. If a radius is missing, the hand is at a right angle to the forearm in a direction pointing toward the face (clubhand). It is not unusual to find associated deformities such as absence of the thumb and the presence of a cervical rib.

When the absence of bones occurs where there is an associated bone, such as in the forearm or in the lower part of the leg, the other bone usually becomes enlarged and frequently deformed. When there is absence of the tibia, the leg is usually shorter and the foot tends to turn inward and backward.

Congenital deformities of this type include short and underdeveloped limbs caused by growth deficiencies. Occasionally, one leg or one arm will be underdeveloped so that it is only about

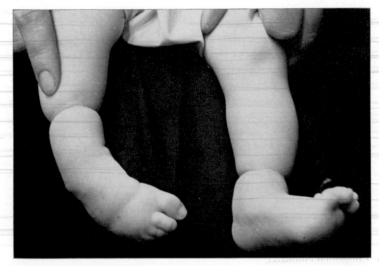

Fig. 149. Amnionic bands and bilateral clubfoot.

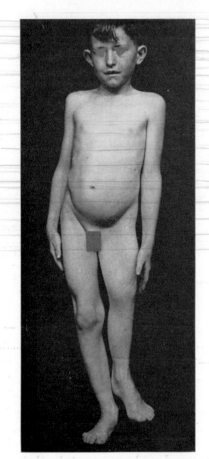

Fig. 150. Congenital shortening of the left femur.

one-half the length of the opposite one.

SPINA BIFIDA

Spina bifida is a defect that may occur in the dorsal or lumbar region of the spine, but occurs much more frequently in the lumbar. In the mild forms it may cause only structural weakness (spina bifida occulta), but in the severe forms there may be complete or partial paralysis of the legs, bladder, and rectum. In the mild forms there may be no obvious deformity, but in the severe forms there may be a sac with a wall of tissue-paper thickness varying in diameter from 1 to 3 or 4 inches in the newborn infant.

Cause. Spina bifida is congenital. During the normal process of development in the embryo the spinal cord is the most posterior structure, but as development takes place the cord is covered by a posterior growth of bone, muscles, and ligaments. The bone growing from each side meets in the center posteriorly, forming the spinous process. In spina bifida occulta the component parts of the process almost meet, but in the severe forms they make little progress

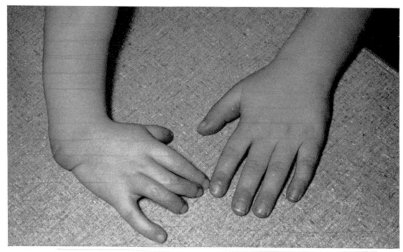

Fig. 151. Congenital clubhand.

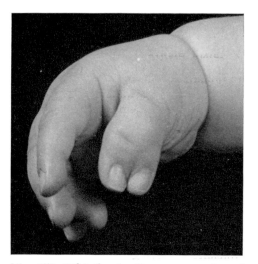

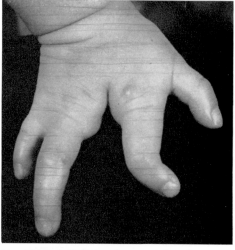

Fig. 152. Bifid thumb. Treatment consists of surgical removal of the accessory thumb.

Fig. 153. A cleft hand. In many cases hands with this deformity are quite functional.

toward meeting. Consequently the spinal cord is left exposed, and nerve development to the limbs is incomplete.

Treatment. Although immediate surgery with an attempt to force closure of the spinal canal was previously advocated, recently the inclination has been to delay surgery and possibly to omit it entirely.

Prognosis. The future of children with

spina bifida is always questionable. They may develop water on the brain (hydrocephalus) and become imbeciles, or they may go through the stages of school life and adult life greatly disabled by the weakness or paralysis in their legs and by the absence of bladder and bowel control. This last causes them continual embarrassment in their contacts throughout school and adult life.

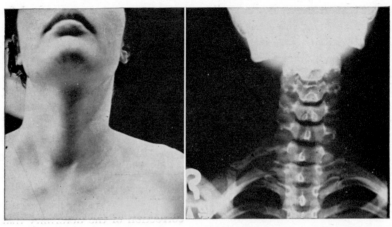

Fig. 154. Cervical rib. The presence of a cervical rib may produce pressure on the brachial plexus and thus cause a radiating pain in the upper extremity. This may be relieved by shoulder exercises and the use of a brace. In some instances surgical resection of the cervical rib is necessary. (From Kenney, William C., and Larson, Carroll B.: Orthopedics for the general practioner, St. Louis, 1957, The C. V. Mosby Co.)

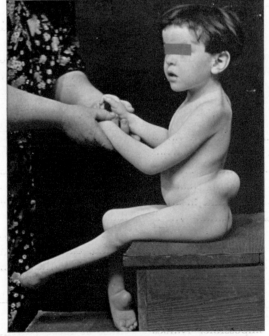

Fig. 155. Spina bifida with meningomyelocele. Note atrophy of the lower extremities and the associated deformities of the feet. (From Kenney, William C., and Larson, Carroll B.: Orthopedics for the general practioner, St. Louis, 1957, The C. V. Mosby Co.)

Braces for the legs or stabilization operations often help locomotion.

Nursing care. The infant with spina bifida manifesta usually is not seen first on the orthopedic service. Such conditions are considered in that early stage to be primarily pediatric and neurologic in nature. However, their congenital malformations are sometimes multiple, or, if deformity has not been present at birth, tendency toward deformity in later years is considerable. Such individuals frequently spend much time on the orthopedic services of hospitals. The patient with the milder form of spina bifida (occulta), who displays but little outward manifestation of the vertebral cleft, may be admitted to the service because of clubfoot or some other deformity, but on the whole this patient does not present many problems in nursing care. It is the patient with sensory and motor involvement from some degree of cord destruction who will be discussed here.

All the problems of nursing care encountered in the patient who has destruction of the cord through disease, tumor, or trauma, accompanied by the inevitable group of symptoms engendered by this condition, are present in the paralyzed patient with spina bifida. Trophic ulcers are a tremendous problem, complicated as they are by incontinence of bowel and bladder. Trophic ulcers have all the menacing features common to pressure areas, and in addition the patient lacks sensation. He is completely unaware of the condition so that there are no warning signals of pain. Furthermore, lack of nutrition to the area, which is caused by impairment of the sensory nerves supplying the muscles and blood vessels in the part, makes healing difficult or impossible. Nurses should remember that in patients with trophic ulcers the blood vessels surrounding the area have become dilated

through failure of the nerve supply that normally regulates blood flow. The blood tends to stagnate, causing the surrounding tissues to become ischemic.

The tendency toward deformity in these patients is so great that frequently children are admitted to the orthopedic wards with hips and knees flexed to a right angle, back extremely rounded, feet inverted to such an extent that the appearance is one of clubfeet that is found to have developed subsequently to birth. Dislocation of the hips is not uncommon, and hydrocephalus frequently adds to the dismaying picture.

The patient with spina bifida is often admitted to the orthopedic ward for correction of the deformity that will enable him to walk with the aid of crutches and braces. Sometimes the immediate cause of his admission may be the grave nature of the trophic ulcers that have baffled the parents' attempts to heal.

Surgery may be performed for correction of the existing deformities. A particularly troublesome deformity is the flexion contracture of the hips. The Soutter operation may be performed for this condition. It consists of stripping the contracted flexor muscles about the hip from their origin on the ilium so that complete extension of the thigh is possible. Aftertreatment is especially important. A bed position that permits extension of the hips, obtained either by the Schwartz or Whitman frame or by the use of a double hip spica cast, is necessary—the purpose being to obtain further extension of the hips or at least to maintain the extension that was obtained at operation.

Early instruction should be obtained from the surgeon in regard to management of these patients. He will realize how serious a problem confronts the nurse and will be able to assist her in planning safe alterations of position. Frequent changes to the prone-lying position must be such as will maintain the extension of the hips. The back, buttocks, and groin must have attention many times a day, certainly as often as the child becomes wet. Wrinkled, compressed, and bluish areas must be meticulously cared for. The child's skin will reflect promptly any letup in nursing care, any wrinkles or crumbs in his bed, or any neglect in changing position.

If a cast is used, the care of it is complicated. It is an extremely difficult task, particularly with girl patients, to avoid a soggy evil-smelling cast. Early attention to waterproofing the entire cast as well as to protecting its edges generously with a durable waterproof material is the first step.

Any apparatus must be considered a menace to the skin of these patients. Vigilant eyes, fingers, and nose cannot be emphasized too strongly here. The patient cannot tell where the pressure is; the nurse must supply this missing sensation by careful frequent inspection of the parts in the apparatus.

Soap and water cleanliness, followed by use of a dusting powder (borated), and freedom from pressure, moisture, and irritating creases in bed are essential in the care of perineum and buttocks. Frequently the most resistant areas of ulceration occur in the groin, as fissures, and beneath the gluteal folds, as large deep-seated sores.

Long leg braces with a pelvic band or girdle are usually prescribed when the child is ready for walking. These, too, must be considered a threat to the integrity of the patient's skin, and the child's body must be carefully inspected for signs of irritation when they are removed. It is not usually considered advisable for patients to remain in these braces for the entire day. Periods of bed rest without braces but in good body alignment should alternate with hours of ambulatory exercise. The problem of keeping the patient dry when he is in his braces can be solved by the use of a rubber urinal or by the use of a Foley catheter when prescribed by the physician. The catheter is connected to a plastic leg bag during the day and to a drainage bag fastened to the side of the bed at night. Wearing a catheter helps to keep the skin dry and prevents breakdown and maceration of the skin frequently found in patients with urinary incontinence. The possibility, however, of urinary tract infection is always present, and aseptic techniques must be used in caring for the catheter. To prevent urinary tract infection there are many things patients and parents must learn to do for themselves. The importance of an adequate or increased intake of fluid needs to be stressed. They must learn

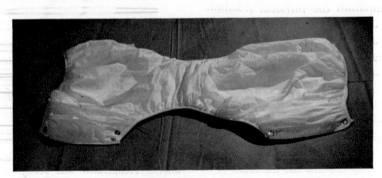

Fig. 156. Side-closing plastic-lined pants with grippers for easy fastening.

the correct method of irrigating the catheter as well as how to replace it when necessary. They need to be aware of the dangers of a catheter that is pinched or clamped off for a long period of time as well as the dangers of a catheter that becomes plugged or does not irrigate properly. The appearance of blood in the urine or a temperature elevation is an indication to seek medical assistance at once.

If a catheter is not worn, the patient will need to wear waterproof pants over layers of diaper cloth. These can be made quite simply from waterproof material with the edges bound with some kind of cloth for better wear. They are best made so that they are opened at the sides as well as the top. It is easier to apply them over braces in this fashion. Tape ties can be sewed to the binding, and these may be tied on the outer aspect of the thigh and hip to secure the garment. Plastic lined pants also may be purchased with grippers at the sides for fastening. When secured for the individual patient these will fit better and are easier to put on.

Parents bring in children who have never walked, hoping that the physician can enable the child to walk. They are grateful when this is accomplished, as it frequently is, but they will not recognize their own part in continuing this progress if they are not permitted to watch the meticulous nursing care that accompanies the physical rehabilitation of the child. The complications that may ensue because of brace pressure on legs must be pointed out. The necessity for preventing recurrence of deformity by watching the child's bed, chair, and walking posture, as well as by the faithful use of such night splints as have been ordered by the surgeon, should be emphasized. The care of the skin, especially around the buttocks and groin, must be demonstrated. The

parents must be urged to assist the child to develop as much self-dependence as he is capable of assuming.

Frequently no more pathetic individual exists on the orthopedic ward or in the crippled children's school than this type of patient. He often feels himself to be an outcast because of his inability to take care of his toilet needs. He has, besides the motor disability that limits him in many ways, the social difficulty that becomes harder to bear as he goes into adulthood. Sometimes his hydrocephalic appearance gives him a look of subnormal intelligence that is not indicative of his actual mental capacity.

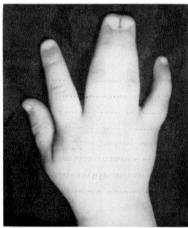

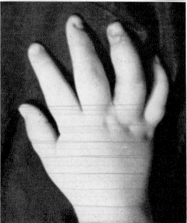

Fig. 157. Syndactylia between middle and ring fingers. Preoperative and postoperative photographs.

SYNDACTYLISM

Syndactylism is a congenital anomaly characterized by the webbing of two or more fingers or toes. The web may be formed by skin alone or by skin and subcutaneous tissue, and in severe cases there may be bony fusion between the phalanges.

The treatment consists in surgical separation of the digits and skin grafting of the denuded areas with free full-thickness skin grafts. The commissure or deepest part of the web is fashioned with a flap of skin from the palmar or dorsal aspect of the web. After skin grafting it is necessary to rigidly immobilize the digits spread apart in a plaster cast or splint for 3 weeks. The best time for surgery is during the second or third year of life.

STUDY QUESTIONS

1. How will a sound knowledge and understanding of the normal infant assist the nurse in providing better care for children with congenital anomalies?
2. What routine inspection might the nurse be expected to give the newborn infant during the initial bath?
3. What nursing problems will confront the mother caring for her child in a hip spica cast? What can the nurse do to help the mother give good nursing care to the child?
4. Why is it important that the following conditions be diagnosed and treated early?
   (a) Congenital dislocation of the hip
   (b) Torticollis
   (c) Clubfoot
5. What symptoms may be observed that would indicate a congenital dislocation of the hip?
   (a) Before weight bearing
   (b) After weight bearing

6. At what sites would you be particularly alert for pressure areas after wedging of a clubfoot cast?
7. Discuss overcorrection as a means of treatment in congenital deformities.
8. List two types of spina bifida and describe each.
9. Be prepared to discuss the nursing care of the patient with spina bifida as related to the following:
   (a) Prevention and healing of trophic ulcers
   (b) Prevention of deformities and secondary contractures
   (c) Care of incontinence
   (d) Problems of the spina bifida patient with braces
   (e) Problems encountered following surgery
   (f) Psychologic, social, and economic factors
   (g) Providing adequate home instruction and follow-up care

REFERENCES

Adams, M. M.: Appraisal of a newborn infant, Am. J. Nursing **55**:1336-1337, 1955.

Allan, J. H.: The challenge of spina bifida cystica. In Adams, J. P., editor: Current practice in orthopaedic surgery, St. Louis, 1963, The C. V. Mosby Co.

Fishbein, M., editor: Birth defects, Philadelphia, 1963, J. B. Lippincott Co.

Bluestone, S. S., and Deaver, G. G.: Habilitation of the child with spina bifida and myelomeningocele, J.A.M.A. **161**:1248-1251, 1956.

Brown, E., and Ward, M.: Toilet problems of seven children with spina bifida, Phys. Therap. Rev. **33**:632-638, 1953.

Conner, E. H.: Our Susan bloomed in plaster, Crippled Child **31**:4-7, 1953.

Craig, W., and Hamara, M. L.: Congenital dysplasia and dislocation of the hips, Am. J. Nursing **56**:1274-1280, 1956.

Deaver, G. G., and McCarthy, J.: Home care for the child with spina bifida, Nursing Outlook **1**:343, 1953.

Diller, L.: Psychology of disabled children, Am. J. Nursing **64**:131-134, 1964.

Ferguson, A.: Orthopedic surgery in infancy

and childhood, Baltimore, 1963, Williams & Wilkins Co.

Grice, D. S.: Talipes equinovarus—diagnosis and treatment, Am. J. Nursing **51**:707-710, 1951.

Hart, V. L.: Congenital dislocation of the hip in the newborn and in early postnatal life, J.A.M.A. **143**:1299-1303, 1950.

Hass, J.: Congenital dislocation of the hip, Springfield, Ill., 1951, Charles C Thomas, Publisher.

Larsen, L. J.: Congenital torticollis, Am. J. Nursing **57**:610-612, 1957.

Larson, C. B.: Common orthopedic problems in children, Pediatrics **17**:786-791, 1956.

Lindsay, M. E.: Nursing the child with torticollis, Am. J. Nursing **57**:612-613, 1957.

Macdonald, M.: Talipes equinovarus—nursing care in the community, Am. J. Nursing **51**:711-712, 1951.

Mercer, Sir Walter, and Duthie, R.: Orthopedic surgery, ed. 6, Baltimore, 1964, Williams & Wilkins Co.

Pediatric Clinic of North America: Pediatric orthopedics, Philadelphia, 1955, W. B. Saunders Co.

Ponseti, I. V.: Early diagnosis of congenital dislocation of the hip, J. Iowa M. Soc. **11**:520-522, 1950.

Putti, V.: Early treatment of congenital dislocation of the hip, J. Bone & Joint Surg. **11**:798-809, 1929.

Ryan, E. K.: Nursing care of the patient with spina bifida, Am. J. Nursing **51**:28-30, 1951.

Second International Conference on Congenital Malformations, compiled and edited by The International Medical Congress, Ltd. 120 Broadway, New York, 1963.

West, J. S.: Congenital malformations and birth injuries, New York, 1954, Association for the aid of Crippled Children.

Williams, B.: Talipes equinovarus—nursing care in the hospital, Am. J. Nursing **51**:710-711, 1951.

Chapter 4

Developmental diseases of bone, including nursing care in structural scoliosis

A number of bone and joint affections occur in middle childhood and adolescence with such regularity in age incidence that they are seemingly related to epiphyseal bone growth. Many of these conditions are self-limited within set time intervals and need treatment only to prevent deformity while the condition runs its cycle. Some are capable of inciting pain and therefore demand treatment. The more common of these conditions will be discussed in this chapter.

COXA PLANA (LEGG DISEASE, LEGG-PERTHES DISEASE, OSTEOCHONDRITIS DEFORMANS JUVENILIS)

Coxa plana at one time was frequently confused with tuberculosis of the hip because the early symptoms are almost identical. Osteochondritis of the hip is a self-limited disease, usually occurring in children between 5 and 10 years of age. Boys are more frequently affected, suggesting possible trauma as one of the instigating causes. Muscle spasm rarely is severe, and motions usually are restricted only in abduction and rotation, as contrasted with tuberculosis or arthritis in which all motions are restricted. In some instances the child will complain of pain in the knee rather than in the hip.

Pathology. Early roentgenograms show small vacuoles on either or both sides of the epiphysis. Following this, during the course of a few months to 1 or 2 years, the head of the femur undergoes degenerative changes in which segmentation first takes place. This is combined with liquefaction over the cartilaginous surface of the joint and flattening of the upper surface of the head of the femur. In 2 or 3 years, when healing finally occurs automatically, the epiphyseal line becomes more horizontal and the head of the femur becomes flattened.

This phenomenon usually does not lead to interference with joint function in early years. It may, however, lead to irritative changes about the hip joint later in life because of the discrepancies in shape between the head of the femur and the acetabulum.

Treatment. During this period of avascular necrosis the head of the femur is pliable and will heal in a deformed position if weight bearing is permitted. It is apparent that the method of treatment must provide protection for the head of the femur during this process of degeneration.

Some investigators recommend complete bed rest and traction during the developmental stages. If begun early this type of treatment gives the best restoration of the normal shape of the

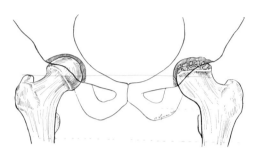

Fig. 158. Legg-Perthes disease. The epiphysis of the left hip is in the middle stage showing extensive segmentation.

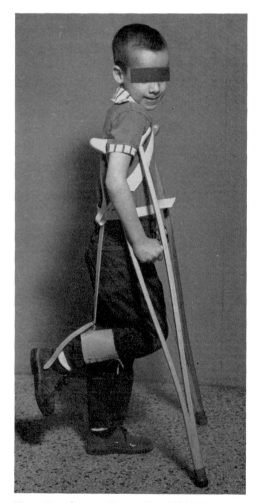

Fig. 159. The Fort harness is designed to prevent weight bearing on the affected extremity. The child wearing this apparatus is taught to walk with crutches, using the three-point gait.

head. However, treatment by bed rest is difficult to accomplish. Because the degenerative changes may continue for 1 to 2 years and regeneration of the head of the femur requires approximately a year, the restriction of bed rest to a child who feels well and has boundless energy requires the utmost in cooperation from parents.

Some physicians (Paul Steele) recommend operation with replacement of the liquefied areas under the head with small bone graft chips from the neck of the femur, some recommend braces to relieve weight bearing, and some recommend the drilling of holes through the neck of the femur into the head of the femur to stimulate bone growth. Others recommend treatment in two long leg casts fastened together in abduction. Some physicians prescribe that the patient be fitted with a leather harness (Fort harness) that prevents bearing weight on the involved limb. The patient is required to walk with crutches. This necessarily places limitations on the child's activities, but does permit his continuing school and living a somewhat normal life.

SLIPPED FEMORAL EPIPHYSIS

Slipped femoral epiphysis occurs in two types of adolescents: (1) the fat overgrown adolescent (Fröhlich syndrome) and (2) the rapidly growing slender type. The condition is more prevalent in boys than in girls and is frequently bilateral. Trauma may play an important part in the precipitation of displacement and symptoms, but undoubtedly there is some underlying deficiency in calcium metabolism and perhaps a deficiency in the function of the thyroid and pituitary glands.

Pathology. The three stages to the disease are as follows:

1. In the preslipped stage the condition manifests itself by the presence of a slight limp to the affected side

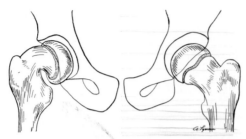

Fig. 160. Slipped femoral epiphysis of the right hip. Note the horse-neck appearance of the neck of the femur and the erect position of the epiphyseal line.

and a slight limitation of internal rotation of the hip. Roentgenograms in the preslipped stage show little or no displacement but light rarefaction of bone on the lower femoral side of the epiphysis.

2. Through trauma or some minor injury during the earlier stages of slipping, the femoral portion of the epiphysis may slide further upward, and further eversion may occur.

3. More extensive slipping of the epiphysis upward with increased eversion of the limb occurs in the more severe or later stages. The bony changes shown by roentgenograms are accompanied by increased limitation of abduction and internal rotation. When such a degree of displacement exists, there is a rather marked limp, but pain is not a prominent symptom.

The condition usually appears during the rapid growth years—between the ages of 12 and 15.

Diagnosis. If seen in a child 7 to 10 years of age, the symptoms and signs present would be similar to those in Legg-Perthes disease. The age of the patient suggests further investigation. The roentgenographic findings are characteristic. There is an active epiphyseal line, below which the bone seems to flow into its deformity. The neck of the femur assumes a horse-neck appearance.

Treatment. The only treatment during the preslipped stages is immediate internal fixation to prevent possible future slipping.

When definite slipping has occurred within a few weeks before observation, manipulation may be done by the Whitman or Leadbetter method. The leg is brought into forced abduction and internal rotation while the patient is under anesthesia. When reposition of the fragments is established, the foot will no longer evert when the heel is rested on the palm of the hand. A cast is applied with the leg in abduction and internal rotation. Nailing with a Smith-Petersen nail is sometimes recommended. Other operative procedures are also used.

When displacement has existed for months, an operation is necessary to restore alignment and improve joint function. This is accomplished by various types of osteotomy through the neck or trochanteric region of the femur.

EPIPHYSITIS OF SPINE (SCHEUERMANN DISEASE, JUVENILE KYPHOSIS, OSTEOCHONDRITIS DEFORMANS JUVENILIS)

As a result of injury that usually consists in forcible acute flexion in a young individual there may be trauma to the anterior joint margin of one of the vertebrae. The lumbar vertebrae are the most susceptible. A small area of bone may be deprived of its normal circulation and undergo degenerative changes. Gradually, it loses its contact with the rest of the vertebrae and becomes encysted.

Symptoms. Symptoms are usually mild and consist of a slight amount of pain on certain motions and possibly an intermittent dull aching sensation in the spine. Roentgenograms show characteristic separation of the vertebral frag-

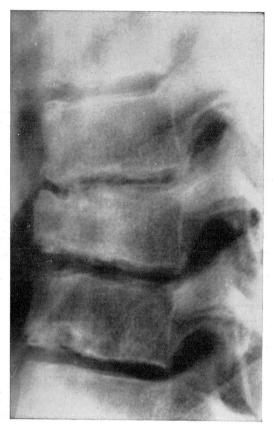

Fig. 161. Osteochondritis juvenilis deformans. Note the wedging of the vertebral bodies and the defects of the anterosuperior and anteroinferior cortical plates. (From Kenney, William C., and Larson, Carroll B.: Orthopedics for the general practitioner, St. Louis, 1957, The C. V. Mosby Co.)

ment with the increased density of necrosis and a surrounding area of rarefaction.

Treatment. Immobilization in a hyperextension plaster of paris body cast for two or three months followed by application of the Taylor back brace will usually lead either to the healing of the process or to the formation of a bridge of bone between the bodies of the adjoining involved vertebrae. Support provided by the cast or brace will help prevent deformity of the spine (kyphosis, round shoulders).

This patient should not be permitted to participate in strenuous sports, and bed rest may be necessary if pain is severe. A firm mattress with bed boards is desirable.

EPIPHYSITIS OF THE TIBIAL TUBERCLE (OSGOOD-SCHLATTER DISEASE, EPIPHYSITIS OF THE TIBIAL TUBERCLE)

Epiphysitis of the tibial tubercle usually occurs in rapidly growing children, most frequently in boys between 10 and 14 years of age. They complain of pain at the attachment of the patella tendon on going up and down the stairs and of acute tenderness and swelling in this region. Roentgenograms may show a small beadlike piece of degenerated bone

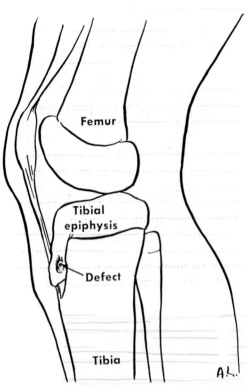

Fig. 162. Osgood-Schlatter disease. Epiphysitis of the tibial tubercle.

under the epiphysis of the tibial tubercle.

Treatment. Mild cases usually respond to protection by a cast or a reenforced elastic knee support. In severe cases operative removal of the small piece of degenerated bone may be necessary.

OSTEOCHONDRITIS OF THE KNEE JOINT

Although osteochondritis may occur in almost any joint in the body, it is comparatively common in the knee. It usually appears under the cartilage of the outer surface of the inner condyle of the knee joint.

Cause. The cause is usually injury in which an unusual motion or strain of the joint occurs. Damage and local disturbance of the supply of circulation to a small area of bone and cartilage within the joint may result. The bone becomes separated from its blood supply and undergoes degenerative changes that separate it from the rest of the bone. This piece of dead bone may break through the covering of cartilage and

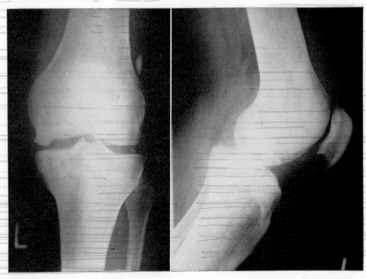

Fig. 163. Osteochondritis of the knee. Note punched-out margin on the medial condyle. The loose body (joint mouse) that arose from the punched-out area is visible in the quadriceps pouch along the latter shaft.

enter the joint. The protective mechanism of the joint attempts to cover this loose bone with cartilage until it finally becomes smooth and may slip from one point to another within the joint, causing lockage when it is caught between the joint surfaces.

Treatment. When the presence of a joint mouse is definitely established by clinical observation and by roentgenogram, it should be removed, even if its presence can be established by roentgenographic findings before it has dislodged.

SCOLIOSIS

Scoliosis is a lateral curvature of the spine. It is called functional or postural scoliosis when there is no abnormality in the shape of the vertebrae and the patient can voluntarily correct the deformity. In structural scoliosis there are changes in the shape of the vertebrae and thorax that make correction of the deformity impossible. The scoliosis is described as thoracic, lumbar, and thoracolumbar, according to the spinal segment involved. Curvatures of the thoracic spine are frequently convex to the right, whereas curvatures of the lumbar spine are more often convex to the left. Scoliosis is usually accompanied by rotation of the vertebral bodies toward the side of the convexity of the curve.

The rotation of the thoracic vertebrae causes the ribs on the convexity of the curve to protrude backward. The ribs on the side of the concavity are more

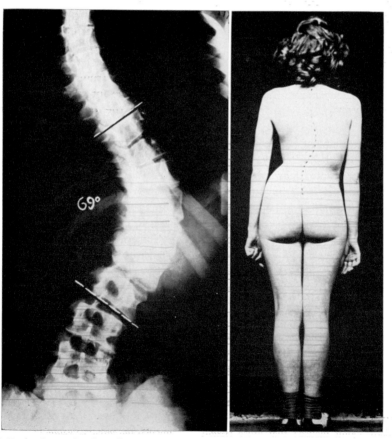

Fig. 164. Right thoracolumbar idiopathic scoliosis.

prominent forward. In severe thoracic scoliosis the thorax is grossly misshapen. Very often the deformity consists of a right thoracic curve associated with a left lumbar curve.

Causes. Functional or postural curvatures are usually the result of faulty posture, weak musculature, and weak ligaments. Postural types of scoliosis rarely develop into structural types.

Structural scoliosis may be caused by infantile paralysis (paralytic scoliosis), congenital deformity of the vertebrae (congenital scoliosis), diseases of the lungs, certain diseases and tumors of the spinal cord and of the ribs, neurofibromatosis, hysteria, etc. The cause of scoliosis is unknown in a large number of cases (idiopathic scoliosis). Poor protein intake is often observed in children with idiopathic scoliosis.

Symptoms. Scoliosis usually develops during the periods of spinal growth. Congenital scoliosis may be detected during early childhood. Paralytic scoliosis develops several months or years after asymmetric paralysis of the trunk muscles. Idiopathic scoliosis, which is the most frequent type, occurs more frequently in girls than in boys and usually has its onset at 10 or 12 years of age. Often the deformity increases until the growth of the spine is completed.

Because scoliosis rarely causes pain until the later stages of the disease, it is frequently unrecognized until the deformity is well established. Scoliosis of the thoracic spine may be detected early by the deformity of the thorax. The ribs are protruded backward on the side of the convexity of the curve and the shoulder on the side of the convexity is higher. Scoliosis of the lumbar spine accounts for asymmetry of the hips. The hip on the side of the concavity of the curve is usually more prominent. Body alignment is often poor, and the thorax is deviated laterally in relation to the

pelvis. The normal contour of the waistline is altered. It is flat on the side of the convexity of the curve and hollow on the side of the concavity.

Diagnosis. Whenever there is a complaint of back trouble, it is important that the patient be properly draped for the examination. The back should be completely exposed from the head to the heels. The range of motion of the spine in all directions should be noted and limitations recorded. The level of the iliac crests should be roughly estimated by pressing the hands into the flanks over them. Accurate measurement of leg lengths should be made from the anterosuperior spine to the internal malleoli. Care should be taken that the position of both hips in relation to the pelvis is the same and that they bear the same relationship to an imaginary perpendicular line extending from the center of the cervical spine through the cleft of the buttocks and down between the ankles. The relative discrepancy in shoulder height should be measured, and a plumb line should be erected from between the heels to the occiput. The line should normally pass through the crease of the buttocks. The amount of lateral deviation of the spine in its various parts should be recorded and compared from time to time during observation and treatment. The range of motion of the segments of the spine should be evaluated. It will be observed that on forward flexion the rotary deformity of the thoracic spine and the thoracic deformity are increased. Roentgenograms of the entire spine taken with the patient in the standing position and in the recumbent position are of value in the diagnosis of the type of curve and shift of body weight. Roentgenograms taken every 3 months will show the evolution of the curve. Many curves increase little or not at all, whereas others progress rapidly.

Roentgenograms taken with the patient bending as far as possible to the right and to the left will give valuable information regarding the correctability of the curve by possible fusion.

An urgent plea is being made for the routine examination of school children for the presence of curvature of the spine and other deformities.

Treatment. A well-balanced diet high in animal proteins should be advised for every child with scoliosis. Unfortunately there is no known medical treatment to stop the progression of the deformity.

Physical exercises under the direction of a competent physical therapist are indicated to improve posture, to develop better muscle tone, and to increase vital capacity. The patient must be taught to be conscious of posture by standing and exercising in front of a full-length mirror. Great benefit may be derived from ballet and modern dancing and should be advised if a teacher is available. By these means the shoulders may be maintained at the same level and the thorax brought into proper alignment with the pelvis. The course of the scoliosis, however, is not often altered by exercises. Daily periods of bed rest, as advised by some orthopedic surgeons, are of dubious value. Corrective plaster jackets may be advisable during periods of rapid increase of the deformity. They should be worn for several months while carrying on the same program of physical exercises. Braces are easier to wear than plaster jackets, but they are less effective.

Fusion of the involved segment of the spine is advised by many surgeons when the deformity is severe. It is well not to fuse the spine until 13 or 14 years of age in order not to interfere with the spinal growth. The curve is first corrected with a turnbuckle plaster jacket that includes the head and one leg. The degree of the curve correction and the extent of the spinal fusion have been previously determined by means of bending roentgenograms. When the desired correction has been achieved, the turnbuckle plaster cast is completed and a window is cut in the back of the cast large enough to allow operative fusion of the spine through it. If the fusion has to include more than six or seven vertebrae, the operation should be done in two stages to minimize shock. The modified Hibbs method of fusion is frequently used, adding bone chips obtained from the ilium or from the bone bank. After spinal fusion the same plaster jacket is worn and the patient is at complete bed rest for at least 6 months to allow for complete consolidation of the bone graft.

Some of the correction obtained after spinal fusion is often lost because the grafts bend or break at the points of maximum stress. Therefore the thoracic deformity is not corrected by the operation, and the vital capacity is often decreased. In idiopathic scoliosis only the severe correctible curves must be fused. Fortunately most of the patients have mild curves that do not need surgical treatment. On the other hand, spinal fusion is often indicated in paralytic scoliosis.

In some cases of severe scoliosis the deformity has progressed to such an extent that correction is hopeless. Pain may be controlled by the use of leather or celluloid jackets. In some instances it is necessary to remove portions of ribs when they impinge on the pelvic bones.

Nursing care

Scoliosis is often discovered in curious ways, but usually it has been present a long time before it is detected. A dressmaker's comment that she cannot get a hem to hang straight because one hip seems to be higher than the other; a teacher's observation of the habitual fatigue and poor posture of a child in the classroom; a girl's complaint that one brassiere strap is always looser than the other; or a child's sleeplessness because of aching pain in the knees or in the low back—these and many similar complaints are sometimes the first hints the parents have that something is wrong with the child's spine.

Sometimes it is not until the child is in the period of rapid growth, between the ages of 12 and 16 years, that the condition becomes so evident it can no longer be overlooked. As with most crippling conditions, early recognition and treatment are vitally important. Parents and the general public need to recognize the fact that it is a dangerous tendency to wait and see if the child will outgrow the condition. This attitude may keep the child from the specialist during the very time when it would be possible to minimize the effect of the curvature. The feeling held by some individuals that scoliosis is a progressive condition and quite hopeless from the standpoint of treatment must be combatted. The child with even a well-established curvature can be benefited greatly by skillful and continued treatment.

Nurses should remember that patients with scoliosis are easily fatigued. All periods of activity should be varied with periods of rest. This should be faithfully observed in the hospital as well as in the home. It is particularly advisable for such patients to assume rest positions for a prescribed period upon return from school. Rest positions are taught by the physical therapist, and they have as definite therapeutic value as exercise itself. Nurses should always be familiar with the rest positions that have been prescribed for their patients. The physical therapist takes the responsibility for teaching these positions, but she will not be on hand to supervise them during a great portion of the day.

Much harm can be done during the period between exercises if the ambulatory patient with scoliosis is allowed to slump in positions contrary to those prescribed for the maximum correction of his curvature. Encouragement from the nurse may be needed to remind the patient of this important feature of his treatment. Parents, too, will need to be reminded of this after the child has returned home. A rest position that is frequently taught is one in which the patient lies on his back with knees flexed, feet flat on the floor (or bed) with arms outstretched, shoulders rotated outward, and elbows flexed at right angles. The patient's body should be in good alignment, with head, shoulders, and pelvis in the same plane.

Not infrequently, the patient is asked to carry out breathing exercises on the ward several times a day. The nurse should be familiar with breathing exercises in order to supervise them adequately. The ribs should be elevated, and the chest wall expanded, beginning with the lower portion of the lungs. The diaphragm should be contracted (lowered) during this process. When the lungs are full the diaphragm is allowed to relax, thus starting exhalation from below. The error most commonly made by the unsupervised patient is in relaxing (raising) the diaphragm in his attempt to elevate the ribs, a situation that actually diminishes breathing space. The diaphragm should not rise until the patient breathes out. If the nurse places her hands on the lower border of the ribs, she will be able to determine the position of the diaphragm during the breathing exercises.

Corrective appliances. The Risser turnbuckle cast and the Milwaukee brace are corrective appliances used on patients with scoliosis.

Risser turnbuckle cast. It is manifestly impossible to describe nursing care for patients in all the varied types of mechanical devices that are used in the treatment of scoliosis. However, the Risser turnbuckle cast and other similar casts have rather general usage, and most nurses will need to be informed about the general features of nursing care for patients in this type of apparatus. The Risser cast usually reaches from the patient's chin and occiput to the knee on one side and to the hip on the other, depending upon the direction of the spinal curvature. It is a thick heavy cast and is usually applied over stockinet and felt or, in some clinics, over sponge rubber. There is considerable strain on the patient during the application of this cast, particularly if he has been bedfast for a long period. The nurse should be prepared to receive an exhausted patient on the ward upon his return from the plaster room. At least three rubber-covered pillows should be in readiness to support the body cast.

After a few days, usually from 3 to 5, the cast is cut through to the stockinet on the side of the concavity. The cut is transverse and reaches from the midpoint on the anterior surface to the midpoint on the posterior surface. On the side of the convexity a wedge-shaped slice is removed, which makes possible the bending of the cast and the spine. After this, a turnbuckle is placed on the side of the concavity and hinges are applied anteriorly and posteriorly at this side of the cast. Now forcible correction of the curve is begun. The turnbuckle is turned each day by the physician until the maximum amount of correction has been secured. A series of turnbuckles are usually needed, begin-

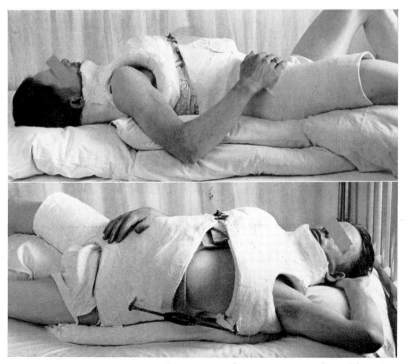

Fig. 165. Turnbuckle cast used for forcible correction of scoliosis. The turnbuckle and hinges are incorporated into the plaster. Each time the turnbuckle is adjusted new points of pressure tend to appear. Prevention of pressure areas and skin breakdown may be difficult.

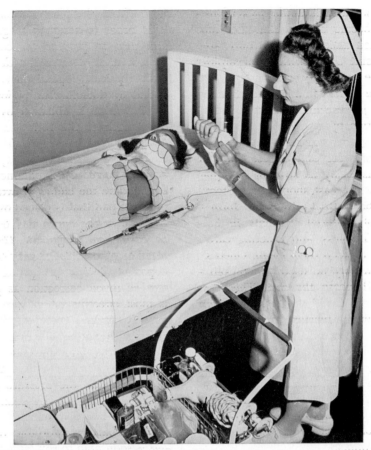

Fig. 166. Turnbuckle cast with petal finish of adhesive tape circles.

ning with a smaller one. This is turned out as far as it will permit and then is replaced by a larger one. In the course of a few days the large wedge-shaped opening on the one side becomes smaller, whereas the opening becomes larger on the side of the turnbuckle.

During the period the patient spends in this kind of corrective cast, nursing care must be skillful and vigilant. Each day alters the position of the patient in relation to the cast, and new points of pressure are bound to occur each time the turnbuckle is adjusted. The procedure is a period of forcible correction, and when such correction is being carried out the skin will suffer if not observed closely.

When the cast is cut, the edges should be beveled to afford greater safety to the skin. The stockinet is then slit and brought out over the edges of the cast. These edges are sealed so that plaster crumbs do not fall off during the process of wedging. Pressure points on ribs must be carefully and frequently explored with the fingers, and, if the pressure becomes excessive, the physician must be notified. He will usually turn back the turnbuckle slightly until the pressure can be relieved. Frequent rubs and slight padding may be used to allay discomfort. Too generous use of padding will increase the bulk of the cast and thereby increase rather than decrease the pressure on the patient. In the Minerva type of distraction jacket, great pressure occurs on the chin that must be watched assiduously. Pressure areas at this point occur with great rapidity and leave unsightly scars. Any complaint of a patient in any type of corrective body jacket should be given prompt consideration by the nurse.

Circular pieces of adhesive tape form a neat finish for cast edges. These do not roll as easily as straight or square edges do. The cast should be protected around the buttocks by some form of waterproof material. Patients in body casts are helpless, and exacting care is necessary to keep them clean. Oiled silk or Pliofilm may be used and tucked in smoothly beneath the cast. This is secured on the outside with adhesive tape or moistened plaster strips so that the loose ends may be slipped out from underneath the cast daily during the bath, washed with warm soapy water, dried, and powdered. It is then replaced under the cast edges and smoothed out carefully so that the skin will not be irritated.

The turnbuckles must not be used as handles with which to turn the patient. They are insecurely applied at best and are likely to break off from the cast if used as handles. Because turnbuckles cause considerable wear on bed linen, it is a good plan to cover them with a small canvas girdle. This can be secured around the cast with tape ties.

Correction of the curvature may require 2 or 3 weeks. Sometimes it may be necessary to apply a new cast in order to obtain complete correction. When the desired position has been obtained, the cast openings are filled in with plaster, and if the patient is to be operated on, a large window will be cut through the back of the cast to provide an unobstructed operative area.

Milwaukee brace. Another type of corrective apparatus used for the patient with scoliosis is the Milwaukee brace. This brace is designed to give support and also to provide for correction of the curvature. It is used with the patient whose primary spinal curve is in the dorsal or dorsolumbar region. Traction on the spine is obtained by increasing the length of the rods connecting the head and chin piece with the pelvic part of the brace. These rods may be lengthened as correction is obtained or to accommodate the child's growth. Also, the pressure pad that is placed over the convex side of the curve may be tightened as correction is gained. The brace is fitted to the child and may be worn for a period of time preoperatively to obtain as much correction as possible. It is most effective when worn in the supine position. Postoperatively (after spinal fusion) the brace is worn for 4 or 5 months, and the child is kept on bed rest during this time. The length of the brace and the pressure created by the lateral pad may be changed by the attending surgeon as necessary. The child is most comfortable on his side and is soon able to roll from side to side by himself. Deep-breathing exercises and exercises of the extremities should be performed faithfully during this period if muscle strength is to be maintained and other deformity prevented. Skin care is a very important aspect of the nursing care. The headpiece causes pressure on the chin, and frequent massage and the use of sponge rubber may be necessary to prevent breaking of the skin. Because this patient spends most of his time on one side or the other, the area over the greater trochanter and the shoulder may become reddened and show signs of breaking if special care is not provided. Bathing of the patient must be done with the brace intact. This takes additional time but can be accomplished much more satisfactorily than if a body cast is being worn. When the

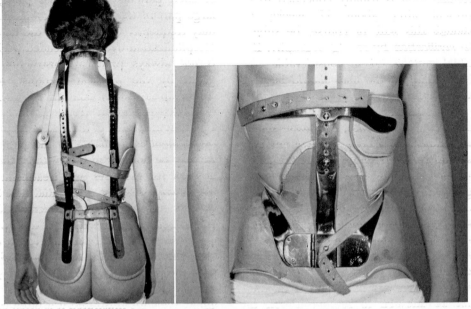

Fig. 167. Posterior and anterior views of the Milwaukee brace. Note provision for adjustment of brace to increase traction on the vertebral column and pressure on the convex aspect of the curve. The anterior view shows the hinge, outriggers, and anterior pad. (Courtesy Dr. Walter Blount, Milwaukee, Wisconsin.)

patient is ready for ambulation, the brace is still worn continuously. Later it is removed at night and then for graduated periods during the day, but it is worn for 6 to 7 months postoperatively.

Nursing care after spinal fusion. Care of patients after spinal fusion has been discussed in another chapter and does not need to be repeated here. If treatment has been that of a corrective plaster cast, it may be of interest to mention that most surgeons perform the fusion operation on the patient in the cast in which the correction has been obtained. They fear to lose correction by a change of cast. If the patient has been in the cast for several weeks, the nurse is usually appalled at the thought of caring for him after surgery in the same cast. A change of stockinet can be accomplished and is a source of great comfort to the patient.

As has been stated, before surgery the doctor will fill in the cut portions of the cast, making it into a solid body jacket. Fenestration of the cast will then be ordered, allowing for preparation of the operative site. Occasionally, on the morning of operation, with the patient under local anesthesia, a No. 20 hypodermic needle will be inserted into the spinous process of one of the prominent vertebrae in the fusion site and a lateral spinal roentgenogram will be taken. This ensures the location of the apex of the curve when the incision is made.

After surgery the patient usually remains in his cast for 3 months, when another cast, sometimes referred to as a semiambulatory cast, will be applied. The period of bed rest depends upon the discretion of the doctor. Immobilization is usually continued for 6 to 12 months. In handling these patients after spinal fusion, it is well to remember that solidification is usually conceded to be present after about 12 weeks, although this will, of course, be subject to verification by roentgenography. If a tibial graft is taken, considerable care in handling of the limb should be used until 8 weeks have elapsed.

If the spinal fusion patient is to be immobilized by a brace, the nurse should remember that a body brace of any type should be fitted snugly about the pelvis in such fashion that the lower band grasps the iliac crests. It should be laced or buckled from the bottom as the patient lies in bed. Saddle soap used sparingly with a little water will keep the leather soft and pliable and in good condition. Naphtha will remove stains. When hinges are oiled, excess oil must not be allowed to remain to soil the leather parts or to catch lint. The laces should be in good condition without knots, or if straps and buckles are used, frayed straps must be replaced as necessary.

If the Taylor body brace is used, the metal and leather section of the apparatus is unbuckled and lifted from the patient's body as he lies prone. The canvas apron remains under the patient. When the patient is to be turned, the brace is replaced on the back and the canvas section is buckled to the metal part before turning is done. The straps should distribute the pull evenly to avoid uneven tension. Shoulder loops are fastened to prevent the shoulders from sagging during the turning. Not all back braces are as easy to apply and remove from the patient as the Taylor. Many require forcible spreading for application. For the most part it is considered preferable to apply back braces to the patient as he lies prone.

General considerations for the patient's welfare. The health features of scoliosis need to be emphasized in any article dealing with the nursing care of such patients. In the first place, a large part of the period of mobilization may frequently take place in the home. Hospitalization over an extended period is not always practical. Instruction is given by the physical therapist, and follow-up is usually done in the outpatient department at frequent intervals by the orthopedist. If a physical therapy department is available to the patient, he may be brought in two or three times a week for exercises and treatment. If this is impossible, it is essential that the parents have a thorough understanding of such exercises as well as of their purpose. One instruction period given at the time the parents come to the hospital to take the patient home is seldom enough. A set of written exercises will help, but unless they are illustrated it is often confusing to the parents. It is advisable for the parents to see the exercises carried out over a period of days before taking the child home. In many states crippled children's services now provide physical therapy follow-up in the home with visits by therapists. The value of this service to this type of patient is inestimable.

It may take considerable ingenuity to keep the child interested in his exercises month after month and year after year. The child sometimes tends to become mechanical and apathetic about his exercises, and the parents, wearying of constant nagging, allow days to go by with no exercise periods. The public health nurse, observing this state of affairs, should consult with the physical therapist. Sometimes new exercises can be substituted for old ones that will stimulate the child to greater interest in their performance. Adequate supervision for these exercises will need to be provided until it is felt that the child has mastered the new set of exercises.

It must be borne in mind that children with scoliotic conditions are at a time of life when appliances are often considered a cosmetic encumbrance, particularly the child with a moderate curve that has not as yet caused him personal embarrassment. The parents, unless firmly instructed on this point, may often succumb to pleas to leave off the braces for parties and dances, and ultimately it may be found at checkup that the child is not wearing his brace half the time. Similarly the patient may often plead to omit his exercises because he is too busy or too tired. The parents should be forewarned that these things are likely to occur. They should be urged to develop emotional control and a firm attitude in these matters for the sake of the child's future welfare. Only persistence in carrying out the doctor's orders combined with a thorough understanding of the long-term nature of treatment and necessity for checkup at regular intervals can be productive of permanent results in scoliosis.

It should be remembered that for his total welfare the child with scoliosis needs more than supervision of exercises and brace-wearing. Fatigue is always to be avoided, and adequate nutrition is particularly important to him, as is careful supervision of his study, rest, and play habits. Tendencies toward weight loss, excessive gain in weight, or periods of rapid growth in height should be observed, and in many instances, these may mean that the child should return to the orthopedic clinic earlier than had been planned. Attention to all these details may mean the difference between success and failure in the child's treatment.

STUDY QUESTIONS

1. What are the symptoms of epiphysitis of the tibial tubercle? The pathology?
2. List two types of epiphysitis.
3. In what two types of individual is slipped femoral epiphysis usually found?
4. What is the treatment for slipped femoral epiphysis?
5. What is the treatment for coxa plana?
6. Give briefly the chief differences between postural and structural scoliosis.
7. Discuss the preventive aspects of postural scoliosis.
8. Distinguish between the terms kyphos, gibbus, scoliosis, and dorsum rotundum.
9. What is the purpose of therapeutic exercise given in the treatment of structural scoliosis?

REFERENCES

Bonfiglio, M., and Batschelet, E.: Slipping of the upper epiphysis of the femur, Am. J. Nursing **53**:1193-1195, 1953.

Bowen, C.: Scoliosis—the nurse's role, Am. J. Nursing **50**:200-202, 1950.

Greenwald, W. F., Jr.: Scoliosis, Am. J. Nursing **59**:817-819, 1959.

Greenwich, J. F.: A new look for the youngster with scoliosis, Am. J. Nursing **59**:814-816, 1959.

Jordan, V., Ohara, Y., Smith, M., and Townsley, J.: Halo body cast and spinal fusion, Am. J. Nursing **63**:77-80, 1963.

Kleinberg, S.: Scoliosis pathology, etiology and treatment, Baltimore, 1951, Williams & Wilkins Co.

Leavitt, D. G., and Leavitt, H. L.: Scoliosis—prevention, control and correction, Am. J. Nursing **50**:198-200, 1950.

Ponseti, I., and Friedman, B.: Changes in the scoliotic spine after fusion, J. Bone & Joint Surg. **32**:751-766, 1950.

Ponseti, I., and Friedman, B.: Prognosis in idiopathic scoliosis, J. Bone & Joint Surg. **32**:381-395, 1950.

Ralston, E. L.: Legg-Calve-Perthes disease, Am. J. Nursing **61**:88-91, 1961.

Risser, J. C.: Application of body casts for correction of scoliosis, Am. Acad. Orthop. Surgeons, Lect. **12**:255-259, 1959.

Chapter 5

Infections of bones and joints

Osteomyelitis, including nursing care, and septic arthritis

OSTEOMYELITIS

Osteomyelitis is of three types: (1) acute infectious osteomyelitis, (2) acute localized osteomyelitis, and (3) chronic osteomyelitis.

Cause. Acute infectious osteomyelitis is usually caused by pyogenic bacteria that reach the bone through the bloodstream. The most common is the *Staphylococcus.* The *Streptococcus* is the next most common. Other organisms that may cause the disease are the pneumococcus, the typhoid bacillus, the colon bacillus, the gas bacillus, gonococcus, *Actinomyces, Coccidioides, Echinococcus, Spirochaeta pallida,* and the tubercle bacillus.

The virulence of the organism frequently determines the severity of the disease. In some instances, especially when the infective agent is the *Staphylococcus* or *Streptococcus,* the disease may be of the violent fulminating type and death may occur within 24 or 48 hours after onset of the infection. Young children are most often affected with the systemic type, and the areas of the body most subject to trauma are the most frequently involved. Boys are four times more susceptible than are girls.

In acute localized osteomyelitis the infection often results from compound fractures or penetrating wounds into the bone. Such infections are rarely virulent and are not usually accompanied by a general reaction in the entire affected bone as is seen in the metastatic infections.

Chronic osteomyelitis occurs in persons whose body has built up considerable resistance to the particular type of organism causing the infection. It is characterized by intermittent exacerbation of pain and inflammation usually brought on by an attempt to throw off sequestra.

The etiology of osteomyelitis presents some factors important to nurses in their health teaching. It is, of course, a well-recognized fact that compound injuries of bone may lead to osteomyelitis, but what is not always so well understood is that any lowering of the resistance or integrity of the tissue may predispose toward the disease. Body resistance lowered by exposure, fatigue, malnutrition, or infected tonsils and teeth seems to be a definite factor in the etiology. Bruises, blisters, deep slivers or splinters, impetigo, sties of the eyelids—all are given consideration as possible etiologic agents by writers on this subject. Any of these types of skin lesions deserve careful attention. The nurse in her teaching should seek to make it understood that a child with extensive skin abrasions should not be allowed to resume normal athletic activities until the lesions are healed. Blisters on the heel—a very common disturbance in the life of young people—should be carefully disinfected and protected from the irritating shoe by felt pads. This cannot be overemphasized. A history of boils is a very common feature in osteomyelitis and they deserve medical attention. Remember that the *Staphylococcus*, chief organism in the common boil, is the same *Staphylococcus* that is the cause of the more serious type of osteomyelitis. It must also be remembered that people with extensive boils carry the same phage type of *Staphylococcus* in their nose in 80% to 90% of the cases; the eradication of the boils cannot be expected unless local chemotherapy is applied to the anterior nares.

Pathology. Acute osteomyelitis usually begins at the end of the long bones, where there is the greatest number of blood vessels. The disease is usually caused by the combination of two factors: (1) local selectivity resulting from trauma and (2) metastatic infection from some source of remote focal infection in the body.

After the bacteria are implanted in the bone they grow and cause pressure and destruction of bone. The pressure serves to spread the infection, which finally breaks through the bone surface and produces elevation of the periosteum. Most of the circulation to the bone enters through the periosteum, and the stripping effect of pus under pressure cuts off circulation to the bone. Death of the bone occurs. The periosteum maintains its circulation and under this stimulation tends to grow and lay down new bone, forming the characteristic involucrum. This involucrum may extend part of the way along the shaft or along the entire distance of the shaft. Within this involucrum of newly formed bone, the dead bone (sequestrum) becomes completely detached and must either be removed by surgery or

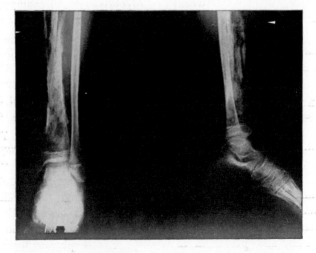

Fig. 168. Chronic osteomyelitis of the tibia. Note destruction of the bone, the sequestrum, and the proliferation of new bone (involucrum). (From Kenney, William C., and Larson, Carroll B.: Orthopedics for the general practitioner, St. Louis, 1957, The C. V. Mosby Co.)

gradually work its own way out by abscess and sinus formation.

Course. The symptoms begin with a feeling of illness, possibly headache, nausea, and a rather rapid increase in temperature. The earliest local symptom is likely to be severe sudden pain, boring in nature, near the region of a joint. Systemically, a chill followed by high fever may introduce the condition. Abruptness and severity of pain are emphasized as the two most notable features of this condition.

In the acute stages it is difficult at times to tell whether the involvement is in the joint or in the neighboring bone. The differentiation can usually be made by the fact that a certain range of painless motion is present when osteomyelitis is near a joint, but when joint involvement is present, any degree of motion is painful. The bloodstream may become infected so that positive cultures of the organism can be obtained, and the leukocyte count may rise to a very high level. Unfortunately, roentgenography is of no value in the early stage of osteomyelitis. Positive roentgenographic evidence of infection may not be found short of 2 or 3 weeks. Even then the findings may be misleading when the progress of the disease has been marked by the administration of the sulfonamides, penicillin, streptomycin, or other antibiotics. Localized swelling and tenderness of the involved area occur within 24 to 48 hours.

Treatment. Surgery and the use of antibiotics offer the best means of treatment. Transfusions, infusions, and supportive care must be included in the care of the patient with osteomyelitis.

In children less than 2 or 3 years of age, when the bone and periosteal tissues are flexible, it may be questionable whether surgical decompression offers any advantage. Incisions and drainage of localized abscesses may be beneficial.

In the average case of acute osteomyelitis the disease usually develops less abruptly. Although some authors have reported series of cases that seem to have been treated successfully by the use of antibiotic drugs alone, without surgery, it still seems logical that relief of pressure within the bone and periosteum by incision and drainage is an advantage. Much should depend on the local and general reaction of the patient within the immediate hours and days following onset of the disease. Immobilization in casts or in splints seems decidedly helpful in most cases, particularly because of the effect of muscle relaxation.

The treatment of chronic osteomyelitis depends largely on the complete removal of all dead bone (sequestra) and the prolonged use of antibiotics. The use of antibiotic drugs at the first sign of bacterial activity will frequently avert the attack.

Nursing care

Nursing responsibilities in various methods of treatment. Perhaps it is significant that methods for treating osteomyelitis have developed during wartime. The first method was the Carrel-Dakin treatment and was used during World War I. The nursing care involved in the Carrel-Dakin treatment is such an important factor and demands so much time and careful technique from the nurse that it has become almost prohibitive because of personnel shortages. The treatment may, of course, be carried out without this meticulous technique, but the results from it are correspondingly uncertain.

A second method that most nurses have read about is the Orr treatment, the closed plaster method of treating osteomyelitis. This treatment had its inception in World War I, but was not used on a large scale until the Spanish

Civil War. Because of the results from its use in World War II it was generally accepted as the treatment of choice for osteomyelitis.

The Orr method has been somewhat modified during the past few years by chemotherapy and the antibiotic drugs, but the principles that Orr laid down are still considered sound and form the basis of modern treatment. Briefly stated, the Orr treatment consists of immediate adequate surgical drainage (sauceriza-tion), the establishment of complete rest for the involved area by the use of a plaster of paris cast that includes the joint above and the joint below the in-fected area, the use of petrolatum pack-ing to maintain drainage of the affected area, and postoperative care in which rest and freedom from the interference of dressings are paramount features.

The Orr technique embodies two principles with which all nurses should be familiar, principles based on respect for the inherent protective abilities of the tissues. The first is that of complete rest. This means that not only are bones and joints immobilized but soft tissues as well. Avoiding the trauma of frequent dressings and protecting the soft tissues around the infected bone against move-ment will often relieve muscle spasm and promote relaxation of the part in the anatomic position. The second prin-ciple is that of asepsis. However, irri-tating antiseptics must not be introduced into the wound because it is felt that strong antiseptics often inhibit nature's powers of eliminating the infection. It has been wisely said that the aim of all good treatment is to aid the healing process of nature, and the Orr technique seeks to do this consistently in osteomy-elitis.

Odor from the closed plaster cast, however, may often present a real problem. Fortunately the effect of the odor on the patient is not nearly as troublesome as it is on members of the hospital staff and visitors. The nurse can give effective reassurance to the family only if she herself under-stands the principles underlying the closed plaster method of treating in-fected bone wounds and the amazing results that have been obtained by use of this method.

On the whole, attempts made to de-odorize these casts have been more in-genious than successful. Commercial deodorizers are partially successful. For the most part, however, there seems to be no substitute for frequent airing of the patient's room.

Although the use of penicillin and other antibiotics has changed the treat-ment of osteomyelitis in some respects, provision for adequate rest of the in-volved area is still considered very im-portant. In the acute stage of the disease the tendency is to institute chemotherapy before resorting to sur-gery. However, the administration of antibiotics does not always ensure re-covery and must often be accompanied by adequate drainage. There has always been controversy over surgery in the acute stage, particularly when bacter-emia and general prostration are pres-ent. It is recognized that the systemic features of the disease may often be of more immediate importance than relief of local symptoms. If surgery is performed in the acute stage, it is usually swift and conservative, consisting of a series of drill holes made through the metaphyseal portion of the bone to evacuate pus and relieve tension. More adequate drainage may need to be sup-plied later. Penicillin may be a life-saving treatment in patients with more severe forms of osteomyelitis accom-panied by septicemia, provided the laboratory tests indicate that the organ-ism isolated is sensitive to this antibiotic. In certain other cases proper choice of another antibiotic may be indicated. The patient is usually given the drug parenterally every 3 hours, and if localized abscesses occur, the drug may be used in the wound as well. Penicillin solution is maintained in the wound by positioning of the extremity, by compression dressings, or by inserting a sterile catheter or polyethylene tube into the wound and permitting the solution to drop in slowly and continuously.

In some instances the organism causing osteomyelitis is found to be resistant to one or more chemotherapeutic agents, but penicillin will be used because it is a powerful bacteriostatic agent. It is particularly fitted to the treatment of osteomyelitis because it is not inhibited by the presence of pus or large numbers of bacteria.

General nursing care of the patient with osteomyelitis. The patient's general condition should be of as much concern as the local condition. Fluids should be given abundantly by mouth if the patient is able to retain them and intravenously if he is unable to do so. Blood transfusions are often part of the early treatment in this disease. The presence of sufficient protein and vitamin C in the diet of these patients is of the utmost importance because both of these substances are vitally necessary for wound healing. Every effort should be made to see that foods containing these are included in each meal even if the patient is receiving only a liquid diet.

A highly important fact to remember in caring for the patient with osteomyelitis is that deformity is a common sequela of the disease. The patient tends to hold the limb in a position that causes the least possible strain on the inflamed bone. Nearby joints are likely to be held in a position of flexion in order to relax muscles. In a patient with osteomyelitis of the lower end of the femur flexion in the hip, flexion in the

knee, and a tendency toward outward rotation of the whole leg may be observed. Drop foot is another feature that develops early. It is customary that as soon as drainage has been established, the physician in charge will have a splint applied to the patient's extremity to hold it in an optimum position. However, if a period of days goes by, during which hot stupes are being used and no splint is in readiness, the nurse must improvise equipment to keep the foot in a normal position. A footboard or box augmented by pillows usually causes the patient very little discomfort. Many writers describe patients in whom a single focus of osteomyelitis is satisfactorily healed but the patient is nonetheless permanently crippled by flexion deformities of the knee and hip and an equinus position of the foot. Contractures of muscles alone may cause the deformity. Although edema is very common in the early stages of osteomyelitis and splinting may be very difficult, some attempt at maintaining optimum joint positions should be made.

Hot fomentations are sometimes ordered for patients with acute osteomyelitis. Unnecessary manipulations must be avoided because of the excruciating pain that the patient suffers on movement. For this reason outer coverings for the packs (dry blanket and waterproofing) should be left in place between treatments. Material for the wet packs should be of lightweight wool flannel or blanketing, not cotton blanketing or bath towels, which tend to be too heavy and do not retain the heat well. The temperature of the water should be approximately 150° F. The stupe should be tested against the inner aspect of the nurse's wrist before she applies it to the patient. The danger of using too hot water is very great because the patient's pain is so severe that he will scarcely be able to tell that the water is too hot. When sterile precautions are necessary because of an opening in the skin, a sterile dressing may be placed on the wound and covered with plastic material so that the moisture from the wet packs will not come in contact with the sterile field.

Laboratory findings play an important part in helping the physician prescribe treatment for this patient. Frequent blood cultures and determination of the blood level of antibiotics may be done. Urinary findings, hemoglobin studies, and white blood cell counts are a necessary part of the patient's management.

Handling of the affected area. The patient with osteomyelitis or septic arthritis is usually extremely apprehensive, and part of this apprehension is caused by his fear of being moved. He may even cry out if the bed is touched. Because it will be necessary for the nurse to move these patients to a certain extent, the manner of handling an acutely inflamed joint or extremity must be brought to mind here.

Persons who have had osteomyelitis or a septic joint tell us that the pain caused by being moved is almost intolerable. The moving of an acutely inflamed joint should not be undertaken without help. All the help in the world, however, will do no good if the principles of joint immobilization are not understood and faithfully carried out. It is not enough that the joint or the part infected is carefully immobilized; the joint above and the joint below must also be immobilized to prevent movement in the infected area. This will be readily understood when the mechanism of muscle action on joints is recalled. The muscles that act to move one joint may also serve as flexor or extensor of the one above or below it. Because this is true, moving a knee in which, or near which, a septic condition exists can be accomplished painlessly only by immo-

bilizing the hip and ankle as well as the knee. This will require three hands. Support should be given under the hip and the knee, and another hand should support the ankle and foot steadily. Every movement of the hands in lifting must be smooth, unhurried, and infinitely careful. Unless these conditions are observed, the patient will lose confidence and will resist bitterly any further manipulation. If he is turned to the side, the limb must stay on the same level with his body and not be allowed to sag as he is turned. His body should be supported by firm pillows, never soft ones. Gentleness in handling is imperative for another reason. Pathologic fractures have been known to occur as early as 10 days after the onset of osteomyelitis. Such fractures are frequently overlooked because the accompanying pain is often wrongly attributed to the concurrent disease.

Complications in osteomyelitis. Besides the drug reactions that may possibly occur from the use of the antibiotics or the sulfonamides, nurses should be alert to any signs that might indicate the progression of the disease to other parts of the skeleton. Any swelling, redness, or pain near a bone must be reported at once. Metastasis to the jaw in severe cases is sometimes overlooked because the nurse and patient may attribute the pain in this area to a wisdom tooth.

Amyloidosis, a waxy degeneration of the liver, spleen, and other organs, is a late and often terminal symptom. It may be manifested by the presence of blood, pus, or albumin in the urine.

As a result of loss of bone substance there is considerable danger of a pathologic fracture during and after osteomyelitis. The extremity that has been involved must be handled with great care even after the period of tenderness and pain has passed. When the patient is allowed to be out of bed, he must be guarded against falls, jerky movements, or any mishap that might threaten the integrity of the weakened bone. Sudden pain, crepitus, or deformity must be reported immediately. A sudden malposition of the limb may be the first indication that fracture has occurred in that area. Pain is sometimes disguised by the general discomfort of trying to walk after many weeks in bed.

Aftercare. In some instances long hospitalization is necessary, and careful follow-up after discharge is indispensable. The duties of the public health nurse in educating the family concerning the need for close observation and supervision of the activities of the patient are manifested. The dangers of neglect and the possibility of deformity, fracture, and stiffness of joints must be carefully pointed out, as must the ever present danger of recurrence. The chronicity of the condition must also be explained to avoid discouragement. Frequent return to the clinic for checkup must be stressed.

Psychotherapy in these patients is important. Impatience, bitterness, and discouragement are to be fought with skill and sympathy on the part of the nurse. Often the patient with osteomyelitis considers himself well on the road to recovery and then develops another abscess that will delay his return to a normal life for a longer period. After this has happened to him several times, a young, active man may very easily develop mental habits of despair and bitterness. A program of occupational therapy designed to stimulate such activity as the patient is capable of is the best antidote for this sort of complication. The patient should be kept as busy as possible with a constructive program of work, diversional as well as practical.

Rehabilitation of these patients pre-sents a real problem. Strenuous work is usually contraindicated because of the tendency of flare-up in the face of future trauma. The danger of trauma or strain must be taken into consideration in rehabilitation. All hazardous occupations risk the patient's future. This should be explained to him and his family by the physician in aiding him to select a future occupation. An attempt to discover and develop latent talents in these patients can be made by the nurse and the occupational therapist during their time on the hospital wards.

Dressings. Another important factor in the care of a patient with osteomyelitis is that of protecting other patients and personnel from the organism causing the infection. Personnel must know and understand the importance of aseptic technique. The value of and the need for proper hand washing cannot be overstressed.

Negligent technique often accompanies the dressing of draining bone wounds in hospital wards. The monotony of changing these dressings over a period of weeks or months may account for this lowering of standards. Nurses should remember that open wounds such as those encountered in patients with chronic osteomyelitis provide almost perfect culture media for bacteria. Cross infection is an ever present danger in such wounds, and cross infection may sometimes mean the difference between recovery and chronic invalidism to the patient. Cross infection may be brought about by many agents, such as dust and lint particles in the air, soaked dressings that come in contact with contaminated bed linen or casts, upper respiratory passages, the fingers of nurses and doctors during dressing periods, and, of course, unsterile instruments and dressing equipment.

Carelessness in sterilizing instruments and in using unwashed hands to apply dressings has been the rule rather than the exception in changing septic dressings. In some instances it has been the custom to remove all dressings before ward rounds in order that the attending physician may see the wound without unnecessary delay. This is a dangerous procedure because contamination and cross infection can so readily take place in a ward where dressings on many infected patients are opened to the air at the same time. The time a wound is exposed to the air should always be kept at a minimum.

In removing dressings from contaminated wounds it is advisable to cut the bandage and remove it in one piece. If the bandage is unwrapped, it tends to lose lint and dust into the air, and this lint may very easily hold bacteria that will infect other wounds in the neighborhood.

Although it is extremely important that all patients with infected wounds be housed in a separate ward, it is also desirable that patients with septic wounds be dressed in a room set aside for this purpose. Greater protection against cross infection is possible if this can be done. Cross infection with a new staphylococcal strain may not be evident unless the antibiotic sensitivities are tested or unless phage typing of the *Staphylococcus* is done.

ACUTE PYOGENIC ARTHRITIS (SEPTIC OR PURULENT ARTHRITIS)

Acute pyogenic arthritis is most frequently a disease of childhood and is caused by pyogenic organisms such as the *Staphylococcus* and *Streptococcus*. According to the virulence of the organism and the susceptibility of the host, the onset and reaction may be mild, medium, or severe. Any joint may be involved, but those most commonly involved are those most susceptible to trauma, such as the knee, the hip, the ankle, the elbow, the shoulder, and the wrist.

Infection commonly results from the combination of trauma and focal infection and enters the joint through the bloodstream or by means of a penetrating wound into the joint.

Symptoms and signs. When the infection is mild, the joint reaction may consist only in the stimulation of synovial fluid production. This is called an effusion.

If the virulence is greater, local reaction is further stimulated and fibrinous material (coagulated white blood cells) may cover the surfaces of the joint.

If the reaction is violent, the joint may be filled with pus under considerable pressure and the symptoms are much exaggerated. The temperature may rise to 103° or 104° F., the joint may become reddened, and a fusiform swelling may occur. Joint irritation is notoriously painful on any attempt at motion. Therefore violent muscle spasm of a protective nature usually accompanies joint irritation and exaggerates the tension and pain. There is usually a marked increase in the white blood cells in the blood.

Treatment. Early recognition and early treatment with antibiotics is the best means to prevent destruction of the joint. If response to antibiotics is not dramatic in 48 hours, surgical drainage must be considered as an emergency measure in the treatment.

Before the advent of penicillin, this type of joint infection was an extremely serious condition. Chemotherapy is now usually begun immediately on such patients, and surgical treatment is used only when necessary. The joint affected is immobilized by means of simple traction or a bivalved cast. Hot fomentations will often be ordered for the joint. Fluids and blood transfusions will be given, and aspiration of the joint under aseptic conditions may be done. If the patient can be brought through the acute phase of this disease, the chances for recovery are good.

In the more severely affected patients, in whom fibrin is deposited on the joint surfaces, more extensive treatment is indicated. Joint washing may be done by using two syringes inserted on opposite sides of the joint. Quantities of physiologic saline solution are flushed through the joint until the return is clear. Then penicillin solution may be injected into the joint. Immobilization should be accomplished by splints or by Buck's extension.

If the joint reaction is severe and there is pus formation, incision and drainage are usually necessary. Drainage may be accomplished by a single or double incision adequate to allow complete exposure of the joint. All fibrinous material is picked out with forceps, and the joint is washed clean with physiologic saline solution. Penicillin solution can then be infiltrated throughout the joint, and the incision is closed. The joint is immobilized in a splint or a plaster of paris cast, and the temperature and symptoms are watched closely.

If there should be continued elevation of temperature or continued pain, it may be necessary to bivalve the cast and inspect the joint. In severely affected patients it may be necessary to open the wound and institute free drainage. Such technique exposes joints to secondary infection and should be avoided if possible.

General treatment should consist in the administration of proper chemotherapy combined with transfusions, infusions, and physical therapy treatments.

Tuberculosis of the bone and joints, including nursing care

The three types of tuberculosis of the bone are the human, the bovine, and the avian. The avian (bird type) is very rare.

Tuberculosis at the end of long bones may manifest itself in the following forms:

1. Encysted tuberculosis in which there is localized destruction of bone surrounded by a wall of thickened bone tissue
2. Infiltrating tuberculosis that is rapid in development and is frequently followed by rapid bone destruction and sequestration
3. Synovial tuberculosis with thickening of the synovial tissue and the formation of rice bodies within the joint

Tuberculosis of the bone usually involves the portion that is in the vicinity of a joint. Occasionally, tuberculous infection in the bone may manifest itself in the form of an irritation of the periosteum and cortical bone, but usually it starts within a joint and extends to the medullary portion of the bone only by secondary invasion from the joint. The original involvement of the joint itself is usually through the bloodstream by means of an infarct or localization of the bacteria at the end of the arterial system. Hence, primary involvement may occur (1) at the end of the long bones or (2) along the periosteum of the long bones.

Clinical picture. Tuberculosis of the joint usually develops as an insidious disease. At the onset there is only occasional pain and muscle spasm about the joint. There might be a slight elevation of temperature without leukocytosis, and a positive intradermal tuberculin test may be present. For an accurate diagnosis of a tuberculous joint, material should be aspirated and injected into a guinea pig as well as cultured for tubercle bacilli. Both of these procedures should be used because one or the other may be positive. In 6 weeks the guinea pig is examined by autopsy, and the presence or absence of tuberculous organisms and exudate is determined by macroscopic and microscopic study. This test is the most accurate way to make a diagnosis of tuberculosis, although the time element is sometimes inconvenient.

Another accurate means of diagnosing tuberculosis in joints is biopsy. Material from the joint surface and synovial tissues can be removed and examined microscopically. If tuberculosis is present, it can usually be demonstrated either through the presence of tubercle bacilli, tubercles, or granulation tissue characteristic of tuberculosis.

The development of the tuberculous process in joints starts in most instances between the ages of 2 and 5 years but may begin later. The disease is not inherited and is usually acquired through association and contamination with older persons who have active or quiescent tuberculous lesions in the lungs.

Tuberculosis of the joints is rarely transmitted to other persons except through very careless handling of dressings from draining sinuses. It must be remembered, however, that the disease is progressive when untreated and does not become checked the minute the surgeon sees it and the diagnosis is made. Also, chest films are necessary to rule out the presence of concomitant pulmonary tuberculosis. Unnecessary exposure of other patients or nursing personnel must be avoided.

Teaching prevention. It is not enough that the nurse recognize the tuberculous patient as a challenge to her manual skill; she must accept the further challenge to educate the public regarding the causes, prevention, and necessity for prompt treatment of this disease.

It seems strange that today there is so much misrepresentation about tuberculosis of the bones and joints. It seems strange, also, that there are still parents with tuberculosis coming in daily contact with their very young children. One physician has stated that pulmonary tuberculosis is as contagious as measles to a child under 4 years of age.

The danger of young children being exposed to adults with tuberculosis cannot be overemphasized. At least the exposure need not be prolonged or repeated. Recent investigation has revealed the danger of young children receiving tuberculosis from servants who have the disease in some unrecognized form. Baby-sitters coming in to relieve the parents in the evening have been shown to present a menace. Because dairy cattle have been placed so well under control, it is now known that practically all tuberculosis in children is contracted from adults. This situation is now as important to eliminate as was the dairy cattle situation a few years ago. Most states require that teachers be examined roentgenographically every year or two. Certainly this should be encouraged to extend to all domestic help and baby-sitters who come in contact with young children.

The prophylaxis of tuberculosis briefly stated is the following: early diagnosis, segregation of infectious cases, and adequate treatment of discovered cases before they become clinically active.

General nursing care. Skill in the care of patients afflicted with skeletal tuberculosis is not determined merely by the dexterity the nurse displays in turning a patient with a tuberculous spine. Perhaps this was true twenty years ago but although the importance of these details is still fully appreciated, there is a broader significance to the care of these persons than that which the nurse gives to the patient in the hospital.

This disease has had its inception early in the life of the patient, perhaps in a household that included an adult relative who had tuberculosis in some contagious form. Perhaps the patient was a member of a family whose housing conditions were such that he was compelled to sleep in the same bedroom or even the same bed with that relative. Recognition must be given the important part that poor nutrition as well as poor environment may have played in his life as a child. The delay in treatment when the first mild symptoms of weight loss, fatigue and anorexia, or disinclination for his usual tasks and games became evident was perhaps engendered through ignorance on the part of parents or wrong advice given those parents by well-meaning friends that resulted in their sending the child to some practitioner of pseudomedicine. This patient in his brace or cast will return to this same unwholesome environment, for patients with skeletal tuberculosis seldom spend their entire period of recumbency in the hospital. Because these things are true, the nurse sees the imperious necessity to train the family in the long-term care of these patients if they are not to return to the hospital 6 months or a year later far worse than they were when first seen. They may have new foci of the disease in other parts of the body, perhaps with draining sinuses, with limbs flexed rigidly into unnatural positions, or, most grave of all, with beginning paralysis of the lower limbs.

The necessity for local rest is manifest to the nurse immediately. Frequently, her concern for the spine or affected extremity is so great that she forgets that tuberculosis is a constitutional disease. Nurses do not always carry over their training in the care of patients with pulmonary tuberculosis to the orthopedic ward and their patients with skeletal tuberculosis. The need for rest that is general as well as local is just as great with these persons and should be borne in mind constantly.

Home care. What instructions are given for the home care of these patients?

Families must first be taught what to observe and then be instructed in the interpretation of their observations. Second, they must be given a definite idea of the principles that underlie all details of the management of the patient at home. Last, they must be instructed carefully in the technique of carrying out these details. This third consideration will most frequently be delegated to the nurse.

The doctor will often instruct the parents of a child with tuberculosis that it is necessary to keep a daily record of temperature and to observe and estimate the amount of food intake, rest, and sunlight that the child receives. He will instruct them in the importance of recognizing any loss of weight or general strength. Signs of setback in these patients often occur so gradually that only by impressing firmly upon the parents' minds the necessity for solicitous observation and the most painstaking care will the patient's future welfare be assured.

Where the doctor knows without question that the status of the family income will not permit proper care for this patient, social agencies will be consulted and community resources called upon. Some doctors feel quite strongly that because of the protracted character of the disease, its tedious course, and the great likelihood of complicating factors and recurrences, the patient should be cared for institutionally until solidification of the joint and quiescence of the disease are assured.

For effective instruction concerning home treatment the nurse should, if possible, employ the demonstration method. Demonstrations of bath and care of cast must be given if her instructions are to have any effect at all on the parents. She must have enough imagination, too, to understand how the home situation will vary from the hospital situation and to suggest means of improvising when equipment will be manifestly lacking. Ability to compute a satisfactory diet for the patient with tuberculosis that takes into consideration the family income is another important feature. Many little details that seem almost too small to be mentioned must be gone into thoroughly in relation to the home treatment of the patient with tuberculosis. Rest periods tend to be curtailed in the home, and substitutions are made for essential foods because the parents thought the substitute just as good.

Instructions will vary with each individual case, but whatever the instructions are they must be given kindly, with an understanding of the magnitude of the problem that confronts the confused parents, and with a genuine desire to help them solve their problems. No greater nursing service is possible than such teaching when one considers the large proportion of home care usually given such patients during the course of their disease. In addition to instructing the patient and parents, the hospital nurse will make a referral to the local visiting or public health nurse. Because most of these patients are instructed to continue with chemotherapy at home, it is essential that a visiting nurse make home visits, administer the drugs, and evaluate symptoms and progress. Cost of drugs must not be forgotten. Prior to discharge inquiry into the cost of the drugs for continued chemotherapy should be made, and, if necessary, appropriate arrangements made with a local authority for supplying the needed drugs.

Surgery. Surgery as an adjunct to modern chemotherapy has come to be the preferred treatment in skeletal tuberculosis. Advantages of surgical treatment are as follows:

1. Biopsy may be performed for diagnostic purposes. With the present-day use of antibiotics this procedure can be performed with little danger to the patient, and, in that drugs used in the treatment of tuberculosis of bone and joint are more effective in the early stages of the disease, it is imperative that a diagnosis be made as soon as possible.

2. It may be used to obliterate joint motion by surgical interference, the operation being called an arthrodesis. This is by far the most common type of operation on tuberculous joints encountered on the orthopedic ward.

3. Evacuation and drainage of an abscess is a surgical process.

4. Decompression when an accumulation of pus has invaded parts of the body that contain vital organs, as may happen when the spinal cord is compressed by inflammatory exudates, may be accomplished.

5. Surgery may be employed to correct an existing deformity. Osteotomies are common in this last group.

Care of the patient after spinal fusion

has been described in another chapter. Joints that have undergone arthrodeses are usually well immobilized in plaster of paris before the patients are returned from the operating room, and their nursing care is the same as that of any surgical patient wearing a plaster cast. However, the systemic nature of the disease that has made the operation necessary should never be lost from the nurse's mind. Care of patients subjected to laminectomy for decompression of the spinal cord will not vary greatly from care given the patient who has had a spinal fusion operation.

Drug therapy. During recent years antibiotics have been used extensively in the treatment of patients with bone and joint tuberculosis. A high percentage of patients treated with isoniazid (the prime drug in the treatment of tuberculosis) have shown marked improvement. This drug is frequently combined with streptomycin. As the result of a high degree of toxicity, dihydrostreptomycin has been discontinued. Para-aminosalicylic acid (PAS) is frequently given with the isoniazid. The toxic effects of PAS are nausea, vomiting, abdominal discomfort, and anorexia. These drugs have their greatest value in the early treatment of the disease before ischemia and bone necrosis have taken place. It is unusual to observe serious damage from streptomycin to the hearing or the vestibular apparatus when the patient has received a total dose of 30 gm. or less per month. An exception to this is observed in older patients and in patients who have renal disease. Iproniazid cycloserine and other antibiotics are available for the patients with more complicated cases. It is important in the presence of relapse of proved tuberculosis that antibiotic sensitivity tests be carried out while the patient is being treated by chemotherapy.

It must be remembered that good nutrition, immobilization, and rest are fundamental in the treatment of the patient with a tuberculous bone or joint. When good general care and surgery as indicated are combined with the use of antibiotics, it is usually possible to shorten the healing period. By shortening the healing period secondary complications, such as renal calculi and joint deformity, may be prevented.

TUBERCULOSIS OF THE SPINE

Symptoms. About half of all cases of bone and joint tuberculosis occur in the spine. The first symptoms are usually stiffness, muscle spasm, and a tendency to reach things on the floor by bending the knees rather than the back.

At first the symptoms may be intermittent and are relieved by comparatively short periods of rest. The intermittent characteristic may cloud the early diagnosis.

Pain may be referred to the limbs, a fact that serves to emphasize the point that examinations should not be made

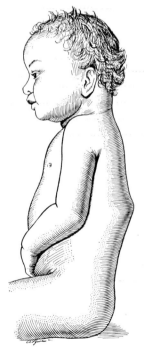

Fig. 169. Tuberculosis of the lower dorsal spine with angulation, or gibbus.

without the complete removal of all clothing. The complaint may be remote from the actual disease.

The lower dorsal spine and upper lumbar spine are most frequently affected, although tuberculosis of the cervical spine and dorsal spine are not uncommon. The greatest deformity develops when the involvement is in the dorsal spine, and its compensatory adaptation to the neighboring uninvolved joints is less effective than in the lumbar and cervical spine.

The characteristic deformity in tuberculosis of the spine is the development of a gibbus, an angulation or pronounced anteroposterior curve of the spine such as is seen in the hunchback. This deformity develops as the result of destructive lesions in the spine and fractures. In some instances, with destruction of one, two, three, or four vertebral bodies, the deformity is so severe that the segments of the spine above and below the destruction become parallel and the anterior margins of the bodies of the vertebrae rest upon each other.

Paralysis in tuberculosis of the spine occurs occasionally. Strangely, it is rarely the result of the mechanical disturbance in the alignment of the spine but rather the effect of abscesses, granulation tissue, and other accompanying factors in the tuberculous disease. For this reason treatment of paralysis usually consists of rest and immobilization. These agents have a tendency to diminish inflammatory factors and relieve nerve pressure. In rare instances it may become necessary to relieve bone pressure by laminectomy.

Treatment. The treatment of tuberculosis of the spine depends considerably on the advance that the disease has made at the time it is first observed and on the age of the patient. It must be remembered, however, that the disease does not halt the minute the surgeon sees it!

Whether or not spinal fusion operation offers the best means of arresting tuberculosis of the spine in young children has been widely debated. Some authorities believe that because of incomplete epiphyseal development, fusion of the spine in younger children does not protect them from further deformity.

It is a well-established fact that tuberculosis of the spine cannot be considered cured until there has been bony union of the vertebrae above and below the diseased process. The time required for this to occur, with or without fusion, is from 3 to 10 years. During this

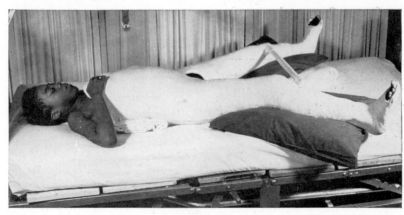

Fig. 170. A complete body cast has been applied to maintain immobilization and good position for this patient with tuberculosis of the spine. Note placement of pillows to support extremities.

period every attempt should be made through casts and braces to maintain as nearly as possible an erect position of the spine.

In conservative management of tuberculosis of the spine treatment consists of immobilization and the use of drugs (streptomycin, para-aminosalicylic acid, and isoniazid). Institutional care, fresh air, sunshine, proper diet, and hygienic surroundings are important factors. Under modern treatment 6 months' confinement in an institution with chemotherapy, then a continuation of chemotherapy for a total of 2 years, is usually indicated.

When improvement in the patient's general condition is apparent—that is, when he has no elevation of temperature and is gaining weight, when there is a decline in the blood sedimentation rate, and when the lymphocyte-monocyte ratio is normal—surgical fusion of the spine may be indicated. Nature automatically fuses the lamina and articular facets when spinal disease has existed over a period of years. Unfortunately, nature's fusion accompanies the destruction rather than precedes it. There is a protective mechanism on her part for the area that has been involved, but she gives no protection to the advance of the disease to other vertebrae. Frequently, as many as four or five vertebrae undergo complete or partial destruction.

Ordinarily, after spinal fusion operations patients are protected for a time by casts that are followed by protective braces for an additional time. When tuberculosis exists in the cervical spine, the cast or brace must extend up to and include the chin and head.

There are many ingenious types of apparatus for obtaining and maintaining correction and immobilization in patients with tuberculous lesions of the spine.

Abscess formation occurs in a fairly large percentage of patients with tuberculosis of the spine. In the cervical region the abscess may develop in the pharynx, causing difficulty in breathing. In the dorsal region it may occur in the mediastinum and may rupture into the lung. In the lumbar spine an abscess may develop between the lumbar muscles or in the gluteal region, or it may follow the course of the iliopsoas muscle and point in the groin. This is the most common form (psoas abscess).

A cold abscess should be opened when pressure is great and spontaneous rupture is likely to occur. Incision may be made through which the abscess is evacuated, and the incision is firmly closed.

The commonest form of surgical attack on spinal tuberculosis is the anterior approach to the spine, so that infected granulation tissue, sequestra, and other necrotic tissues may be removed. Drainage of an abscess is common when the abscess is progressive and not controlled by antibiotics. Approach to the abscess is usually made through costotransversectomy. If there is a great deficiency of bone at the conclusion of the operation, bone grafts can be added to bridge the gap between the vertebral bodies.

Nursing care

Because tuberculosis of the spine (sometimes called Pott's disease after Sir Percival Pott who first described the syndrome over 150 years ago) is most frequent in occurrence of the skeletal tuberculous lesions, the care of these patients will be dealt with in full. Patients with tuberculosis of the other joints of the body need the same general care. Usually, the local care of the other types of skeletal tuberculosis is somewhat simpler for the nurse because their immobilization is most commonly accomplished by circular or bivalved plaster casts.

Bedridden patients. In cases of spinal

tuberculosis the nurse must employ her best technique of cast care. She must constantly be on the alert for abscesses that have begun to drain beneath the cast, and her sense of smell is the best agent for discovering these. She must depend upon the patient's weekly weight chart, a record of his appetite and rest habits, his pigmentation from heliotherapy treatments, and his general appearance of well-being and absence of symptoms of recurrence (undue fatigue, night cries, irritability, or apathy) to assure her of his progress.

Local rest can be accomplished in a number of ways, and each orthopedist has a particular apparatus he prefers. It may be a Bradford frame; it may be a plaster jacket applied from shoulders to hip or sometimes including the legs to the knee; or it may be a bivalved plaster bed of some type, extending from occiput to knees but divided into an anterior and a posterior section to permit care and sunlight to the patient's skin. The aim of all this apparatus is rest—"Rest, uninterrupted, enforced and prolonged," a trilogy of treatment promulgated many decades ago by a great orthopedist, Hugh Owen Thomas of Liverpool. In patients with tuberculosis of the spine, even in this era of early mobilization, such unqualified rest is considered essential.

The care of the patient in the hospital and later in the home will vary somewhat according to his type of apparatus. Hyperextension frames have been used in the treatment of spinal tuberculosis for many years. However in recent years, with early diagnosis and the use of drugs, the orthopedic surgeon may per-

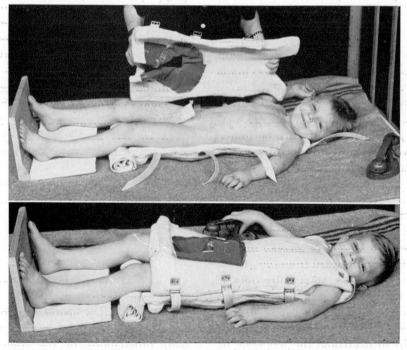

Fig. 171. The plaster shell or plaster bed is frequently used to immobilize the spine after fusion. Each half is lined with stockinet. The straps and buckles make it possible to remove either half for bathing and skin care. Before the patient is turned the straps are buckled tightly. (Courtesy Iowa State Services for Crippled Children.)

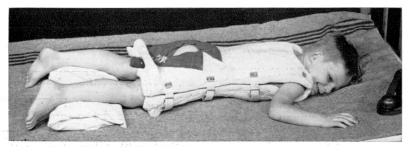

Fig. 172. Prone position. The anterior and posterior halves may be buckled in place to prevent the child from rising up and turning. Note the waterproof material placed about the perineum and buttocks. (Courtesy Iowa State Services for Crippled Children.)

mit the patient to have more freedom than was prescribed previously. A straight Bradford frame may be used to restrain the child and ensure maintenance of a horizontal position. This is important because the upright or vertical position will cause increased pressure on the diseased vertebrae. For the adult patient recumbency on a firm mattress may be the prescribed restriction.

Care to the patient's back is important. If he is thin and emaciated, pressure areas will demand close attention. The gibbus, or knuckling that occurs at the level of the diseased vertebra, is often the site of severe pressure areas. Because the patient lies on this spot over a long period, it can readily be understood why this pressure necrosis occurs. Occasionally a bursa will have formed on this gibbus, and it may be hot and indurated. Hot wet dressings are sometimes ordered.

If no inflammation is present, a good massage with lanolin or alcohol may be given, working outward from the gibbus. A semicircle of felt, sufficiently thick to extend beyond the gibbus, may be secured to the skin with narrow strips of adhesive (avoiding the gibbus area) and will help to overcome the tendency toward serious decubitus. Care to the back should always include the back of the head, so often a point of denudation and pressure.

Children with tuberculous spines should not be allowed to feed themselves because feeding oneself in so complete a state of recumbency is fatiguing. Tuberculosis is one disease in which fatigue is to be avoided at all costs. The fatigue incident upon feeding himself often causes the tuberculous child to eat less than he needs, and in this way double damage is done. The child should be fed slowly, with careful observations of his eating habits. His diet, carefully planned for high caloric intake and high protein and vitamin content, should be urged firmly, but understanding of the child's capacity should aid the nurse to use her discrimination in judging when he has had sufficient. Between-meal nourishment should always be included in the tuberculous child's diet. It should be planned to be nutritious without filling him to such an extent that he will be unable to take his next meal. Milk should be rich and plentiful, and the child must not be allowed to develop finicky habits incident to his dislike of certain vegetables and other wholesome foods.

Restraints are a matter of importance in the nursing care of children afflicted with tuberculosis of the spine. They must be efficient in maintaining the position prescribed by the doctor, but on the other hand, they must inflict no unnecessary restraint upon the child.

In tuberculosis of the lower dorsal and lumbar spine it is frequently necessary to restrain the child's feet by some loose bands around the ankles secured to the frame. This is seldom necessary, however, in tuberculosis of the upper spine, and, as has been stated, any unnecessary curtailment of activity for the child is to be avoided. Restraints to maintain position may be of the vest or jacket variety, in which a canvas garment for the upper part of the body is equipped with webbing straps and buckles.

Because the chronicity of this disease is one of its most outstanding features, early consideration must be given to the education of the child. Present educational methods have been adapted very satisfactorily to bedside teaching, so that the long treatment required by this disease does not need to interrupt the child's schooling. Most communities have arrangements wherein such children are given the advantage of a specially arranged plan of study to suit their needs. The child should not lose the interests common to his age, nor must he face a future in which he is forced to return to school at a much lower level than his age justifies.

Occupational and diversional therapy are most important. Limitation of activity with these patients, of course, must be considered because the child's position makes many occupations impossible for him and also because fatigue must be avoided. However, such persons can be taught many useful crafts and be permitted to enjoy these during certain periods of the day. Many inclinations are developed and many natural gifts and talents are discovered that may play an important part in the patient's future rehabilitation. Because of the unnatural position, the possibility of eyestrain from reading and handwork, should always be a matter for consideration. Lighting must be carefully supervised.

Ambulatory patients. A new set of duties supervenes for the nurse when the patient's period of recumbency is over and healing and calcification have progressed to such an extent that the orthopedist feels he may be allowed up for short periods with some type of ambulatory support. Limitations of time designated by the doctor must be rigidly adhered to. Too often the ambulatory patient on the busy orthopedic ward is forgotten in the rush to care for a patient more seriously ill. Periods of activity for the newly ambulatory tuberculous patient should never be prolonged or vigorous during the first weeks. Appetite must be observed lest it begin to decrease as a result of fatigue from overactivity. Weight should continue to be checked weekly. Evidences of any loss of progress should be reported to the physician. The same observations for beginning abscesses or pressure sites are as necessary now as they were during the period of recumbency.

The type of support may be an ambulatory cast, jacket, or brace. Commonly used in spinal tuberculosis is the Taylor body brace. The Taylor body brace, or modifications of it, is in common use in most hospitals. It consists of two thin flexible steel bars that form a support for the vertebral column, one lying on either side of it, which fits the curves of the back perfectly. A pelvic band made of steel and leather is fastened at the bottom of these supports. Another crossbar attaches at the scapular level. Straps fastened to the vertical bars go over the shoulders, under the axillae, and return to their original attachment, making a sort of loop. In the front a canvas apron supports the chest and abdomen and is fastened to the brace by tape-webbing straps and buckles. These secure the brace tightly to the chest and abdomen. It should always be remembered by the nurse applying these braces that the pelvic band must closely encircle the pelvis slightly below the iliac crests. If this is done, the brace will be in the proper position with regard to the rest of the body. Whatever the type of body brace used, both bracemaker and physician advise that you fasten the brace around the pelvis first if the patient is lying down, and this should always be the case while fitting tuberculosis patients.

COMPLICATIONS IN TUBERCULOSIS OF THE JOINTS

The symptomatology of complications in tuberculosis of the joints should be known to the orthopedic nurse. The most frequent causes of death are given by Steindler as meningitis in the child and recrudescent tuberculosis of the lungs in the adult. Chronic, reasonless irritability in the young child who has tuberculosis of a joint should be a point of observation on the part of the nurse. Symptoms of this nature may occur many weeks before evidences of lethargy, headache, neck rigidity, or convulsive states are manifested. Rapid loss of weight in the adult, severe night sweats, temperature elevation, anorexia, and debility may indicate oncoming miliary tuberculosis.

Steindler states that tuberculosis of the kidney occurs more often with bone tuberculosis than in the pulmonary tuberculosis. Renal complications may be manifested in urinary disturbances— cystitis, hematuria, and the like. An accurate measurement of intake and output is indicated for the tuberculous patient in whom this sort of complication is suspected. Periodic urinalyses are usually ordered by the doctor. Although gastrointestinal upsets, distention, constipation, and nausea may be the result of retentive or reclination apparatus, they should be reported if they become obstinate or persist over a long period.

In this connection it might be well to mention here that retropharyngeal abscess complicating tuberculosis of the cervical spine is often manifested by dysphagia or dyspnea. These symptoms have special significance and must be reported as soon as they are observed. Spasm of the muscles of the thigh and a tendency toward flexion and lateral rotation of a limb that is accompanied by great pain on motion may suggest to the doctor that a psoas abscess is in the process of formation long before a fluctuating mass may be seen in the groin.

Sudden weakness or trembling of the legs may be the first indication of further breakdown in the affected vertebrae. It is a very grave symptom, often a forerunner of paralysis, and must be reported to the physician in charge without delay.

TUBERCULOSIS OF THE HIP

Tuberculosis of the hip constitutes the second largest group of tuberculous joint involvement.

Symptoms and signs. The disease usually begins at an early age (1 to 3 years) with a limp of gradually increasing severity. The hip becomes slightly flexed, abducted, and externally rotated, and the child has a tendency to walk on the toes of the affected side. Night cries are frequently present. These are caused by a definite mechanism. The muscles relax in sleep, and the joint is unprotected. In the subconscious state body movements may occur and the joint may become irritated. There is an immediate violent spasm of the muscles that causes severe pain by bringing the irritated joint surfaces together and the child cries out as he awakens.

As the disease progresses, the destruction of the head of the femur and possibly of the acetabulum increases and the deformity changes. Adduction and

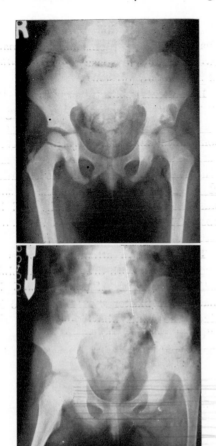

Fig. 173. Roentgenograms of a tuberculous hip. In the top picture the head of the left femur and the joint space are still well defined. As the infectious process continues, the joint cartilage is destroyed, calcium is deposited, and eventually motion in the joint is destroyed.

internal rotation develop, whereas the flexion deformity remains.

Diagnosis. The usual methods of clinical and laboratory diagnosis of a tuberculous joint are used. In persons afflicted with the more advanced cases the characteristic destruction as shown by roentgenograms is in itself almost positive proof of the disease.

The symptoms are more severe than they are in Legg-Perthes disease and slipped upper femoral epiphysis and less

severe than they are in acute pyogenic arthritis of the hip.

Treatment. During the early stages and in younger children, recumbent treatment is combined with the use of drugs. It is hoped that with rest (local and general), good food, and hygienic surroundings, combined with chemotherapy, joint motion may be saved. Immobilization of the joint may be maintained by plaster splinting or by traction.

In patients with more severe cases fusion of the hip may be necessary. There are several methods of accomplishing fusion, but all successful methods consist of some form of bone graft between the femur and the pelvis, and growth of this graft leads to solid bone formation between these two structures and the elimination of joint function. Tuberculosis seems to lose its affinity for

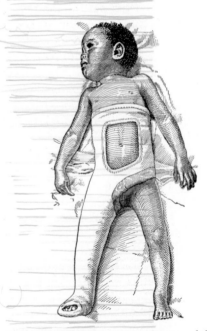

Fig. 174. Plaster spica cast for immobilization of a young child with tuberculosis of the hip. (From Shands, A. R.: Handbook of orthopaedic surgery, ed. 4, St. Louis, 1952, The C. V. Mosby Co.)

a joint when motion and friction are eliminated. After fusion operations a plaster of paris cast is applied from the chest to the toes of the affected side. The position of the hip joint is of considerable importance. There should be from 10- to 20-degree flexion and, if there has been some destruction, about 5-degree adduction to give the best weight-bearing line. Approximately 6 to 8 months are required for bone healing after hip fusion. This must be determined by roentgenography.

TUBERCULOSIS OF THE CARPAL AND TARSAL JOINTS

When tuberculosis affects joints that communicate with each other and are partially separated by cancellous rather than cortical bone, the progress of the disease may be very rapid and destruc-tion may be very difficult to control. The characteristic symptoms and signs (pain, swelling, muscle spasm, and limitation of motion) are present.

In patients with tuberculosis of the distal joints of the limbs the swelling is usually fusiform or pear-shaped, and sometimes abscesses develop relatively early. There is usually some redness and tenderness but only moderate elevation of temperature. The diagnosis is sub-stantiated by roentgenography and biopsy. The roentgenogram is character-ized by destruction without repair.

Treatment. An attempt at conserva-tive treatment with drugs and immobili-zation in plaster of paris should be made. The plaster should extend to in-clude the joints above and below the affected area. In the wrist resection of the carpal bones with operative fusion

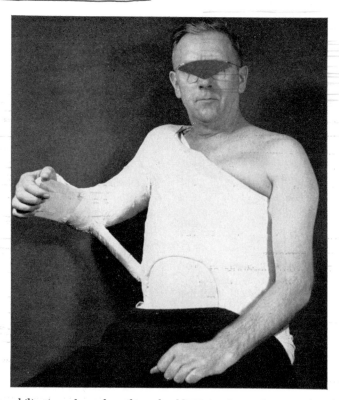

Fig. 175. Immobilization of a tuberculous shoulder joint by application of a shoulder spica cast. Note abducted and flexed position of the shoulder.

of the metacarpals to the radius may accomplish a cure.

If the bones of the foot are involved, local curettage of the affected areas followed by immobilization may lead to improvement if combined with complete rest and general hygienic treatment. Frequently, however, from an economic standpoint and considering the future health of the individual, amputation well above the area of involvement is the treatment of choice.

TUBERCULOSIS OF THE KNEE AND ELBOW, SYNOVIAL TYPE

The synovial type of tuberculosis affects the knee and elbow more frequently than any other joints. It is often amenable to treatment by immobilization in the milder cases and synovectomy in the more severe cases. Joint tuberculosis is the most common type, and when the diagnosis has been proved, drug therapy should be instituted. Operative fixation of the joint may also be necessary. This is best accomplished by the removal of all hypertrophied synovial tissue and the cartilages of the joint sur-

faces and by supplementary fixation of the joint by penetrating bone grafts.

TUBERCULOSIS OF THE SHOULDER

Type 1—Tuberculosis sicca. Tuberculosis sicca is an inactive form of adult tuberculosis that causes marked limitation of motion but comparatively little pain or other symptoms. The diagnosis is made by the history and by roentgenography.

Type 2—Destructive tuberculosis. Although insidious in origin, destructive tuberculosis shows the typical fusiform swelling about the joint, and there is extreme pain and muscle spasm on any attempt at motion. Roentgenograms show extensive destruction in the head of the humerus, and eventually there is collapse.

Treatment. If the disease has not advanced too far, an attempt should be made to fuse the shoulder joint in a position of approximately 70-degree abduction. Frequently these cases are not suitable for fusion, and a removal of the head of the humerus may be necessary to effect a cure.

STUDY QUESTIONS

1. How has the use of antibiotics changed the treatment and nursing care of the patient with osteomyelitis?
2. Describe precautions you will take when dressing a draining wound:
   (a) To protect the patient
   (b) To protect other patients in same ward
   (c) To protect yourself
3. What will you teach the patient regarding the dressing of his wound?
4. Describe the method of handling an acutely inflamed joint that will cause the least pain.
5. Discuss the importance of early diagnosis and treatment of active pulmonary tuberculosis as it relates to the prevention of bone and joint tuberculosis.

6. Discuss the treatment and care of a child with a tuberculous spine:
   (a) General health measures and treatment
   (b) Specific treatment and nursing care pertaining to the spine
   (c) Teaching of patient and family
7. For what particular complications should the nurse be on the alert when caring for a patient with skeletal tuberculosis? What are the symptoms of such complications?
8. Define the following terms: Brodie's abscess, cold abscess, ankylosis, arthrodesis, fusion, gibbus, involucrum, kyphos, night cries, saucerization, and sequestrum.

REFERENCES

Bickel, W. H., Young, H. H., Pfuetze, K. H., and Norley, T.: Streptomycin and tuberculosis of bone and joint, J.A.M.A. **137**:682-687, 1948.

Ferguson, A.: Orthopedic surgery in infancy and childhood, Baltimore, 1963, Williams & Wilkins Co.

Frenay, Sister Mary Agnes: Drugs in tuberculosis control, Am. J. Nursing **61**:82-85, 1961.

Kelley, W. O., and Poole, H.: Skeletal tuberculosis—medical surgical treatment and nursing the patient with skeletal tuberculosis, Am. J. Nursing **57**:332-336, 1957.

Kilham, B. A.: Nursing patients with osteomyelitis, Am. J. Nursing **50**:19-20, 1950.

Mercer, Sir Walter, and Duthie, R.: Orthopedic surgery, ed. 6, Baltimore, 1964, Williams & Wilkins Co.

Miller, J. A.: The drama of tuberculosis, J.A.M.A. **115**:1272-1277, 1941.

O'Brien, R. M.: Osteomyelitis, Am. J. Nursing **50**:17-19, 1950.

Orr, H. W.: A new method in the treatment of osteomyelitis, Am. J. Nursing **28**:755-758, 1928.

Shands, A., Raney, R., and Brashear, R.: Handbook of orthopaedic surgery, ed. 6, St. Louis, 1963, The C. V. Mosby Co.

Smith, A. D.: The treatment of bone and joint tuberculosis, J. Bone & Joint Surg. **37-A**:1214-1222, 1955.

Smith, M. H.: Practical management of tuberculosis, Pediatric Clinics of North America, Philadelphia, 1956, W. B. Saunders Co.

Weiss, M.: Chemotherapy and tuberculosis, Am. J. Nursing **59**:1711-1714, 1959.

Chapter 6

Metabolic disorders of bone

BONE METABOLISM

To understand metabolic disorders of bone, a brief discussion of factors controlling normal bone metabolism is necessary. This discussion will include the constituents, normal metabolism, and abnormal metabolism of bone.

Constituents. Bone is composed of water, solid, and chemical constituents.

Water makes up 75% of the bone in the newborn infant and 15% of the bone in the adult.

The solid part of bone is the matrix, the ground substance of bone that is composed of complex proteins laid down by osteoblasts (cells that produce bone).

The chemicals of bone are chiefly calcium and phosphorus, made up mostly of calcium phosphate 80%, calcium carbonate 13%, and magnesium phosphate 2%. These chemicals are deposited in the matrix of bone to give it rigidity and make it strong. It is important to note that bone is constantly made in the amount necessary to resist stress. When stress is lacking, bone resorption will take place by the action of cells called osteoclasts. The calcium and phosphorus of bone structure comes from foods ingested and absorbed through the gastrointestinal tract. Milk and milk products are the best sources of calcium. The acid medium of the upper gastrointestinal tract, along with the adequate presence of vitamin D, is most favorable to calcium absorption. The vitamin D does not necessarily need to be ingested because the body is capable of synthesizing it if exposed to sufficient sunlight. The actual deposition of calcium and phosphorus is complicated and not completely understood, but it is certainly aided by the enzyme systems and follows certain chemical laws. The amount of calcium circulating in the blood serum maintains a constant level that is somewhat regulated by the parathyroid hormone. The calcium is carried to the bone by the blood serum and is deposited in the protein bone matrix that forms the solid portion of bone. The calcium and phosphorus necessary to bone metabolism have another role in body chemistry, namely, regulation of acid-base balance.

In patients with kidney disease in whom acidosis may exist, the calcium and phosphorus are excreted in more than normal amounts to control acidosis. In such circumstances the bone is depleted of its calcium in order to maintain the most important calcium-phosphorus equilibrium. By testing the amount of calcium and phosphorus in the blood serum and the amount of calcium excreted in the urine, it is possible to get some idea of the abnormalities in bone metabolism.

Abnormal bone metabolism. Any interference with the normal regulatory mechanisms of intake, absorption, utilization, or excretion of calcium can lead to metabolic bone disorders. The diseases caused by altered bone metabolism can be divided into two general groups as follows:

1. Lack of mineralization of bone, which can be the result of:
   (a) Insufficient intake of calcium, phosphorus, or vitamin D
   (b) Insufficient absorption of calcium, phosphorus, or vitamin D
   (c) Insufficient utilization of calcium, phosphorus, or vitamin D
2. Demineralization of bone, which can be subdivided into:
   (a) Excessive amounts of hormones affecting calcium and phosphorus, such as parathyroid, thyroid, and sex hormones
   (b) Chronic acidosis or ketosis—kidney dysfunction
   (c) Malignant disease affecting bone
   (d) Atrophy of disuse or immobilization of bone

RICKETS

Rickets is a bone disease of childhood as a result of an insufficient amount of calcium available for deposit in bone. It can be caused by inadequate calcium intake in the diet, but more commonly it is the result of inadequate vitamin D. Vitamin D is necessary for proper calcium absorption from the intestine and also is needed to aid in the deposition of calcium in the bone.

This disorder results in soft bones that deform if not checked and will also interfere with growth. The treatment is to provide adequate intake of calcium and vitamin D. (Fig. 176.)

Resistant rickets is caused by a defect in the utilization of vitamin D and will

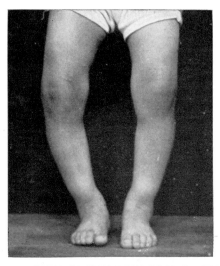

Fig. 176. Bowlegs (genu varum) that are the result of active rickets. If the rickets is brought under control, the bowlegs will correct themselves by further growth.

require more than normal amounts of vitamin D intake to control calcification of bone.

OSTEOMALACIA

Osteomalacia is identical with rickets but occurs chiefly in adults. Therefore it does not result in dwarfism and marked deformities. The commonest deficiency is inadequate calcium intake. Occasionally, osteomalacia results from poor absorption in persons who have steatorrhea. It can occur after repeated pregnancies if the intake of calcium has not been equal to the increased need of calcium for the growth of the fetus.

RENAL RICKETS

In kidney dysfunction bone can be demineralized as a result of calcium being drawn from the bone reservoir to bolster any drop in serum calcium. This occurs when the calcium and phosphorus of the serum must be utilized to regulate the acid-base equilibrium through urinary excretion.

There are several kinds of renal rickets

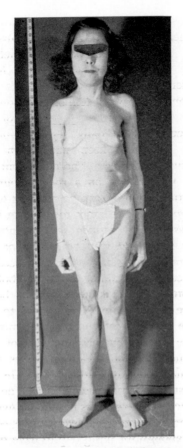

Fig. 177. Fanconi syndrome. This patient in her early 30's shows deformities of the legs and the dwarfing that occur in metabolic bone disease when the primary defect is in the kidney.

dependent upon the specific kidney dysfunction, such as the Fanconi syndrome, cystine rickets, and rickets associated with nephrosclerosis. The treatment of this entire group depends upon the control of the kidney dysfunction. (Fig. 177.)

HYPERPARATHYROIDISM

A hormone from the parathyroid gland has a regulatory effect on the amount of circulating calcium in the blood serum. It acts to maintain a constant level of serum calcium, but the serum calcium rises when an excessive amount of parathormone is present. This constitutes hyperparathyroidism and is found associated usually with tumors of the parathyroid.

If the condition is allowed to go on indefinitely, the kidneys are damaged because they excrete more calcium than normally. Kidney stones are frequent as a result. Calcium is drained from the body stores, namely bone, to make up for the excessive loss of calcium in the urine. This can become so marked that cysts are formed in the bones. Osteitis fibrosa cystica is a term sometimes used to describe the syndrome of hyperparathyroidism. The treatment is removal of the parathyroid tumor.

PAGET'S DISEASE (OSTEITIS DEFORMANS)

Paget's disease is a disease of the bone in which there is overactivity of osteoblasts and osteoclasts, building and destroying bone in an unaltered chemical pattern. High levels of phosphatase occur and are an index to the rapidity and amount of new bone being formed. The cause of this disease is entirely unknown, and the treatment is limited to the correction of deformities that occur. People afflicted with this disease are usually past middle age, and the bones involved may be few or many.

The bones become broader and weaker than normal and are easily fractured. The fractures heal readily. In the generalized form the patient becomes shorter and, because the skull expands may require a larger hat. In rare instances the involved bone may show malignant changes.

HYPERVITAMINOSIS D

Hypervitaminosis D is caused by an excessive intake of vitamin D. It is included here to warn and to point out that excessive doses of vitamin D can cause harmful chemical changes related to calcium and phosphorus metabolism.

Serum calcium is increased, and calcium deposits in the soft tissues occur. The kidneys can be irreparably damaged by calcific deposits and must excrete large amounts of calcium in the urine. The treatment is to lower the vitamin D dosage.

OSTEOPOROSIS

Osteoporosis (porous bone) refers to bones that show demineralization. This condition is the result of various causes, the more common of which are disuse, senility and a lack of estrogenic hormones in the postmenopause period.

Disuse. Normally, the trabeculae of the bone withstand the stresses placed upon them, such as in bearing weight and muscular activity. The bone grows and mineralizes to withstand the demands placed upon it. This accounts for the fact that a football player grows a thicker and more dense tibia than a less active person. Should these stresses be removed by a sedentary life or prolonged bed rest for the treatment of a chronic ailment, the bones respond by

becoming less calcified and showing thinner cortices. At times the loss of bone substance can be great, such as after prolonged immobilization in a plaster cast. This is known as the atrophy of disuse, a form of osteoporosis.

Senile osteoporosis. In persons of advanced age the daily replacement of bone may not keep pace with the wearing-out process. The bones will appear washed out on a roentgenogram, and the condition can be referred to as osteoporosis. The exact mechanism that allows this to happen is not entirely clear but could well be a part of the general slowing of metabolic processes, particularly pertaining to the metabolism of protein that is necessary in bone. There is no treatment other than to improve protein, calcium, and vitamin D intake and to increase activity of the patient with the idea that stress will stimulate bone formation. (Fig. 178.)

Postmenopausal osteoporosis. The incidence of osteoporosis in females five to ten years beyond the menopause is common enough for this group to have been

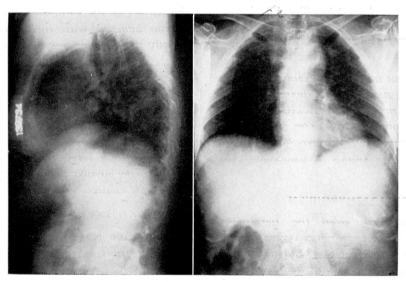

Fig. 178. Osteoporosis. This is a metabolic disorder of elderly persons (females especially) in which calcium in the bone is depleted and the bone matrix fails to produce replacement bone. The result is a weakening of the structure.

given special consideration. This is because this group will respond to hormone therapy. Studies have indicated that lack of estrogenic hormones has an effect on protein and calcium metabolism to such an extent that osteoporosis of rather severe degree can occur. The resultant weakening of bone is likely to be greatest in the vertebral bodies, and it is common for these to collapse under normal stresses. When collapse occurs, the spine becomes painful. The treatment is identical with that for senile osteoporosis, with the addition of estrogenic hormones.

REFERENCES

Bick, E. M.: The physiology of the aging process in the musculoskeletal apparatus, Geriatrics **10**:274-277, 1955.

Howorth, B. M.: A textbook of orthopedics, Philadelphia, 1952, W. B. Saunders Co.

Lonergan, R. C.: Osteoporosis of the spine, Am. J. Nursing **61**:79-81, 1961.

Luck, V. J.: Bone and joint diseases, Springfield, Ill., 1950, Charles C Thomas, Publisher.

Lyford, B.: Implications of osteoporosis, J. Am. Phys. Ther. A. **42**:106-110, 1962.

Weinberg, M.: Osteoporosis: diagnosis and treatment, J. Am. Geriat. Soc. **4**:429-437, 1956.

Chapter 7

Arthritis, including nursing care

Rheumatism is a general term that includes disorders in which pain and stiffness of the muscles or skeleton are prominent features. It ranks second only to mental and nervous diseases as a cause of time lost from work.

Arthritis is a form of rheumatism in which the joints are the structures primarily affected. It has been estimated that four and one-half million people in this country have arthritis and that 190,000 of these are totally disabled. Over one-half of the disabled persons are less than 45 years of age. With the associated social, economic, and emotional burdens on the families of arthritic patients the importance of the nursing care of the patient with arthritis becomes obvious.

Arthritis is a chronic disease causing varying degrees of disability, frequently quite severe. Unfortunately there is no cure for most of the forms of arthritis. The desired goal in the care of the patient with arthritis must be to help him function efficiently as a human being and as a member of society. It follows, then, that the treatment program must consider the patient's physical health, emotional health, and social problems that may be present, especially as they relate to family members and economic situation. If the treatment program does not, it is inadequate and will fail to achieve the goal that common sense tells us is the only logical objective. Indeed this should be the desired goal in the care of any patient, no matter what his ailment may be.

The described objective in the care of the patient with arthritis cannot be adequately achieved by any one person. The combined efforts of a number of specially trained persons—the patient's personal physician, consultant physicians, nurses, physical therapist, occupational therapist, social worker, and vocational counselor—will be needed at various times. The overall program is directed by the physician who has the responsibility for the patient's long-term care and who must know all of the facets of the patient's problems.

The physician who has the primary responsibiilty for the patient's care must attend not only to his medical needs, but also must assist the patient in other areas. The role of the nurse, as will be shown, is very important in the total program of treatment. The physical therapist has close contact with the patient and similarly contributes a great deal. Many patients have disabilities that make it difficult or impossible for them to perform everyday tasks that we take for granted in our lives, such as putting on shoes or socks. The occupational therapist can help the patient by showing him ways of adapting to his disabilities, by demonstrating techniques for simplifying everyday tasks, and by providing devices to aid the patient in

223

performing these activities. The social worker can help in working out family problems, in providing contact with special service agencies, and frequently in providing moral support to the patient who has emotional problems contributing to his disability. The vocational counselor contributes a real service when he helps the patient find a new occupation after that patient can no longer continue at his previous work because of his disability.

There are numerous types of arthritis. The following three types are relatively common. The other less common types usually resemble clinically one of these three, and the principles of nursing care can be applied accordingly.

RHEUMATOID ARTHRITIS

Rheumatoid (atrophic) arthritis is a chronic systemic disease of unknown cause. It is to be emphasized that it is a generalized or systemic disease and not strictly a joint affliction, although the joint involvement is the major clinical feature. Varying degrees of deformity and destruction of joints commonly occur, causing varying degrees of disability. The joint damage may be so severe in some instances as to result in complete invalidism. Rheumatoid arthritis occurs more commonly in women than in men, in a ratio of two or three to one. It may occur at any age from infancy to advanced old age, but most often between 20 and 60 years of age.

The prominent symptoms of rheumatoid arthritis are stiffness, especially upon arising in the morning, and joint pain and swelling, involving multiple joints. The joint swelling is caused by the inflammation of the joint capsule and by the accumulation of fluid within the joints. There is a definite tendency for involvement of the same joints on both sides of the body, and the arthritis usually involves more joints as time goes on. Although any joint in the body may be involved, there is a predilection for the small joints of the hands and feet. The wrists, elbows, ankles, and knees are commonly involved also.

As a result of the chronic joint inflammation, important anatomic changes may occur resulting in limitation of joint function. Involvement of the joint capsule and supporting ligaments may cause weakness, stretching, or rupture of these structures resulting in instability. When the instability is severe, partial dislocation of the joint, referred

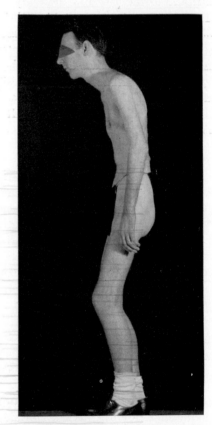

Fig. 179. Strümpell-Marie arthritis. Typical posture in ankylosing arthritis of the spine. Hip and shoulder joints may also be involved. (From Smith-Petersen, M. N., Larson, C. B., and Aufranc, O. E.: Osteotomy of the spine for correction of flexion deformity in rheumatoid arthritis, J. Bone & Joint Surg. 27:562-571, 1945.)

to as subluxation, may occur. In other instances there is scarring of these tissues resulting in limitation of motion. This is termed contracture of the joint capsule or ligament. When scarring occurs within a joint, limitation of motion also occurs and is called ankylosis. It may be so severe as to result in a completely motionless joint. Actual destruction of cartilage and bone within the joint is a common occurrence in rheumatoid arthritis. When severe, it may result in greatly impaired joint function. Muscle weakness is common and may contribute to the patient's disability.

The course of rheumatoid arthritis usually is one of periods of increased disease activity alternating with intervals of decreased disease activity. There may be great variation in the intensity and duration of the periods of increased disease activity from time to time. It is very difficult, therefore, to predict the course of the disease in an individual patient. A small percentage of patients with rheumatoid arthritis will have a mild course with little disability. Most patients will have varying degrees of disabiilty that increase with the duration of the disease. These patients remain largely independent of others for self-care and are usually able to pursue occupations not requiring vigorous physical activity. Severe incapacitation will occur in relatively few patients.

Ankylosing spondylitis, also known as rheumatoid spondylitis and Strümpell-Marie arthritis, is a chronic form of arthritis affecting primarily the sacroiliac joints and spine. Frequently it leads to severe ankylosis or limitation of motion of the back (Fig. 179). It affects men approximately four times more frequently than women and usually occurs between 16 and 40 years of age. Pain and stiffness of the back are the com-

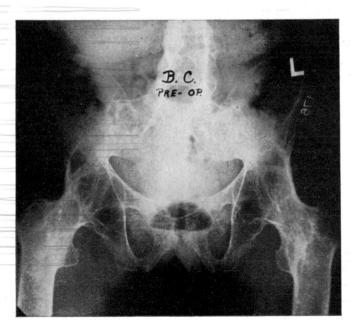

Fig. 180. Strümpell-Marie arthritis. Both hip joints, both sacroiliac joints, and the zygapophysial joints have been destroyed and have undergone bony ankylosis. Note the calcification of the vertebral ligaments. No motion in this portion of the back and in the hips is possible. (From Kenney, William C., and Larson, Carroll B.: Orthopedics for the general practitioner, St. Louis, 1957, The C. V. Mosby Co.)

mon symptoms of this disorder. In-volvement of the extremity joints occurs in some patients and is usually less severe than in typical rheumatoid arthritis. The course of ankylosing spon-dylitis is variable just as in rheumatoid arthritis. It is usually a progressive disease involving more of the spine with the passage of time.

Treatment and nursing care

General considerations. Because rheu-matoid arthritis is a chronic systemic disease, consideration must be given to the care of the patient's general health as well as to the treatment of the joint problems. Adequate rest, relief of pain, prevention of deformity, proper nutri-tion, treatment of other diseases when present, and assisting the patient to understand his disease and develop a proper attitude toward it are the im-portant general features of treatment. There is no cure for rheumatoid arthritis and it must be clearly understood that all treatment is directed at maintaining good general health and helping the patient to function at his best possible level.

Years of experience have shown that a successful basic treatment program for rheumatoid arthritis must include ade-quate rest, relief of pain, and a regular exercise program. Patients with rheuma-toid arthritis require 8 to 12 hours' sleep each night and, when the disease is more active, frequent rest periods during the day. In the event of an acute flare-up of the arthritis, several days of bed rest are helpful in reducing joint inflammation and systemic symptoms. Remaining in bed, however, for pro-longed periods of time is undesirable because it leads to increased muscle weakness and limitation of joint motion.

No drug has been found to be more desirable than aspirin for relief of pain. It is the basic ingredient of the drug

therapy portion of the treatment pro-gram. Aspirin often controls the pain satisfactorily when given in adequate dosages—eight to sixteen or more 0.3 gm. tablets daily. Many patients will not require any other medication. In other patients additional drugs are needed but the aspirin is continued as the basic drug.

Physical therapy in the form of heat applied to the joints and a daily exercise program is of fundamental importance in the treatment of rheumatoid arthritis. Heat, usually applied with a hot moist pack or a paraffin bath, is helpful in re-lieving stiffness and pain in muscles and joints. Therapeutic exercises are of vari-ous types, but basically accomplish two things: (1) maintenance or improve-ment of muscle strength, and (2) main-tenance or improvement of the range of joint motion. Special exercises may be prescribed at times but the objectives are still the same.

Other factors must be considered in the basic treatment program for patients with rheumatoid arthritis. Adequate nutrition is accomplished by a balanced diet having sufficient caloric intake to maintain normal weight. Overweight, even of moderate degree, is deleterious and should be corrected by diet. The adverse effect of obesity must be clearly explained to the patient, and the im-portance of weight reduction should be strongly emphasized. Special diets, sup-plements, or vitamins have no value in the treatment of rheumatoid arthritis. Treatment of other diseases when pres-ent should be done to improve the patient's general health.

Because rheumatoid arthritis is a chronic disease and the patients often have pain and are limited in the per-formance of their daily activities, it is common for them to become discouraged and to develop a poor outlook for the future. Moral support for the patient is a very important aspect of treatment and can mean the difference between success and failure of the overall program. It is very important that the patient develop the proper attitude toward his disease. Obviously, a give-up or hopeless reaction on the part of the patient is undesirable and when severe may be a major factor in causing disability. On the other hand, failure to acknowledge the limitations placed on him by the disease can cause the patient much difficulty too. Those patients who adopt a realistic attitude toward their disease, live within the limitations imposed by it, and follow advice for treatment definitely do better than those who do not. Physicians, nurses, and others concerned with the patient's care have a great deal of responsibility in this regard because it is from them that the patient derives many of his ideas and attitudes concerning his illness. Those who care for the arthritic patient must have a realistic but hopeful approach to the patient and his disease. Because of her frequent contact with the patient, the nurse has ample opportunity to benefit the patient in this area. Attitudes

of pity or unconcern will certainly have an undesirable effect.

Prevention of deformity is of the utmost importance, for when severe it may be the major cause of disability in an arthritic patient. Many components of the treatment program contribute to this aspect of therapy, such as resting an inflamed joint, medication to relieve pain, and physical therapy treatments to maintain joint motion and muscle strength. Braces or splints to support the joints may be indicated. Some are used only when the patient is resting or sleeping and others are used only when the patient is up and about. Shoes that give proper support are important in preventing or alleviating foot deformities.

An often neglected but very significant area for the prevention of deformity is the arthritic patient's bed in which he spends one-third to one-half of his time. The mattress must be firm with a bed board between it and the spring. The pillow should be thin so as to cause minimal flexion of the neck (Fig. 181). Pillows should never be placed beneath the knees because this will very likely

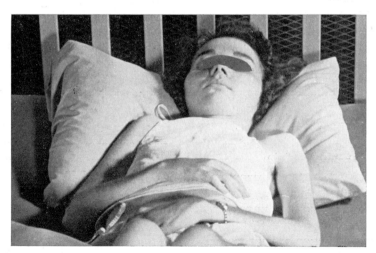

Fig. 181. Position frequently assumed by arthritic patients. Shoulders adducted, elbows and wrists flexed.

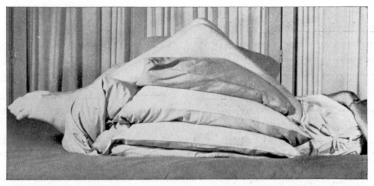

Fig. 182. Permanent flexion contractures of the knees and hips caused by the continuous use of pillows to support the knees in a flexed position. A common deformity in arthritis.

lead to the development of flexion contractures of the hips and knees (Fig. 182). This is a serious deformity. A pillow placed between the knees to separate the legs slightly, however, is definitely helpful in preventing adduction deformity of the hips. The bed should be relatively high because many arthritic patients have weak leg and hip muscles. The use of a footboard on the bed to prevent contracture of the heel cord (drop-foot deformity) and to keep the bed covers off the feet is important. Maintaining proper body alignment when resting is helpful in preventing deformity. The arthritic patient should lie with the joints extended as far as is comfortable a good portion of the time. Sandbags or a trochanter roll placed along the lateral aspect of the lower extremity help to maintain a neutral position of the hip joint. This prevents external rotation of the limb, an undesirable position for the patient with acute hip involvement.

Daily nursing care. Many aspects of daily nursing care that the nurse learns to do routinely require modification or individual attention with arthritic patients. Such simple things that are ordinarily done without thinking, such as going to the bathroom, turning in bed, or even moving an extremity, may be an ordeal for an arthritic patient because of pain or disability. He frequently requires a great deal of time. To hurry him or become impatient will only cause him unnecessary pain or dissatisfaction with the nurse. This will retard or prevent the nurse from developing satisfactory rapport with the patient. In the morning especially, or after a period of rest, the arthritic patient moves slowly because of the stiffness that is so characteristic of the disease. Pain is also frequently increased at these times. It is very worthwhile for the nurse to listen to the patient for often he has learned special ways of taking care of his needs that make it easier for him. Because there is an infinite variety in the types and degrees of disability in arthritic patients, care must be individualized according to the patient's needs. It is important to determine what the patient can and cannot do by himself. He should be expected to do those things of which he is capable, but he will require assistance in others. There is a distinct tendency for some patients to grow increasingly dependent on others, even for those things which they can do for themselves. This, of course, is to be discouraged and the patient should be led to do more and more for himself as his therapy progresses.

Standard nursing care activities such as bathing, shaving, brushing teeth, and making up beds are necessary parts of the patient's care and are not to be ignored. Because of disability, assistance may be required but should be given only if needed. The patient should be encouraged to establish a daily routine for performing self-care. Because arthritic patients may spend considerable time in bed, special attention to skin care is important. Cleanliness, and skin lotion when necessary, is most helpful. Careful attention must be given to pressure points located over bony prominences, such as the elbows, spinous processes of the vertebrae, sacrum, trochanters, ankles, and heels to prevent decubitus ulcers. Soft foam-rubber pads will offer some protection for these areas, but the most important preventive measure is frequent change of position. Observation of the patient performing his daily activities will give clues for making his efforts easier or less uncomfortable. A trapeze can be placed over the patient's bed to aid him in turning and in getting in and out of bed. The patient with troublesome weakness or pain in the legs will benefit from the use of a chair with a relatively high seat. It is much easier for him to get in and out of such a chair than from a low one. Armrests give additional assistance in getting in and out of a chair. If troublesome hand deformities are present, eating utensils with modified handles may be beneficial. Likewise, a chair in the shower to enable the patient to sit down while bathing, a bath sponge on a long handle, a long-handled shoehorn, or a rod with a hook at one end to help in putting on socks may be very helpful to the patient.

Many routine daily activities present potential injury hazards for the arthritic patient because of his weakness or instability. The bathtub and shower should be provided with handrails and nonslip floor mats. Wheelchairs, when the brakes are not applied, can be treacherous and all patients should be firmly warned of this. The rubber tips of crutches and canes are essential for safe use of these walking aids. Without them, or when they become worn, the danger of a serious fall is always present. Therefore, they should be checked frequently. Stairways must have handrails. Some of these precautions may seem unnecessary or obvious, but for the arthritic patient they are very important.

Special forms of treatment

Drugs. No matter what medications are used in the treatment of rheumatoid arthritis it must be remembered that none are curative. They are useful only to aid in the relief of pain and stiffness, and probably none has an effect on the disease itself. Therefore, these medications are never a substitute for the basic treatment program, but are additions to it and are of less importance than the basic program itself. Because pain in active arthritis is caused by inflammation, it follows that most of the drugs are used to suppress inflammation. Medications that have this effect include aspirin, phenylbutazone, the antimalarial drugs chloroquine and hydroxychloroquine, gold, and the various cortisone-like drugs that are frequently called corticosteroids or steroids.

Phenylbutazone is an anti-inflammatory drug of relatively low potency. It may be helpful in some patients when aspirin is not quite sufficient. Bone marrow depression or a decrease in the white blood cell count may be caused at times by this drug. Therefore, appropriate blood examination must be done periodically to detect these complications early if they should occur.

Two drugs, chloroquine and hydroxychloroquine, used in the treatment of malaria have been found to be beneficial in some patients with rheumatoid arthritis. Whether they will be helpful in an individual patient cannot be predicted. The beneficial effect, when it occurs, usually appears after approximately 3 months of treatment. After this period of time if it is felt that there has been a beneficial result, treatment is continued with a lower dosage. Chloroquine has clearly been shown to cause eye complications. One form of eye complication leads to visual impairment. Blindness also has resulted. For this reason it should no longer be used for the treatment of rheumatoid arthritis. Hydroxychloroquine is a similar but chemically slightly different drug. Serious eye complications have not yet been reported, but caution is required in this regard and eye examinations by an ophthalmologist should be done periodically. The drug is given in the same manner as chloroquine.

Gold has been used in the treatment of rheumatoid arthritis for approximately 30 years, and we have learned a great deal about the use of this drug. It is not beneficial in all patients, and treatment may have to be carried out for 3 to 4½ months before the beneficial effect is noted. If no benefit is noted after approximately 20 weeks, during which time a weekly intramuscular injection was given, it is usually not helpful to continue the drug. If it has been found that the gold has been beneficial after approximately 4 months of weekly treatments, the injections are given every 2 weeks for 2 to 3 months. Treatment can be continued with injections every 3 to 4 weeks after this as long as necessary. Gold has definite toxic properties that may appear as a skin rash, bone marrow depression, decrease in the white blood cell count, or abnormal substances in the urine. In nearly all instances of toxic reaction,

stopping the drug results in disappearance of the abnormality if done at the onset of the reaction. For this reason examination of the skin, blood, and urine should be done before each dose is given. Two preparations of gold are commonly used, both given intramuscularly. Gold sodium thiomalate is in aqueous solution. The trade name is Myochrysine. Gold sodium thioglucose is prepared usually as a suspension in oil. The trade name is Solganal. The common dosage schedule is 10 mg. in the first injection, 25 mg. in the second injection, and 50 mg. in each injection thereafter.

The cortisone-like drugs, or steroids as they are often called, have been used in the treatment of rheumatoid arthritis for more than ten years, and a great deal of experience has been gained in their use. They are potent drugs, both with respect to their effect of suppressing the inflammation of rheumatoid arthritis and their effects on many aspects of body metabolism. These metabolic effects are undesirable and may cause serious complications. Many types of steroids have been developed, but none is clearly superior to the others. Prednisone—one of the earlier types to be developed—is as effective as any other, has the benefit of a number of years of experience, is available in small-size tablets, and is less expensive than most of the other steroids.

The complications of steroid therapy are varied when large doses are used for prolonged periods. These complications include excessive weight gain, salt and water retention, high blood pressure, diabetes, peptic ulcer with all of its possible complications, osteoporosis that may lead to spontaneous fracture of bones, and mild to severe emotional changes—including psychosis. A rare but very serious complication of rheumatoid arthritis is the development of blood vessel inflammation that causes, among other things, severe muscle weakness or even paralysis and may lead to death. It is believed by most authorities that this is related to large doses of steroids. These complications frequently have severe effects on the patient's health, and may constitute serious illness by themselves. When added to the disability of rheumatoid arthritis, they may incapacitate the patient. Small doses of steroids usually improve the patient's symptoms. The incidence and severity of complications increase with an increase in the dose of steroids. Therefore, the drug should always be given in the smallest dose that adequately controls the patient's symptoms. The recommended maximum dosage of prednisone is 8 mg. per day.

Steroids are also frequently used in the treatment of arthritis by injection into the joints. It has none of the risks associated with systemic steroid therapy. The results, while good in most instances, are quite different than when steroids are given orally. Injection of a steroid into a joint gives improvement in that joint only, whereas systemic steroid treatment suppresses inflammation in all joints. Injection of a steroid into the joints is most often done when one or a few joints are significantly more inflamed and painful than the others. The beneficial results are temporary, lasting an average of 10 to 14 days. A joint may be safely injected repeatedly at frequent intervals if indicated. The only major complication of this method of treatment is that of introducing infection into the joint. If strict attention is paid to aseptic technique, avoidance of this catastrophe can be virtually guaranteed. Hydrocortisone TBA (hydrocortisone *tert.*-butylacetate) and prednisolone TBA are the two most effective preparations for joint injection. The average dose is 25 mg. of either preparation, ranging from 15 mg. to 50 mg., depending largely on the size of the joint.

Braces, splints, and traction. As a result of the weakening and stretching of the joint capsule or supporting ligaments, or because of severe destruction of cartilage and bone within the joint, troublesome instability of the joint may be present. This may cause severe pain or result in a joint that is too unstable to function properly. The use of a movable brace to give added support to the joint can be quite helpful at times. They are most often used for support of knees and ankles.

During treatment for relief of joint contractures, the use of a rigid support that places a mild, steady stretching force on the contracture is of definite benefit. Such a support is referred to as a splint. Splints are most frequently used on the knees, but can be used for contractures of other joints (Fig. 184). Splints are also of benefit when used to support an acutely inflamed and painful joint. In this instance the support gives relief of pain and aids in the prevention of a contracture. Recent development of effective rigid splints for support of unstable wrists and knuckle joints of the hands offers promise for effective relief of this difficult problem. Such splints can be worn when working.

Proper application of braces and splints to the extremities is important for their proper function and for the prevention of pain and pressure sores. In this respect the nurse has an important responsibility to the patient using these devices. Early recognition of these problems will prevent unnecessary discomfort or a troublesome complication for the patient. The nurse should become thoroughly familiar with the proper use of braces and splints.

Occasionally, when severe contractures are present, traction is used in an

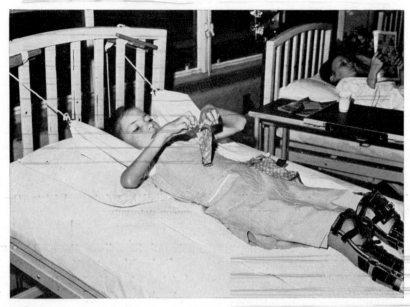

Fig. 183. Method of maintaining abduction of arms without interfering with activity of hands.

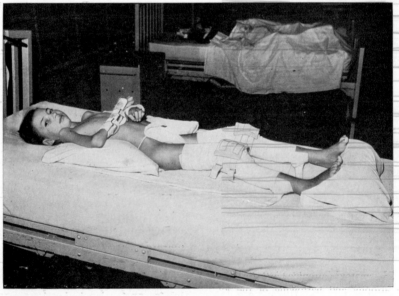

Fig. 184. Rest position with pillow under dorsal spine. Adducted position of arms is undesirable for long periods and should be alternated with positions of abduction and external rotation. Note night splints applied with Ace bandages to prevent flexion contractures of the knees. Bars attached at the ankle area prevent rotation of the limb.

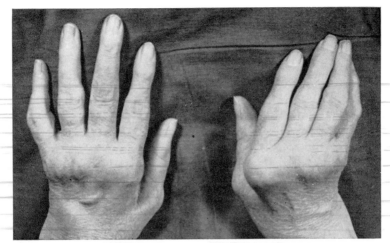

Fig. 185. Arthritic hands. Note the enlarged metacarpophalangeal joints and the spindle-shaped fingers as a result of the swelling of the proximal interphalangeal joints. The ulnar deviation of the fingers on the right hand is a common deformity.

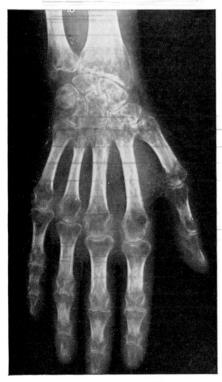

Fig. 186. Rheumatoid (atrophic) arthritis showing bone atrophy and narrowing of the joint space. (From Kenney, William C., and Larson, Carroll B.: Orthopedics for the general practitioner, St. Louis, 1957, The C. V. Mosby Co.)

attempt to relieve them. This may be applied either to the skin or to the skeleton. A patient in traction requires meticulous nursing care in order to prevent complications. One of the most common is pressure sores resulting from contact with either the bed or the traction apparatus. Because of pain, stiffness, and his resulting reluctance to move, the arthritic patient is quite vulnerable to decubitus ulcers. Therefore, his care requires strict attention to details on the part of the nurse. Important are such simple things as frequent changes in the patient's position in bed, providing at all times clean bed linens that are kept smoothly in place, minor adjustments in the position of the traction apparatus, and protective sponge-rubber padding over pressure points when necessary.

Surgery. Surgical treatment of rheumatoid arthritis is indicated in many patients. Operations are performed for removal of swollen synovial tissue in joints and about tendons, repair of severely weakened or ruptured ligaments and tendons, and release of severe contractures. Joints that have severe destructive changes may require insertion of a prosthesis (an artificial joint or joint portion), a repair procedure (arthroplasty) or, at times, bony fusion. The principles and details of nursing care pertaining to both arthritic and orthopedic surgical patients must be applied simultaneously in these patients and may be a challenging task.

DEGENERATIVE ARTHRITIS (OSTEOARTHRITIS, DEGENERATIVE JOINT DISEASE)

Degenerative (hypertrophic) arthritis, as the name implies, is the result of joint deterioration, specifically of the joint cartilage and underlying bone. This process results in varying degrees of joint destruction, but usually not of great severity. The weight-bearing joints of the lower extremities are most often affected and usually only one or a few joints are involved. The cause of degenerative arthritis is not known, although there is clearly an association with the aging process of joint cartilage. It is not a systemic disease but is confined to the joint. The onset of this disease is usually during middle or old age.

The major complaint of patients with degenerative arthritis is that of joint pain upon weight bearing or motion which is relieved by rest. There frequently is also stiffness of the involved joint that is relieved by a few minutes or less of activity. The joint may appear to be normal on examination. Frequently, however, there is grating on motion and there may be bony enlargement. Accumulation of fluid is not uncommon, but it is not usually a large amount.

When degenerative arthritis with significant pain has been present for a relatively long period of time, mild to moderate contracture of the joint capsule often occurs along with muscle

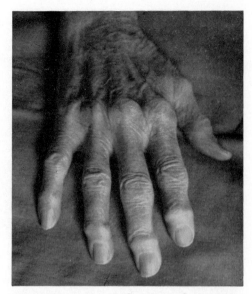

Fig. 187. Heberden's nodes. In hypertrophic arthritis the distal interphalangeal joints may become painful and deformed. (In atrophic arthritis the metacarpophalangeal joints and the proximal interphalangeal joints are involved.)

weakness. This results in limitation of joint motion. Although relatively uncommon, severe joint destruction when it does occur may result in marked limitation of motion and more severe pain.

One of the most common sites of occurrence of degenerative arthritis is in the distal finger joints, those nearest the finger tips. The bony enlargement of these joints has been given the name of Heberden's nodes (Fig. 187). The cause for involvement of these small nonweight-bearing joints is unknown. Women are affected approximately twenty times oftener than men and there is a definite hereditary factor in this form of arthritis. Frequently there are no symptoms. It is not uncommon, however, for these patients to have mild aching pain. Hand function is seldom significantly affected.

The course of degenerative arthritis

usually progresses very slowly. The severity of symptoms parallels fairly closely with the amount of use of the involved joint. Most patients have mild to moderate restriction of activity, largely because of pain. Relatively few patients have severe limitation of physical activity. A patient rarely will be severely incapacitated because of degenerative arthritis.

Traumatic arthritis is degenerative arthritis occurring in a joint that has been previously injured. The injury may have been in the nature of infection, repeated dislocation, fracture, or another type of arthritis. There is an interval of time, months or even years after the injury, before the degenerative arthritis appears. It may be mild or severe, depending upon the severity of the previous injury and other factors.

Treatment and nursing care. Because degenerative arthritis involves only a few joints, patients with this form of arthritis are usually more easily cared for than those with rheumatoid arthritis. Occasionally patients with severe involvement, for example, of both knees or both hips, will have considerable disability. The presence of other diseases affecting their general health may cause, in conjunction with their arthritis, disability more severe than would result from the arthritis alone. In a patient with a heart disease that limits his physical endurance, the presence of moderately severe degenerative arthritis in a hip or knee may cause walking to be much more laborious with the result that endurance is further reduced. Very often patients with this form of arthritis are elderly and may require modification of care and treatment routines.

The basic principles of treatment are the same for degenerative arthritis as for rheumatoid arthritis, including rest, relief of pain, and physical therapy. Because degenerative arthritis is not a sys-

temic disease, these patients require no more bed rest or sleep than if they did not have arthritis. Rest of the involved joints, however, is very desirable because it provides for relief of pain. Usually this can be accomplished by resting in a chair. Some patients, however, must lie down for relief of pain, especially when the hips are involved. Frequent interruption of activity with short rest periods is much more effective than occasional long periods of rest.

The need for medication to relieve pain is usually not great. Two or three aspirin tablets three or four times daily usually is sufficient. At times, when aspirin alone is not adequate, the addition of phenylbutazone for a 5- to 10-day period is often helpful. The other drugs used in the treatment of rheumatoid arthritis have no value in this disease. Specifically, steroids, the cortisone-like drugs, should never be given orally. Injection of a steroid into a joint with troublesome pain, however, is frequently helpful in relieving symptoms. The same doses are used as in rheumatoid arthritis.

A large proportion of patients with hypertrophic arthritis are cared for in the home. Mild degrees of the condition are very common among the population beyond middle-age. These persons will usually be hospitalized only when reconstructive surgery is necessary, although they may enter the hospital briefly for corset or brace fittings or for periods of physical therapy.

The health supervision the nurse can give in the home may be an important detail. Health supervision will include attention to details for improvement of the patient's posture and general habits of working, sitting, and standing. Constant sitting for patients with hypertrophic arthritis of hip or spine is a bad practice. It often leads to flexion contractures of hips, adduction of hips, and a tendency toward dorsal kyphosis. Within the limits of the patient's tolerance, activity is to be encouraged. These are not patients who are to be encouraged to assume a life of idleness or sedentary occupation when other activity is possible.

If shoe corrections have been prescribed, nurses should check frequently to see that these do not become worn down and useless. Shoe corrections provide support and comfort to pronated feet, which are common in this condition, and they may have a great deal to do with improvement in posture. If a brace or corset has been ordered, frequent inspection of the apparatus and supervision of its application is important. If postural exercises have been prescribed, the nurse should have a full understanding of these so that she may be able to assist and encourage the patient in their performance.

Another point of importance in which the nurse may play an important role is that of giving reassurance. Worry is not an uncommon feature encountered in patients having this condition. They should be brought to understand that hypertrophic arthritis does not tend to cause rigid joints and that it does not go from one joint to the other as does rheumatoid arthritis. When the patient understands this, a great burden is sometimes lifted from his mind, particularly if he has a secret fear of becoming a helpless cripple, having perhaps seen a friend or relative crippled with rheumatism.

Physical therapy plays an important role in the treatment of this form of arthritis. The objectives are the same as in rheumatoid arthritis. This aspect of the treatment program is a major factor in preventing increasing disability by maintaining muscle strength.

Local treatment may consist of heat in some form, such as baking, diathermy, and hot moist fomentations. These latter may be given as in poliomyelitis and have often been found to afford considerable relief from pain and muscle spasm. Massage may be ordered to the muscles above or below the affected joints. Exercises must be taken cautiously because they tend to be followed by exacerbation of symptoms. Complete immobilization, on the other hand, must also be avoided because of the danger of disuse atrophy.

The use of a cane or crutches is often helpful in relieving pain by decreasing the amount of weight borne by the joint. Contractures causing limitations of joint motion are not uncommon. Frequently contractures can be greatly improved with exercises and, at times, night splints. Occasionally surgery will be required. Marked joint destruction associated with severe pain or limited motion, or both, may require surgical treatment. This is usually in the form of an arthroplasty, a repair of the joint.

GOUT

Gout is a disease resulting from the abnormal metabolism of uric acid. In gout there is an increase in the amount of uric acid in the body that is reflected in an increase in its concentration in the blood. The clinical picture of gout is characterized by this elevation of blood uric acid concentration along with recurrent attacks of acute severely painful arthritis. In some patients with gout, deposits of uric acid known as tophi occur in various places in the body (Fig. 188). Approximately 95% of gout cases are men. There is no doubt of a hereditary factor in this disease. In approximately one-half of the cases a history of gout in family members can be obtained. The age of onset, determined by the first attack of acute gouty arthritis, is usually between 20 and 60 years of age.

The typical acute attack of gout begins rather abruptly. There is severe constant pain and the joint becomes swollen and red. The usual attack lasts for 3 to 10 days when untreated.

For unknown reasons the large joint of the great toe is involved much more commonly than any other joint. Other joints in the foot, the ankle, and the knee are also commonly affected. Any joint in the body, however, may be involved.

The course of gout is quite variable,

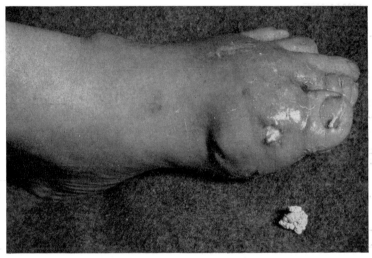

Fig. 188. Gouty arthritis with involvement of the first metatarsophalangeal joint, urate crystals, and a draining sinus from a large tophus.

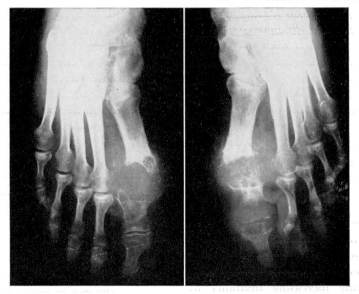

Fig. 189. Gout. Note the predilection for involvement of the first metatarsophalangeal joint. (From Kenney, William C., and Larson, Carroll B.: Orthopedics for the general practitioner, St. Louis, 1957, The C. V. Mosby Co.)

from one or a few attacks during a lifetime to a progressively severe disease with marked crippling, when untreated, in some patients. Most patients, however, fall between these two extremes. With proper treatment attacks of acute gout are infrequent and crippling deformities do not occur.

Treatment and nursing care. Few patients with gout require hospitalization for orthopedic treatment. Medications are available that are very effective in controlling the disease. Colchicine is the traditional drug of choice for treatment of the acute attack. It is given in the dose of one tablet (0.5 mg. or 0.65 mg.) every hour until the attack improves; until nausea, vomiting, or diarrhea occurs; or until a total dose of twelve tablets has been taken. Relief of the attack is almost always striking. Phenylbutazone is equally effective for relief of the acute attack, or may be combined with colchicine in a stubborn attack. It is given in a dose of 800 to 1000 mg. on the first day, followed by reducing dosages over a period of one week. Colchicine is also important for prevention of recurrent attacks, and the

dose is usually two or three tablets daily. Probenecid (Benemid) is an equally important drug used in the treatment of gout. Its function is to increase excretion of uric acid by the kidney, reducing the total amount of this substance in the body. It has no effect on the acute attack of gout. In order for it to be effective, probenecid must be taken regularly every day. Severe dietary restriction, once a standard part of the treatment program, is no longer advocated because it does not contribute greatly to reducing the amount of uric acid in the body. Avoidance of foods high in purine content—such as liver, kidney, sweetbreads, sardines, anchovies, and meat gravies—is a reasonable measure.

When properly treated, gout rarely causes deforming arthritis. The untreated or inadequately treated patient, however, may develop a variety of deformities and contractures of joints. In addition, there may be severe destruction of multiple joints in the late stages of chronic gouty arthritis. These problems require the same principles of treatment and nursing care as in other forms of arthritis.

STUDY QUESTIONS

1. What is the basic objective in the care and treatment of a patient with arthritis? What are the roles of the various people who may be involved in the patient's care?
2. What are the principles that guide the nurse in her care of a patient with arthritis?
3. What is the fundamental difference between rheumatoid arthritis and degenerative arthritis?
4. What are the basic ingredients of a treatment program for a patient with arthritis?
5. To what details of care and arrangement of the patient's bed must the nurse give her attention? What is the objective?
6. What are the two ways in which rest is beneficial to a patient with rheumatoid arthritis? How does this differ in a patient with degenerative arthritis?
7. Contractures are to a large degree preventable. What important contributions can be made by the nurse in this regard?
8. The patient with arthritis who lives within the limitations imposed by his disease does better than those who do not. How may the nurse help the patient to adopt this attitude?

REFERENCES

Arthritis and related disorders, J. Phys. Ther. A. **44:**574-619, July, 1964.

Bland, J. H.: Arthritis medical treatment and home care, A book for family use, New York, 1960, The Macmillan Co.

Brooke, J. W.: Arthritis and you, New York, 1960, Harper & Brothers.

Crain, D. C.: Help for ten million, Philadelphia, 1958, J. B. Lippincott Co.

Ellison, A.: The function of corrective therapy in the treatment of rheumatoid arthritis, J. A. Phys. & Ment. Rehab. **9:**196-197, 1955.

Flatt, A.: The care of the rheumatoid hand, St. Louis, 1963, The C. V. Mosby Co.

Glomset, D. A.: Current trends in the management of arthritis, J. Iowa M. Soc. **46:**285-289, 1956.

Goldring, D., Behrer, M. R., and McQuater, F.: Rheumatoid arthritis in children, Am. J. Nursing **56:**1437-1439, 1956.

Jaschik, E., and Olsen, C.: Nursing care of the arthritic patient at home, Am. J. Nursing **55:**429-432, 1955.

Jessar, R. A., and Hollander, J. L.: Types of arthritis and their medical treatment, Am. J. Nursing **55:**426-429, 1955.

Lamont-Havers, R. W.: Arthritis quackery, Am. J. Nursing **63:**92-95, 1963.

Lowman, E. W.: Arthritis, general principles, physical medicine rehabilitation, Boston, 1959, Little, Brown & Co.

Lowman, E. W., Lee, P. R., and Rusk, H. A.: Total rehabilitation of the rheumatoid arthritic cripple, J.A.M.A. **158:**1335-1344, 1955.

Manual for Nurses: Arthritis and related disorders, issued by the Medical and Scientific Committee, Arthritis and Rheumatism Foundation, 23 West 45th Street, New York 36, N. Y.

McDermott, I. K., and Wensley, E.: We can help arthritic patients, Nursing Outlook **3:**582-585, 1955.

Miale, J. E., and Plotz, C. M.: Nursing care of patients with rheumatoid arthritis during therapy with cortisone, Am. J. Nursing **53:**290-293, 1953.

Phelps, A. E.: Your arthritis: what you can do about it, New York, 1953, William Morrow & Co.

Rossman, I. J., and Schwartz, D. R.: The family handbook of home nursing and medical care, New York, 1959, Random House.

Strike back at arthritis, issued by the U. S. Department of Health, Education, and Welfare Public Health Service in collaboration with The Arthritis and Rheumatism Foundation. Superintendent of Documents, U. S. Government Printing Office, Washington, D. C.

Talbott, J. H.: Gout and gouty arthritis, Nursing Outlook **2:**540-543, 1954.

Talbott, J. H., and Ricketts, A.: Gout and gouty arthritis Am. J. Nursing **59:**1405-1408, 1959.

Young, H. H., Ward, L. E., and Henderson, E. D.: The use of hydrocortisone acetate in the treatment of some common orthopaedic conditions, J. Bone & Joint Surg. **36-A:**602-608, 1954.

Chapter 8

Poliomyelitis, including nursing care

CAUSE

Prior to the use of the Salk vaccine, and now the Sabin vaccine, there were a few cases of poliomyelitis in every community every year, and occasionally the disease would appear in epidemic form. Since the widespread use of the vaccine, the number of cases reported has been reduced drastically, and epidemics have been eliminated. Because of the lack, however, of epidemic control in many countries, this chapter on the care of poliomyelitis patients has been retained partially in its detailed form.

The condition occurs most commonly in the late summer months, although epidemics have occurred in the early winter months. Young children are most often affected, but there seems to be no age limit to the susceptibility to infection.

One theory is based on the probability that it is a common childhood disease but that paralysis occurs only in the severely affected persons. It is postulated that immunity against the disease is developed in many instances without the entire clinical picture being present and without knowledge that the person has had the disease. This is borne out to some extent by clinical studies in large epidemics in which it appears that only about 10% of those who are examined show some laboratory and some clinical evidence of the types that develop paralysis.

The infectious organism is known definitely to be a virus that is minute enough to pass through the Berkefeld filter, but it has never been demonstrated microscopically. Three strains of the poliomyelitis virus have been isolated. An attack of poliomyelitis does not develop immunity to more than one strain of the virus.

PATHOLOGY

The destructive lesions in poliomyelitis are in the anterior horn cells of the spinal cord. The motor system of the body consists of three groups of cells: (1) those in the brain that initiate the motions, (2) those in the medulla and ganglia that coordinate the motions, and (3) those in the spinal cord (the anterior horn cells) that transmit the impulse to the muscle cells.

The anterior horn cells are distributed in groups throughout the entire spinal cord but are concentrated in the groups that supply nerve impulses to the upper and lower extremities. These groups of cells are arranged more or less in small groups supplying individual muscles,

240

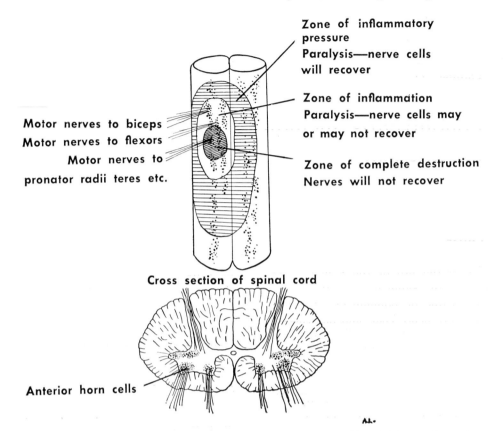

Zone of inflammatory
pressure
Paralysis—nerve cells
will recover

Zone of inflammation
Paralysis—nerve cells may
or may not recover

Zone of complete destruction
Nerves will not recover

Motor nerves to biceps
Motor nerves to flexors
Motor nerves to
pronator radii teres etc.

Cross section of spinal cord

Anterior horn cells

Fig. 190. Schematic drawing of spinal cord showing the method of attack of poliomyelitis.

such as the deltoid, the biceps, the gluteus maximus, the quadriceps, etc.

During an attack of poliomyelitis the following may occur: (1) There may be several areas where complete destruction of cell, either by local activity of the disease itself or the destructive effects of the toxins formed, may cause an actual degenerative process of varying size and degree. (2) Waste products and edema may endanger the vitality of a major group of cells around the destroyed area. (3) Beyond this are large inflammatory changes that temporarily incapacitate a much larger group of cells. This accounts for the degree and speed of recovery of the functional power in muscles.

In the completely destroyed areas there will never be any return of muscle power. In the intermediate zone the cells may recover or disintegrate according to the demands placed upon them. Rest is the important factor. The cells damaged by relatively mild inflammatory change only will recover under almost any condition.

The rapid recovery that takes place within 1 to 3 weeks after an attack of poliomyelitis is because the muscles are innervated by the cells that have been impaired temporarily by the inflammatory process.

The recovery that may or may not take place in the following weeks or months is directly related to the number of cells destroyed or not destroyed by the edema and waste products of the disease activity.

The permanent paralysis is directly related to the number of cells destroyed by the local activity of the disease.

Improvement continues in patients with poliomyelitis (infantile paralysis) for at least several years. Any improvement after a few months, however, is not the result of any further recovery of the nerves but rather to improved function of the muscle fibers whose nerves of stimulation have already recovered.

There are two other types of involvement with poliomyelitis. The bulbar type consists of an involvement of the nerve cells high up in the spinal cord. If the inflammatory condition reaches the vital centers, the condition is fatal. If the damage is not sufficient to cause death, a relatively complete recovery usually occurs within a few weeks or months. These patients may require the use of the respirator during the more active stage of the disease because of the paralysis of the intercostal muscles and the diaphragm. Poliomeningitis manifests symptoms that are frequently very similar to other forms of meningitis, including delirium, stiff neck, strabismus, and incontinence. Actual paralysis of the muscles is not usually present. There may be flaccidity or spasticity of the extremities.

SYMPTOMS AND SIGNS

The disease usually begins rather abruptly with a headache and an intestinal disturbance. There may be an elevation of temperature from 99° to 102° F. There is usually some evidence of spinal cord irritation that is recognized by stiffness of the neck with some resistance and pain in the back when attempts are made to raise the head from the bed. Paralysis, when it develops, usually occurs somewhere between the third and seventh day after the onset of the illness. In some cases, however, the initial symptoms are so mild that the disease is not recognized until paralysis

has set in. The patient may fall because of weakness of a limb.

In those persons in whom paralysis does not develop, all symptoms may disappear within 2 or 3 days. It is unwise, however, to give any statement regarding the severity of the disease until 48 hours have elapsed after the disappearance of all fever because apparently mild cases may subsequently become severe. When paralysis develops, there may be pain on movement of the limbs and joints or on pressure upon the muscles involved. After the acute symptoms, the patient is usually quite comfortable except for this.

HOW POLIOMYELITIS IS DIAGNOSED

The early symptoms of poliomyelitis are not such as will point definitely to the disease in a nonepidemic period. Headache is present in a large percentage of the patients who are old enough to complain of it. Fever is not excessively high, ranging usually from 101° to 103° F. Nausea, vomiting, and constipation or diarrhea may be present. Stiff neck and back are common. Many physicians have commented that the early symptoms tend to be flu-like in character (the characteristic minor illness), but a head cold is not considered a common early symptom of poliomyelitis. Sore throats occur in a low percentage except in the bulbar type of the disease, when they are considered to be of neuritic origin. Considerable soreness of peripheral areas to touch is commonly found, and spasm of the posterior neck muscles, the back extensor muscles, and the hamstring muscles is thought to be highly significant in diagnosing the disease.

All these symptoms may disappear after 24 hours. Sometimes there is an interval of a week or more before further symptoms appear. Formerly, this type of

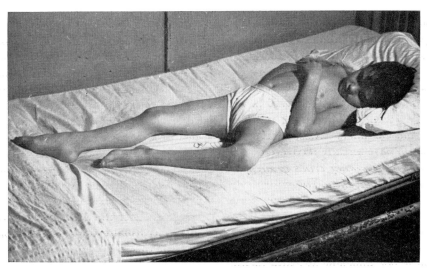

Fig. 191. Frog position often assumed by child with poliomyelitis during the acute illness. (From Steindler, A., and Greteman, T. J.: Care of infantile paralysis in the home: a handbook for parents, Iowa City, Iowa, 1938, Children's Hospital.)

onset was referred to as dromedary but is now called Bactrian, named after the Bactrian two-humped camel.

Patients with fully developed cases of poliomyelitis almost invariably show muscle tenderness and rigidity in the back, neck, and hamstring muscles. The tendency for the patient to assume what has sometimes been called the frog position has long been considered characteristic of the disease. Because sacrospinalis spasm and hamstring spasm are present in a large number of patients, whether they be severe or so mild that paralysis does not develop, it is easy to understand why flexion of the knees and hyperextension of the back and neck are often observed.

Diagnosis is confirmed by the spinal tap and identification of the virus (one of three strains now known). Many recently identified viruses such as the ECHO group can cause symptoms, exclusive of paralysis, that simulate the acute stage of poliomyelitis. A spinal fluid examination that reveals a slight increase in pressure, a clear appearance, and a cell count of from 10 to 300 or slightly higher is considered very significant. The cell count, if performed early enough, shows a predominance of polymorphonuclear leukocytes, but these are succeeded within 24 to 48 hours by lymphocytes. Spinal sugar is normal; nurses will remember that it will be about one half the amount of the blood sugar. Chlorides are normal, and the Pandy test for spinal globulin may be positive, 1 to 4 plus. The total protein is usually increased, and an elevation of 45 mg. per cubic millimeter or above is thought to be significant. The virus has not yet been found in the spinal fluid, nor has it been isolated in the bloodstream.

If laboratory facilities are available, the poliomyelitis virus should be looked for, by the use of suitable culture techniques, in the stool of the patient or in throat washings.

Some patients have none of these systemic symptoms. They may, however, have them in so minor a degree that they are overlooked as having any significance. There is also the patient who apparently has no symptoms at all until he actually becomes paralyzed. What prodromal symptoms he has are mild or disguised by another condition. One adult patient told of the onset of the disease as being so mild and localized that he thought it was a return of a myositis of the shoulder that he sometimes had seasonally. Another patient, a young woman in the seventh month of pregnancy, recognized nothing until she returned from a shopping trip and became paralyzed an hour later.

CURRENT THEORIES REGARDING SPREAD OF THE DISEASE

Because it has been established that the virus may leave the body of the patient (or healthy carrier) in the discharges of the bowel or the nose and throat, it seems safe to assume that person-to-person contact must play a large part in the spread of the disease. Although the upper respiratory passages are no longer considered the primary routes of infection, nevertheless, the exact manner in which the virus enters the body is not completely understood and care should be used in handling the discharges from the nose and throat of any patient suspected of having poliomyelitis. The virus has repeatedly been recovered from the throat of patients during the first 3 to 5 days of the disease. For this reason it would seem advisable for nurses to be masked when caring for these patients during the acute stage and while working directly over the patient. This procedure is necessary in order to prevent contamination by droplet transmission. Nurses should disinfect all discharges from the nose and throat as carefully as those from the gastrointestinal tract.

It is now an accepted fact that the virus of poliomyelitis remains in the gastrointestinal tract sometimes over a period of weeks, and, therefore, considerable attention must be given to the matter of disinfecting stools. The nurse working in the area of communicable disease where these patients are cared for should seek definite instruction as to the disposal of excreta. The process will vary somewhat from state to state, according to rules set down by the state board of health. Where an efficient sewage disposal system is available, of course, fecal disinfection is not necessary. When possible, it is advisable to use disposable diapers for young children during an epidemic.

Present-day knowledge indicates that there are three strains of the poliomyelitis virus that cause the disease in human beings. Immunity from infection from one strain of the virus does not necessarily assure immunity from the others. Furthermore, the virus has been noted to be extremely variable in its activity in different hosts and to alter considerably with the changes in and around these hosts. The time factor, for instance, from exposure to the onset of the disease seems to be exceedingly variable, and it has been stated by some investigators that an outbreak lasting several weeks may possibly be the result of the exposure of all victims at the same time.

It has been known for quite some time that fatigue and chilling seem to play a definite part in the etiology of the disease. The explanation of this is not entirely clear, but it is thought by some authorities that the spinal cord may be invaded by the virus in the early stages of the disease—that it is, in fact, present in the spinal cord approximately as early as it is in the intestinal tract. Strenuous work, exercise, or chilling may be the factors needed to activate the virus or to lower the body's defenses against the disease so that immediate paralytic symptoms appear. Parents should be instructed to insist on proper rest habits for their children during epidemic seasons and to guard against overexertion and chilling.

HEALTH TEACHING AND THE PREVENTION OF POLIOMYELITIS

At the present time, the nurse's most important responsibility pertaining to poliomyelitis lies in the area of prevention. Helping parents understand the necessity of having members of the family receive the poliomyelitis vaccine, and providing them with information of immunization programs available in their community are vital if this disease is to be prevented. The oral vaccine is available at a minimum cost, and every child and adult should receive this protection against poliomyelitis. Additional teaching done by the nurse is based on a few rules of hygiene dictated by our present-day concepts of the disease. Because in many cases it seems unquestionable that the virus is ingested, all foods should be protected from filth, flies, dirty hands, and animals. If food is to be eaten raw, it should be well washed. Hands should be carefully washed not merely before meals but before eating any food. Milk should be certified or pasteurized, and the water supply should be from approved sources. Because one of the nurse's chief duties is to prevent the spread of misinformation, it should be pointed out at this time that modern epidemiologic evidence does not seem to indicate that infected milk or water has ever been the source of an epidemic.

The necessity for having adequate rest and of avoiding strenuous exercise and chilling should be emphasized in health teaching.

POLIOMYELITIS VACCINE

The method by which poliomyelitis is spread from person to person is not known. During the past few years, however, there has been considerable progress in immunization against this disease. The incidence of poliomyelitis since the advent of the Salk vaccine has declined to the point where no cases were reported in the state of Iowa during 1963. The Salk vaccine is produced from the killed virus of the three poliomyelitis strains, and all three types are combined. It is necessary to inject the vaccine four times, over a period of 7 months. Booster injections have to be given yearly to insure protection against polio. The Salk vaccine is rapidly being replaced by the Sabin live virus vaccine that can be taken by mouth. It is made from live virus modified (weakened) for the purpose of producing immunity without producing chronic illness, much like the smallpox vaccine. The Sabin oral vaccine has been given to more than 70 million people in Russia, Mexico, Czechoslovakia and Yugoslavia with excellent results. Several hundred thousand doses have been used in the United States with complete safety.

Only one type of virus can be given at a time when using the oral vaccine. If all three types of virus are mixed into a polyvalent vaccine, it is possible that type I and III may be suppressed by an overgrowth of type II. The oral vaccine usually produces an intestinal barrier against infection and eliminates the vaccinated person as a carrier. This cannot be accomplished with killed virus vaccine. The oral vaccine may be given to persons of all ages. It is safe for newborn infants, but if the first dose is given before the age of 6 weeks, it may be necessary to give a booster dose when the child is a year old. After the age of 3 months, each monovalent vaccine can be given at intervals of 6 weeks; never less than 4 weeks. Definite side effects or symptoms clearly attributable to the feeding of the Sabin oral vaccine have not been reported.

ISOLATION OF THE PATIENT

The incubation period for this disease is now thought to be rather brief, but it appears that in some instances it may be as long as 35 days. The average period, however, is usually considered to be from about 4 days to 2 weeks. As in other infectious diseases, a short incubation period has been noted to be significant of a more severe involvement. The period of infection is now thought to be about 3 days before and 3 days after the onset of prodromal symptoms.

The patient is usually isolated for approximately 2 weeks, although in some localities it may be longer. The fact that recent investigations have established the presence of the virus in the gastrointestinal tract for many weeks after the onset of the disease makes the whole question of quarantine a very involved problem. The extent of isolation varies in different localities and in different institutions. Rigid isolation precautions may be the rule in some instances, whereas group isolation may be the rule in others. The nurse may work in some localities where segregation, scrupulous attention to cleanliness, and the disinfection of excreta are the only precautions observed. The general tendency, however, is still toward careful isolation of these patients.

Poliomyelitis is usually considered as customarily attacking only one member of a family. This has never been consistently confirmed by experience. Although it is true that often only one member of the family becomes paralyzed, it is suspected that other members of the family are affected and that they probably became infected through a common source. In most of the victims paralysis does not develop, and, therefore, it is not recognized that the other family members have manifested the disease by mild symptoms, such as those of a summer cold, influenza, or similar indispositions.

TREATMENT

Treatment of poliomyelitis is divided into three stages: acute, convalescent, and reconstruction.

During the acute and febrile stage, rest is all-important. A firm bed and relaxation of the affected extremities in a position of physiologic rest has been the treatment of choice. This consists in maintaining the shoulders in slight abduction, the elbows flexed or extended, and the wrists at slight dorsiflexion. In the lower extremities the knee and hip are flexed a few degrees, and the foot is held in a position at right angles to the leg.

Warm moist packs may be applied to the involved parts. Passive exercises performed by a physical therapist help maintain a normal range of motion. This treatment seems to have the advantage of eliminating stasis in the muscles, thereby preventing spasm and contractures, maintaining flexibility, and making the patient more comfortable; but, unquestionably, nothing can effect the recovery of the nerve cells in the anterior horn of the spinal cord.

Deformity should be prevented during the convalescent stage, but if it occurs or if weaknesses persist the limbs must be protected by braces or the deformities corrected by operation, or both.

Nurse's responsibility. Until a few years ago, treatment of the paralysis in poliomyelitis was based upon principles of constant protection of the weakened muscles. All nursing procedures had to be adapted to this feature of treatment. Weakened muscles were protected against the strong, normal antagonistic muscles at all times lest they be stretched out like old elastic. The weakened muscle was kept as short as possible to protect against stretching—that is, the origin and insertion of the affected muscles were brought as close together as was possible and kept that way during a long course of treatment and bed rest. This was accomplished by the use of splints and later by braces. Aside from this one common feature of immobilization for muscle protection,

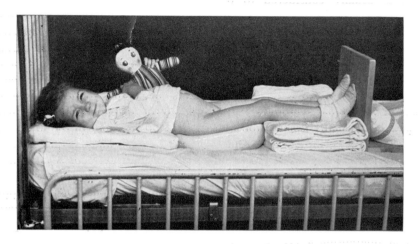

Fig. 192. Arrangement of bedpan for child not on frame so that support of back and legs is maintained. (From Steindler, A., and Greteman, T. J.: Care of infantile paralysis in the home: a handbook for parents, Iowa City, Iowa, 1938, Children's Hospital.)

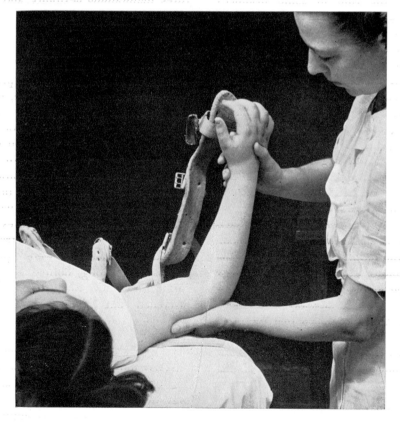

Fig. 193. Manner of lifting a paralyzed arm from splint. Note support given to elbow and wrist. (From Steindler, A., and Greteman, T. J.: Care of infantile paralysis in the home: a handbook for parents, Iowa City, Iowa, 1938, Children's Hospital.)

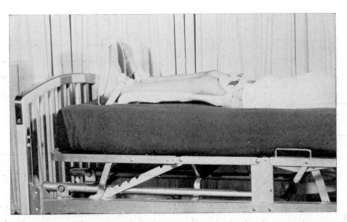

Fig. 194. Toronto splints frequently used in convalescent poliomyelitis to maintain good position of the lower extremities. The crossbar at the ankle (not visible in the picture) prevents external rotation of the limb. Note space for the heel, a likely spot for decubitus ulcers if permitted to rest on the bed.

there was no universal agreement as to the care of the patients. Mobilization varied in degree and type from complete rigid immobilization in circular casts to the use of splints for only part of the day while complete range of joint motion was carried out during physical therapy treatments.

Muscle tenderness, a fairly constant symptom, was of great concern to patient and nurse. Because of this tenderness, physical therapy was usually not begun until the end of this period, although there were exceptions to this rule and some doctors ordered daily warm baths or packs soon after quarantine was over, or, in some cases, before. Heat and massage, passive and active exercises, were seldom begun while any muscle tenderness existed. Muscle stimuluation by electricity had some advocates, but it was not in general use. Improvised splinting by use of pillows, sandbags, towels, boxes, and the like were usually employed for muscle protection until the period of quarantine was over. After that, permanent splints, such as bivalved casts, wire splints, or specially constructed metal and leather apparatus, were employed.

External heat for the elimination of muscle tenderness was used in many localities for years. Some institutions routinely applied hot moist packs for this. Others used dry heat in some form. Some disregarded this feature, although it was generally admitted that heat was a very necessary adjunct to treatment. Patients themselves commented gratefully on the effects of the heat in alleviating their pain.

The position of the body for protection against deformity was known as the neutral or the anatomic position. The entire body was kept in one plane—shoulders aligned above pelvis, legs straight—on a firm unsagging bed. The feet were kept at right angles, turning neither in nor out and maintained thus by splints, pillows, sandbags, or boxes. The knees were usually relaxed somewhat with a small roll of toweling. Some abduction of the legs was usually ordered because the adductors of the legs were thought to be stronger than the weak abductors, which were therefore given the benefit of protection. The arms were usually kept at about 75 to 90 degrees of abduction to protect the very important muscle of abduction, the deltoid, which was found frequently to be affected. Unless muscle checking revealed a badly paralyzed triceps, the elbow was kept flexed.

Patients with severe involvement were usually kept recumbent for several months. Atrophy resulted, and sometimes when immobilization was uninterrupted stiffness of joints and surrounding structures occurred. This varied, of course, with the extent and kind of treatment that had been given. Certain consistent tendencies toward deformity were observed, but in the hands of experienced, conscientious workers and medical personnel deformities could be avoided and gratifying return of function occurred. The widespread opinion in the public mind that no treatment for poliomyelitis had evolved before the past few years is erroneous.

Most of the previously mentioned methods of treatment carry over into present-day methods. Attention to body alignment is still important; on the whole, it has not varied much, except that the arms are at the sides, not abducted, and no support is placed at the feet during the acute stage. Physical therapy and mobilization activity may be started earlier if the patient's condition warrants. Thus tight muscles, limitation of joint motion, and atrophy of uninvolved muscles are prevented. It is extremely important to handle the patient with the utmost gentleness and skill. Fatigue must be solicitously avoided no matter what system of treatment is used.

GENERAL NURSING CARE

The poliomyelitic patient is almost invariably irritable, hypersensitive, and apprehensive, and everything possible should be done to regulate the environment for his comfort. A quiet room, free from noise, drafts, and glaring light,

should be provided, and all handling of the patient whether psychologic or physical should be skilled and gentle. Every effort should be put forth to reassure the patient as to his condition and his treatment. He must be told in advance about new features of his nursing care that might be a source of alarm to him. The initial treatments must be performed with the utmost gentleness; otherwise, no amount of reassurance will establish confidence.

The patient's bed should be the proper height to make caring for him as easy as possible for the nurse or mother. Blocks for elevating the bed in the home may need to be prepared for this purpose. The bed should be made firm with boards beneath the mattress. A footboard should be prepared for the foot of the bed. It should be higher than the patient's feet to prevent bedclothing from resting on the toes. The footboard should be separated from the mattress by two blocks of wood wide enough to provide a trough for the patient's heels, which should not be allowed to rest on the mattress. Portable footboards or boxes are more suitable for children's wards because the child in the full-size bed tends to squirm about considerably if he is out of line with his ward mates, as he will be if his body must be pulled down so that his feet can contact a footboard at the foot of the bed. Foot supports frequently will need to be altered to meet the needs of the individual patient, with the angle sometimes increased or decreased to accommodate weak or paralyzed muscles.

The mattress should be covered with a waterproof material, and blankets rather than sheets are used to make the bed because they are more absorbent and less likely to chill the skin. Chilling in poliomyelitis is always to be avoided because it tends to increase muscle spasm. A drawsheet is placed beneath the hips, and another beneath the head. Upper covers should never press on the toes or upon sensitive portions of the extremities. A cradle may need to be provided to eliminate this, although the footboard may prove sufficient for the purpose. A pillow should not be used during the acute stage, but if the neck muscles are in spasm some support may be needed for this area. A small rubber air ring partly inflated or a child's white cotton stocking stuffed with cotton and made into a ring may be used for this purpose.

Observations to be made on admission. Nurses should be alert for early manifestations of respiratory or bulbar involvement when the patient is admitted. Shallowness of breathing, increased breathing rate, rigidity of the chest or abdominal muscles, an exaggerated thoracic cleft, or ballooning of the abdomen should be reported to the physician immediately. Any signs of hoarseness, inability to swallow, or a nasal twang to the speech (resembling the speech of a patient with a cleft palate) may be indications of pharyngeal muscle involvement. These are extremely important signs, and the physican should be notified without delay.

Nurses should seek information from the parents regarding the child's bowel and bladder function. Temporary impairment of these organs is not uncommon, and constipation and retention will need to be dealt with very early in the course of the disease. Intake and output should be carefully recorded during the acute period.

The observations of the nurse are of great importance not only when the patient is admitted but throughout the course of the disease. Nurses should learn to inspect the patient's body intelligently before applying packs or, if baths are given, when giving the bath. With a little practice they will be able to detect increase or decrease of spasm in various muscles. Any position that is maintained by the patient over a long period should cause the nurse to suspect the presence of muscle spasm in that area. Abnormal skin creases or grooves, prominence of tendons, hypersensitiveness to touch, or limitation of motion are significant findings and should be recorded.

RELIEF OF MUSCLE SPASM

Methods of using heat to relieve muscle spasm vary greatly in different localities. Nurses must be guided entirely by the physician's preference in using this treatment as well as by the patient's tolerance. Parts to be packed and frequency of packing should be prescribed by the physician as any other treatment would be prescribed.

General nursing needs must never be neglected because of the attention that must be given to packing. Packing is not the end-all of treatment in poliomyelitis and should never be thought of in that light.

Oil or lubricant is not used to protect the skin because there is no danger of burning if the packs are wrung dry enough. Baths are usually not given during the stage of acute muscle spasm, and back rubs are omitted. These two features of nursing care tend to increase spasm in affected muscles and are, of course, dispensable. Local baths after the use of the bedpan will be sufficient.

Technique of applying packs. In applying hot fomentations for treatment of the muscle spasm, certain principles should be borne in mind. The fomentations should be hot, not lukewarm. They should be wrung completely free of moisture. This cannot be done safely by hand or by stupe-wringer. If a hot pack machine is not used, packs should be wrung through a tight wringer twice.

Packs should not cover joints, for they must not give the patient any sense of being unable to move. They should cover the entire muscle, not merely the muscle belly.

Gentleness in handling to avoid pain and apprehension is necessary whether one is aiming to prevent stretching of paralyzed muscles or further spasm in the affected ones. It must be remembered always that the pain in the initial stages of the disease is intense, and that the patient's response to it is one of dread and sometimes hysteria. Crying, protesting, and lack of cooperation in patients with this disease have a very real cause. It is urged that the first manipulation the patient has at the nurse's hands be particularly gentle so that no defense response may be set up against further treatment.

During and between packing periods strict attention should be paid to the bed position of the patient. During the period of painful spasm, however, it is generally permissible to allow the patient to lie in the position that is most comfortable to him. This is permitted until packing has relieved some of the spasm and pain.

Prone and lay-on packing. There is an increasing tendency to use lay-on packs to alternate with pin-on packs, particularly when spasm persists in certain areas of the body. These packs have the advantage that the patient need not be turned or manipulated during their application. Prone packing is particularly adaptable for stubborn spasm of the muscles of the back and thighs. The patient is placed in the face-lying position in good bed posture, with supports to areas where tightness exists, and the packs are applied by laying them on the parts without pinning. No special packs need be cut for this because the back, thigh, and calf packs are used. They should completely cover the posterior area of the back and should be tucked in at the sides.

The term continuous hot packs is misleading, and this fact should be clearly explained to parents and volunteer workers. Light cradles, hot-water bottles, or heating pads are not used with the packs. It is not desirable that the packs remain at the same temperature during the entire period they are on the patient. The gradual cooling of the packs is considered to have a tonic effect on the muscles. Hot moist packs are beneficial in that they tend to increase the blood supply to the part during the early period following their application; but, as they cool, the blood vessels contract and in this way assist markedly in the elimination of fatigue products from the muscles. This will not occur if the packs are kept at the same temperature all the time they are on the patient. Furthermore, the skin of most persons will not tolerate continuous hot moist packing, particularly if the packs are used both night and day. Maceration of the skin or sudamina tend to occur after a few days of such treatment, and itching may become excessive because of the constant contact with wool. The skin needs periods of freedom from both wool and moist heat for maintaining its integrity.

If parents and volunteers are not informed of these facts, they will sometimes change packs more frequently than ordered and will place hot-water bottles along the packs to keep them hot, feeling that this will hasten the child's recovery.

Precautions to observe during packing. Any patient who is receiving hot applications needs careful nursing observation. If the atmosphere is of high humidity, prostration may occur rather easily. A seriously ill patient may become prostrated from the use of heat at any time. Careful checking, therefore, should always be made of the pulse, temperature, and amount of perspiration. Any irregularity or threadiness in the pulse, alteration of depth or rate of breathing, cyanosis, or pallor indicates that treatment should be discontinued until the doctor can be contacted.

Immersion of the patient in a hot tub daily, or even oftener, is becoming a preferred method of treating muscle spasm in many localities. This is true particularly in areas where the disease affects small children. Young children tolerate these tubs better than hot moist packs in humid summer weather.

Physical therapy. In order that the patient's treatment may be closely coordinated, nurses should have a clear concept of what the physical therapist is seeking to accomplish. In some localities all of the physical therapy treatment of the poliomyelitic patient, including hot packing, is considered the responsibility of the physical therapy department. Hot packing, however, is usually done by the nursing service. Early passive joint movement to all joints may also be part of the nursing duties after demonstration has been given by the physical therapist. Passive joint movement is usually done several times during the day, and it is felt that it is sometimes more convenient for the nurse to do this because of her frequent contacts with the patient. Every effort is put forth to maintain complete range of joint motion in all joints from the earliest days of the disease. All passive motion must be kept below the pain level, with the possible exception of those done following administration of a muscle relaxant. Then, upon specific instruction from the physician, the range is sometimes carried beyond the point of pain.

Massage is seldom given in the acute stages of the disease because of its tendency to increase spasm. Warm pool treatments or hot tub baths are sometimes given several times during the week as part of the physical therapy treatment. Intensive packing of tight or contracted muscles, followed by forcible stretching, may be done after the acute period of pain and spasm is over.

BULBAR INVOLVEMENT

The term bulbar is used to designate involvement of the brain stem, which has the following parts: the medulla, pons, and midbrain. Strictly, the term bulbar should probably be applied only to involvement of the medulla, or bulb, but it is now used to indicate all types of involvement above the spinal cord.

There are apparently many types of bulbar involvement. Three of these will be discussed briefly. The largest group is that in which the nuclei of the cranial nerves are affected. If the tenth cranial nerve is not involved, this type may not be a serious threat to life, although facial palsy and paralysis of the external ocular muscles may result. If the tenth cranial nerve (the vagus nerve) is affected, however, abductor paralysis of the vocal cords may present an extremely grave complication. Laryngoscopic examination may reveal that the vocal cords are adducted to the midline, with almost complete occlusion of the airway. Prophylactic tracheotomy is usually performed to prevent obstruction in breathing when this type of involvement is anticipated. It is now felt that even a short period of anoxia has a profoundly deleterious effect on nerve cells and may be a large factor in hindering recovery. Furthermore, it has been noted that an obstructed airway accompanied by the deep, almost gasping inspiration necessary to get oxygen into the lungs may result in acute pulmonary edema, a frequent and often fatal complication of bulbar paralysis.

The patient developing this complication will usually present a picture of progressive toxicity. He is likely to be apprehensive, excited, and overactive. He will reveal shortly symptoms of dysphagia and dysarthria, and oral secretions will be found to be pooling in his throat. Immediate treatment will be necessary to save his life. Treatment will usually consist of tracheotomy and oxygen administration, combined with constant and skillful nursing.

Another very grave situation, and one for which nurses caring for poliomyelitis patients should always be alert, is involvement of the respiratory center in the medulla. This may be a late complication and has been known to occur as long as a week after other bulbar symptoms have been recognized and treated. It may occur even after tracheotomy. Sudden disturbances of the mechanics of respiration with variations in depth, rhythm, and rate, and periods of apnea may be noted. This is considered to be an indication of oxygen starvation and will often require the use of the respirator as well as increased oxygen concentration. For limited periods, oxygen may have to be used in a 100% concentration.

In addition to alterations in the respiratory pattern, the nurse might be aware of personality changes in the patient. He may become stubborn, demanding, and uncooperative. Cerebral anoxia is said to be the cause of this personality change.

Combination spinal cord and bulbar involvement is not uncommon in epidemics. The respirator may be needed for these patients during the early stages of the disease, but great care will be taken to ascertain that the air passages are open before placing the patient in the machine. If there is blocking of the airway, tracheotomy will be necessary, or the action of the machine may result in severe pulmonary damage.

A patient who has had a tracheotomy and who must also be placed in the respirator is a nursing problem of considerable magnitude. The most expert and conscientious type of nursing service is indispensable. The respirator may be tilted at intervals (approximately 30 degree angle) to promote drainage of secretions and to aid somewhat in extending the neck so that the area operated upon is free from contact with the collar. Signs of edema, however, must be watched for whenever the foot end of the respirator is elevated. Modifications have been made in respirator collars to accommodate patients with tracheotomy. One such modification is a 20-inch sponge-rubber collar with a depressor that can be clipped on to push the collar down from the patient's chin. The sloping front respirator is also helpful in the care of these patients.

Nursing care in bulbar involvement. Medical treatment and nursing care in bulbar poliomyelitis are based on four considerations: preventing asphyxia, averting exhaustion, maintaining adequate nutrition, and checking secondary infections.

The onset of the bulbar type of paralysis may frequently be so abrupt that no symptoms at all are noted until the development of a nasal voice and difficulty in swallowing become apparent. The disease in these patients is usually severe and fulminating and may result in death within 12 hours.

Usually, certain early symptoms may predict such involvement, and the nurse should be familiar with them. Symptoms do not always descend on the patient within an hour's time. There are often significant prodromal manifestations that should give their warning. Restlessness, wakefulness, an increase of mucus in the throat, difficulty in swallowing, drawing back of the head, rigidity, and an expression of apprehension are significant and should be reported without delay.

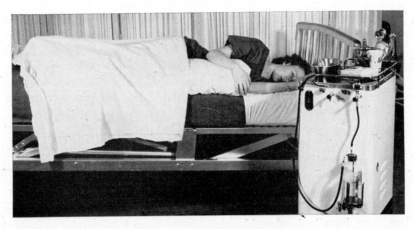

Fig. 195. In bulbar poliomyelitis nursing measures are directed toward keeping the airway open and free of mucus. The foot of the bed is elevated to provide a postural drainage position. The patient is placed on his side, and the position of the head and neck must permit · drainage of secretions. Suction apparatus with rubber catheter and oxygen equipment are kept available.

Choking, exhaustion, and cyanosis are late symptoms; the physician should be notified before they occur. Meanwhile, elevation of the lower end of the bed may prevent choking from an accumulation of secretions in the throat and is usually considered an immediate nursing duty in these cases.

The bulbar form of paralysis may also manifest itself in foamy saliva, tenacious sputum, crowing respiration, nasal voice, hoarseness, limited excursions of the ribs, and inability to expectorate mucus. Somnolence may also occur. The patient tends to breathe shallowly, fearfully, lest he choke in the process.

These cases are often swiftly fatal, but if the patient can be carried through the acute period until fever has subsided he will usually survive. The situation during the acute stage is analogous to suffocation or strangulation. Once this constriction is moved, the patient tends to recover. Danger of fatigue is great because if the patient relaxes for a moment he is likely to be wakened by choking attacks caused by pharyngeal secretions. Fear of this keeps him constantly awake and apprehensive. Sedatives are some-

times ordered to prevent exhaustion, but the nurse will recognize the urgent necessity to check the respiratory rate of her patient after the administration of morphine. Marked decrease in the number of respiratory excursions per minute should be reported.

Tube feeding is not usually considered advisable during the stage of acute distress because of the danger of vomiting. Nasal feeding is attended by risk in any situation, but when it is complicated by pharyngeal edema and the hyperirritability of the patient with bulbar poliomyelitis it seems too great a responsibility for the nurse to assume.

When nausea subsides, it is usually considered safe to begin oral administration of fluids, but fluids should be given guardedly, a teaspoonful at a time, to prevent aspiration. Milk is contraindicated because it seems to form a tenacious phlegm in the throat.

Nursing care for these patients will usually include postural drainage by elevation of the foot of the bed to a 20- to 40-degree angle, placing the patient on his side, sometimes with the head slightly over the side of the bed. The prone position is usually considered un-wise because it may somewhat restrict chest movement. Suctioning is per-formed to prevent choking on the oral secretions that collect in the throat. It must be done with great gentleness and skill. A soft rubber catheter is used, and the suctioning is done only as often as is necessary, for sometimes the procedure serves to excite the patient and exacer-bate his symptoms. Some physicians prefer constant to intermittent suction because of this factor. Because fluids accumulate most heavily in the side of the throat on which the patient lies, the suctioning catheter should be aimed at this area.

To eliminate the possibility of aspira-tion, food and drink are usually with-held as long as there is nausea. Parenteral feeding or transfusions of whole blood may be given. Care is exercised, however, to limit the amount of fluid given by vein because there appears to be some evidence that too liberal use of fluids may be inadvisable, particularly when cerebral edema may already be present.

Oxygen may be ordered, and it may be given by tent, mask, or nasal catheter methods. If it is administered by catheter, it will be necessary to allow each nostril periods of rest from contact with the tube to prevent irritation of the mucous membrane.

Mortality in bulbar involvement is high, but if the patient survives the acute stage of the disease he tends to recover with remarkably little residual involve-ment. Occasionally, however, a weakness may occur in the throat muscles, often accentuated by fatigue or overexertion. This can usually be overcome by careful attention to the patient's rest habits and by modifying the diet so that numerous small meals are given instead of infre-quent large ones. Food should be ground and tenacious fluids avoided.

Nursing care after tracheotomy. Tra-cheotomy has been performed quite fre-quently in recent years on patients in whom paralysis or spasm of the muscles of the larynx threaten to occlude the airway and has unquestionably saved the lives of many patients.

The patient with poliomyelitis who has had a tracheotomy needs the same care to the tube and wound as a patient who does not have poliomyelitis. Nurses have learned these techniques in other services, and they will not be repeated here, except to reiterate general prin-ciples. The nurse must be alert to wipe mucus and tracheal secretions from the tube as soon as they appear and to use the suction machine when necessary to prevent coughing and restlessness. It is, however, usually considered advisable to avoid too frequent suctioning when oxygen is being given through the tube. Suctioning interferes with continuous oxygenation. Extra catheters for suc-tioning and for oxygen administration must, of course, be available. Skill in removing and cleaning the inner tube when it is necessary is important. Some-what greater emphasis is placed on air humidification in poliomyelitis than is necessary for other types of patients. Unless the air is moist, the mucus in the trachea tends to become viscid and re-sistant, and suction will be very difficult. Orders may be written to inject small amounts of saline solution (5 to 10 ml.) into the tracheotomy tube prior to suc-tioning. This helps to loosen mucus and facilitates more adequate suctioning. Humidifiers must be kept in the patient's room if oxygen is not being given. It is felt, however, that it is much more satis-factory to administer moistened air and oxygen combinations through a trache-otomy inhalator.

The nurse must be constantly alert for signs of further complications of the dis-ease, such as paralysis of the extremities, of the chest muscles, of the respiratory center, or signs of incipient polioencephalitis.

The patient will need gentle handling and constant reassurance. The importance of the nurse's continued presence at his bedside can hardly be overemphasized. A calm attitude and quickness to understand the patient's needs contribute immeasurably to his comfort and security.

To prevent sepsis in the trachea and lungs, penicillin, nebulized in a saline solution, may be ordered for administration through the tracheotomy tube. Penicillin is also sometimes given intramus-cularly as a prophylaxis against secondary infections.

Involvement of the muscles of respiration. In the spinal type of poliomyelitis or in the combined spinal and bulbar type, weakness of shoulders and arms is sometimes an early sign that impairment of the muscles of the chest (pectorals) and those of respiration (intercostals and diaphragm) may take place. The nurse must be alert for signs of approaching respiratory embarrassment when caring for a patient with obvious involvement of the upper extremities.

The patient may be asked to take a

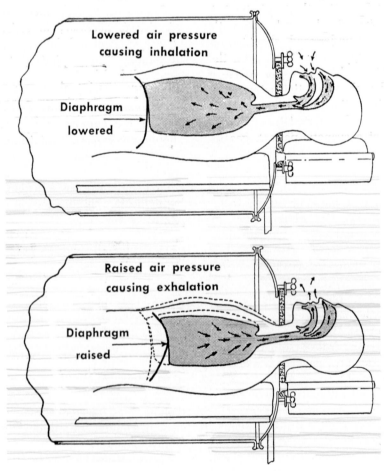

Fig. 196. Diagrams illustrating mechanism of respirator. (From Norcross, Mary E.: The Drinker respirator, Am. J. Nursing **39:**1063-1068, 1939.)

deep breath and begin counting. If he is unable to count to ten without taking another breath, some disturbance of the respiratory muscles has probably occurred, and the physician should be notified immediately.

Anxiety, restlessness, and apprehension are also prodromal symptoms. Attempted use of the auxiliary muscles of respiration, a jutting forward of the chin and prominence of the sternocleidomastoideus muscles or of the platysma, dilatation of the nostrils on inspiration, and cyanosis are late signs. The nurse should have detected and reported earlier symptoms before these occurred.

Principles underlying the use of the respirator. Operating the respirator is in reality quite simple and, once the mechanism is understood, should cause no panic in any nurse. The reason that panic exists at these times, of course, is the speed with which the patient must be put into the respirator and the machine must be started to work. The spectacle of a cyanotic patient, gasping for breath, perhaps already breathless, is one that demands firm self-control and a pair of quick, unfaltering hands. It demands a calm confident manner and expression, and also the ability to keep the patient from being alarmed additionally by the panic of those around him.

Each year finds newer improved models of the respirator, therefore no attempt will be made to describe other than the actual nursing care of the patient. For assistance in operating the machine, the nurse is referred to the directions that are usually permanently attached and plainly visible on the machine itself.

Some review of the mechanics of respiration is necessary in order to adequately understand the operation of the respirator. The respiratory function is accomplished by inspiration and expiration. When the individual breathes in, the thoracic cavity enlarges by contraction of the muscles of inspiration, the diaphragm and intercostal muscles. The

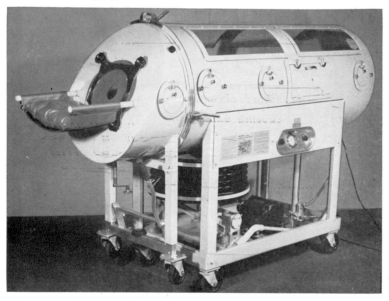

Fig. 197. Respirator modified for the care of the patient with tracheotomy. (Courtesy Warren E. Collins, Inc.)

contraction of the intercostal muscles lifts the rib cage, the contraction of the diaphragm depresses the floor of the chest, both thereby increasing the chest capacity. This enlarged chest cavity returns to normal more or less passively. Expiration is considered almost entirely passive by some physiologists. It is the result of the relaxing of the intercostal muscles and diaphragm, as well as to the returning upward pressure of the abdominal walls now free from the pressure of the contracted diaphragm. When paralysis of the diaphragm and intercostal muscles is present, all this is obviously impossible, and it is in these patients that the respirator has made its greatest contribution.

With the patient's body in the airtight chamber of the respirator, but with the head outside, the respirator bellows upon expansion will cause the air pressure in the tank to become lower. Because it is a physical fact that air pressures tend to equalize themselves, air from the outside will rush into the lungs through the nose and throat, expanding the lungs and thereby lessening the pressure in the chest, and equilibrium of air pressure will be restored. The contracting bellows immediately increase air pressure on the body in the tube, the chest cavity is compressed, and the patient exhales. This constant rhythmic procedure aerates the lungs in the manner of natural respiration but with no effort on the part of the patient.

Actual positive pressure is seldom ordered, and negative pressure somewhere between 14 and 18 cm. of water is usually considered optimum. Too much pressure in either direction is unsafe and may damage lung tissue considerably. Furthermore, it is exceedingly unpleasant for the patient. Hyperventilation of the lungs has been known to be the cause of pulmonary emphysema, as well as emphysema of a more superficial

nature. Alkalosis and tetany sometimes occur from this, and nurses should be prompt to report spasm of the wrists or feet or twitchings of the face, legs, or thighs; these will be particularly significant if negative pressure in excess of 20 cm. has been used over a considerable period in an attempt to overcome persistent cyanosis or other respiratory difficulty.

Weaning the patient from the respirator. It is now felt that early weaning from the respirator may be vital to the patient's ultimate recovery. When the physician has decided that this may safely be attempted, nurses should do their utmost to promote the patient's gradual independence from the machine. The problem will have to be approached differently with each patient, but a few suggestions may be of assistance for the nurse who has no previous experience in this matter.

It has been found that some patients prefer to begin this weaning process by having the motor turned off for short periods several times during the day. The machine is not opened during the first few times this is done, and the patient is never left alone during these periods. His full cooperation is necessary if a mental block is not to be set up against the whole weaning process. The patient will gradually extend this period of independence, sometimes reaching to several hours, before the carriage is removed from the machine. With the carriage out of the machine, the patient may suffer what he believes to be a setback, because usually he will not be able to maintain his independence for as long a period as when the machine was closed. Tolerance for this, however, can be built up rather quickly if continual encouragement and assurance are given. The nurse must be prepared for unpredictable and apparently reasonless periods of panic in which the patient is totally unable to stay out of the machine for the accustomed time.

Patients usually have their greatest difficulty in attempting to remain out of the respirator during the night. Long after they have attained almost complete independence from the machine during the day, they are sometimes unable to sleep out of it, and they must be returned before they are able to sleep. Considerable skill and experience are necessary in handling this situation, and the nurse must be guided by the physician's advice before urging that the patient attempt to sleep out of the machine when he is manifestly unwilling to do so.

Rocking bed. A rocking bed has been used by some physicians to assist the patient in gaining independence from the machine. The mechanism of this bed consists of a seesaw motion, and inhalation occurs more or less passively as the head is elevated and the abdominal viscera are shifted downward. Then, with the feet up and the head down, the viscera move upward against the diaphragm and assist in exhalation. These oscillations are regulated so that they are at the rate of normal breathing. However, no matter what method is used to wean the patient from the respirator, it is always extremely important to watch the patient carefully for signs of fatigue. Even a mild degree of fatigue is undesirable, and the patient should be returned to the machine before he becomes excessively tired.

It should be mentioned that, although the patient may have worked up an independence of an hour or two, this cannot be depended upon in an emergency. If the electric current fails, for instance, the patient's endurance may be less than

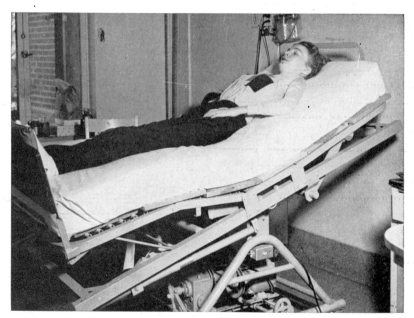

Fig. 198. The rocking bed may be used to promote early weaning of the patient from the respirator. Each day, or several times daily, the patient is placed on the bed for increasingly longer periods. The length of time tolerated is determined by the patient's facial expression, pulse rate, and color. Nursing activities can be performed with the bed in motion. Liquid or food is given when the head of the bed is highest. During this phase the abdominal viscera tend to move downward, favoring movement of the diaphragm and inhalation of air.

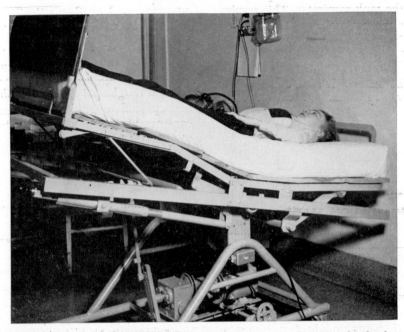

Fig. 199. As the head of the bed lowers, the viscera shift upward against the diaphragm and air is exhaled. At this time, when air is going out through the larynx, it is easier for the patient to speak. The patient learns to inhale as the head of the bed rises and exhale as the head of the bed lowers.

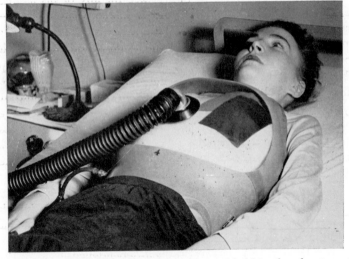

Fig. 200. The chest respirator is placed over the chest and held in place by straps that encircle the patient's body. The rubber edges must fit snugly about the chest wall if the person is to receive benefit from the respirator.

2 minutes, because it is complicated by a kind of panic.

Chest respirator. In some instances it is possible to use a chest respirator to replace the tank respirator. This respirator gives the patient more freedom and greatly facilitates nursing care. Various kinds of material may be used for the chest covering. The edges, which must fit snugly against the chest wall, are made of rubber. The shell is held in place with tape-webbing straps. Considerable care must be given to the skin that comes in contact with the rubber because it tends to break down easily.

CHRONIC POLIOMYELITIS— RECONSTRUCTION STAGE

Poliomyelitis is said to have reached the chronic stage after the muscles have made their maximum recovery, usually from 18 months to 2 years. A great deal of the progress, however, that has been made during the convalescent stage can be lost if careful medical and nursing supervision are not provided thereafter. Weight bearing and other similar activities place considerable strain on muscles, and even patients who have had very minor involvement may develop unsuspected weaknesses at this time unless a close check is kept on their progress. This fact is perhaps not clearly realized at present, because many persons have read so much about new types of treatment that they tend to believe that any progress they have made is irreversible in nature.

Emotional aspects. The treatment of poliomyelitis in the early weeks is dramatic enough that the full import of the patient's disability does not always become apparent to him for some time afterward. Progress during the first weeks tends to be more rapid than it will be after 6 months' time has elapsed. A gradual awareness of the permanent nature of his handicap may in some instances, particularly with the adolescent and the young adult, be the cause of major depressions and personality changes. Indifference, apathy, or self-pity may replace the patient's original attitude of hope, courage, and determination to recover.

The nurse should be forewarned that these things are likely to happen, that this is a rough spot over which she must be expected to guide the patient with considerable permanent involvement. She should be able to warn parents and relatives that such an occurrence is a natural reaction. To limit this period and to cut it down to its minimum by sympathetic, intelligent advice should be part of the nurse's skill.

Management of these situations demands early recognition of their likelihood. Although the nurse's attitude like that of the patient must be based on faith and optimism, statements made must be guarded. The patient should very gradually be brought to accept his handicap from the first days of his paralysis, to plan his life in terms of it, rather than in terms of complete functional recovery. This is the only honest course for any of his associates to take. It is kinder than unguarded optimism and cheeriness that break down under the strain of long-deferred hope. It goes without saying that such principles of mental hygiene as the nurse herself applies in her relationship to her work with the patient must be given to the family of the patient to guide them in their understanding of the patient's problems. That this takes ingenuity is an understatement. The nurse may be instrumental in helping the parents of a child patient to plan in relation to the patient's homecoming such alterations of environment and living as will make self-dependence possible for him. The importance of friendship and relationship with young people of his own age must be pointed out so that the parents may make special efforts to see that friendships he enjoyed in school are continued while he is homebound.

The patient's problem is a very real one. Faced in the cold light of day and robbed of the mitigating factors that attend the early illness with its dramatic fight for survival, the outlook may be very black indeed. It is a situation that the newly crippled person realizes, however dimly, that he has to face alone. The pattern of his life is smashed. He must re-collect the fragments and make what he can of them, and the task may look hopeless, the effort not worth the while.

It is impossible to lay down a schedule of treatment for this situation. To meet it adequately, the nurse's preparation must be broader than she herself perhaps realizes. Besides her courses in orthopedics, sociology, community health, and mental hygiene, all of which should have perfected her ability to some degree in this regard, she needs a deep-seated interest in people and their problems. She needs to know what community resources for education and rehabilitation may be available to help this person. He will not know of them, for three months ago he was a healthy person with no knowledge or need of such services. If ever there was an urgent necessity for broad information on these points it is at this time when the nurse earnestly accepts the challenge to assist a young newly crippled individual attacked by all the forces of pessimism and personal disintegration.

The student should know the ways in which the physical therapist and the occupational therapist keep the patient interested in making further effort toward physical reclamation. They must do this day after day in their work. There is more skill in this than the student will realize unless it is occasionally pointed out to her. Facile encourage-

ment, more or less mechanical, will not accomplish much. The patient soon learns to detect patent signs of insincerity in the nurse.

Nurses can do much to provide diversional activity for these young people in the hospital if they will remember the things they liked to do at that age and find some means of encouraging the patients to develop like interests. To encourage hobbies in her patients, the nurse should have a few of her own that she may offer to explain to the patient. Many nurses initiate such hobbies by contributions of their own. Stamp collecting, postmark collecting, and match-folder collecting are cheap and interesting and might provide a beginning for a pack-rat career.

Where it is possible, a ward-governing body may be developed. Such groups can have more functions than might be apparent at the outset, and they often do much to improve ward spirit and morale. Complaints, requests, plans for activities and parties, and welcoming committees for new patients are functions that can be worked out of the original self-governing group. Great pride in this matter has been observed in wards where such a democratic system of ward regulations is carried out over a period of time.

General health supervision. Nurses who supervise the care of patients after poliomyelitis should aim to assist their patients in the daily requirements of living in the home, such as bathing, dressing, getting out of a chair, going to the toilet, and other similar activities. It will often take considerable planning and ingenuity to make it possible for the severely affected patient to do some of these things, but certainly no service can be more important. To achieve these ends, adaptation in home equipment may often be necessary. Nurses will frequently be able to secure help and advice from members of the family who have an aptitude for mechanical construction and carpentry. Consultation with a physical therapist or an occupational therapist will often give the nurse valuable hints she needs for attaining some of her objectives.

Frequent inspection to detect habitual faulty positions in sitting, walking, or standing should be made during the period when functional activity is being resumed. The public health nurse should be alert for incompletely extended hips, for tendencies to stand in the back-knee position, and for deviation of the spine as a result of poor habits of sitting and standing. She should observe unequal growth of the legs or feet that might indicate overuse of one extremity because of a disguised weakness in the other. The parents should be instructed to observe signs that the unaffected parts of the patient's body are becoming weakened because of overuse and fatigue. No matter how mild the involvement from poliomyelitis, patients must be taught to avoid fatigue for a long time after their recovery. Periods of rather strenuous activity will often reveal weaknesses in muscles that were never originally thought to be affected. Periods of bed rest should always follow periods of prolonged or strenuous activity. The afterlunch nap of an hour should be part of the patient's daily program. It should be taken in a darkened, ventilated room, free from the distraction of radio or toys.

The child with only a short leg brace or splint often tends to sit or lie for long periods with the leg rolled outward because of the weight of the apparatus. The mother's attention should be called to this position that is often the cause of troublesome deformity at the hip level when the child begins to walk.

The danger of eyestrain should be borne in mind, particularly in the older patient, who spends so much of his time reading or doing handwork requiring

close attention. Attitudes denoting eyestrain, squinting, frequent headaches, reddened lids, or holding the work too close to the eye should be reported to the physician. Glasses can probably relieve much of this strain.

The child's eating habits should have close attention. He needs vegetables and milk. He should not be allowed to make excuses in his eating. Because of relative inactivity combined with normal appetite, these patients tend to gain weight easily. The diet may need to be limited sensibly, but it should not be limited in essential features for a growing person. Parents need instruction in this matter, or they will not realize that plenty of good food does not particularly mean whipped cream, pork chops, and desserts in abundance. The child's functional disability will be greatly exaggerated by a substantial gain in weight, and weakened muscles will undergo further strain from having to support it.

Constipation may become a chronic problem, particularly if the patient has had too many cathartics early in the course of the disease. Regularity by habit should be maintained with these children as far as possible. Although standing orders for cathartics usually exist on orthopedic divisions, it is well for the nurse to seek advice from the physician about persistent constipation in these children rather than to administer cathartics routinely.

In a ward full of crippled children it is easy for the nurse to lose her individual approach and, in the pressure of work and responsibility, to keep at the child about position, attitudes, habits, and the like until he becomes surly and disobedient at the slightest provocation. This is mismanagement in its way as serious as the mismanagement of muscles. Consideration of the patient as an individual is necessary, and his individual problem, which is bound to be a little different from that of the child in the next bed, must be given consideration. If he seems unruly and twists and turns in bed despite all of your pleas, perhaps you can arrange his bed so that he may see different parts of the ward at different times of the day.

On the whole, younger children tend to adjust to their condition much more easily than older ones, which is not difficult to understand. The older patient will be affected by periodic spells of gloom and depression, accompanied in some cases by definite refusal of cooperation. These patients need some definite assurance of advancement. It is the long period of confinement, the inactivity, and the limitation of body motion that bring on these periodic spells of depression.

Braces

Application of braces. When braces are ordered, a considerable outlay of expense is involved. A respect for the cost and skilled labor going into these braces is a healthy virtue for the nurse to develop in the patient. Their care is part of the teaching the student nurse does for the family. Knowledge of their purpose, the correct way to apply them, recognition of the purpose of each part, and the necessity for keeping them intact are essential.

Nurses may encounter some resistance to the use of braces at present. This is because of the unwise publicity given to the dispensability of braces in certain systems of treatment. Many persons honestly believe that to walk in any manner, however hazardously, without braces, is preferable to walking with them. The patient who has a strong dislike for braces can rationalize his determination not to wear them by resource to many arguments he has read in the press against their use. Nurses will need to be well informed about the reason

for the prescribed braces to present the case for them intelligently.

Braces are frequently necessary to permit the patient to walk without undue strain or fatigue. They are also used to prevent or overcome mild deformity or tendencies toward deformity. The ultimate purpose of orthopedic surgery is to restore the patient to normal living. Braces are only a step in this direction. The ultimate aim is to eliminate, if possible, the use of braces either by further development of the patient's own remaining powers or through some type of reconstructive surgery.

Braces should be applied with the patient lying in good position in the bed. The prone position is recommended for the application of the combined body and leg brace frequently used in chronic poliomyelitis. Pelvic bands should fit just below the iliac crests. The trunk part of the brace must be observed to be certain that the fastening is in the midline of the body; any minute variation of this will make the fitting of the entire apparatus faulty.

The use of cotton shirts beneath these jackets is essential both for the patient's comfort and for the cleanliness and long life of the brace. Oiling of the skin tends to stain leather portions of the braces, and these stains are very difficult to remove. When incontinence is present, the upper portion of the leather thigh cuff sometimes may be protected with waterproofing. Although it is desirable, it is not always possible to get the bulky diapers and rubber pants beneath the brace, and these have to be applied outside, leaving the leather portions near the groin exposed to frequent wetting.

All straps on braces should be securely fastened, but care should be taken as the child puts on weight or grows that constriction of circulation does not develop because of the straps. Nurses new to orthopedic services will need instruction in the application of each of the more complicated types of braces, particularly the corrective scoliosis braces, the different kinds of clubfoot braces, and the Taylor spine brace. Automatic locks should be explained and their use demonstrated. The student deserves to have this instruction from her head nurse rather than from the patient, from whom she too often gets poor instruction.

Lacings or shoestrings used on braces should be kept in good condition, without knots and changed as they become frayed. If the tips fall off, new ones can sometimes be constructed by collodion applied in successive layers. Frayed straps should be reported to the doctor or bracemaker if he is available. Felt padding or metal bars may be cleaned with cleansing fluid, ether or benzene.

If arm splints are used, they should be inspected frequently to see if the splint is actually maintaining the arm in the position designed. Patients wearing arm splints have a tendency to lift the shoulder by contracting the strong upper trapezius muscle, thereby robbing the upper arm of the support of the splint. It may be necessary to take a little time to instruct the patient to relax the trapezius muscle so that the arm may rest in the splint as prescribed. If weakened shoulder or back muscles are present and no splint is worn, the weight of the arm in the splint should not be allowed to pull the shoulders downward in undesirable postural attitudes. Some provision to eliminate this pull may need to be devised. If the patient is bedfast, canvas hammocks may be suspended from an overhead bar that will support the arms and prevent the pull on weakened shoulder muscles. If the patient spends considerable time sitting, the arms may be supported by armrests constructed of pillows, pads, or boxes, which may be placed on the desk or table top or on the arms of the chair. It is sometimes possible to improvise an upright support with an overhead bar to a wheelchair. Hammocks or cuffs may be suspended to this bar to support the hands and arms for part of the day. It is usually permissible for the patient to use his hand and elbow functionally in eating, writing, or holding a paper if there is no involvement in these areas even though weakness is present in the shoulder muscles. Too constant use of the forearm, however, may put more strain than is desirable on the shoulder, and frequent periods of rest from activity are advisable.

Long leg braces may be of the caliper type, fitting into the patient's shoe. With this brace it is especially important that the shoe be well fitting and of a type proper to good functioning of the foot. Another type of long leg brace is made with a footplate that is worn inside the shoe. The shoe must be wider to accommodate the footplate.

Braces may have different kinds of locks at the knee. The most common is known as the sleeve lock. This lock slides up and down over the hinge, releasing it or holding it fixed in the position of extension. The automatic lock is one that the patient must learn to operate. When the patient is ready to sit, the spring that controls this lock is released by pressure on the seat of the chair. The patient is then able to bend the knee.

Care of braces. All joints and locks on the braces should be oiled weekly with 3-in-1 oil, or a similar lubricant, and surplus oil removed immediately so that it does not stain the surrounding leather. Lint should be removed from screws before they are oiled. Saddle soap and small amounts of water cleanse leather parts satisfactorily, although cleaning fluid such as benzine may be used. Leather should be polished after the use of saddle soap. This both refurbishes and

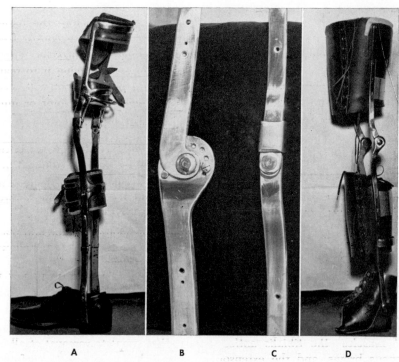

Fig. 201. **A**, Long leg caliper brace with an automatic knee lock. **B**, Set or fixed lock. **C**, Sleeve lock. **D**, Long leg brace with footplate and no knee lock.

imparts a certain amount of water resistance to the leather.

Missing parts (screws, laces, hooks, straps, pads, or felt lining) should be reported as soon as they are noticed. The patient will learn respect for his apparatus by the nurse's prompt attention to such details. The shoes attached to his braces, usually by caliper through the heel, must be inspected frequently for signs of wear and abnormal pressure. Children tend to outgrow shoes and braces with alarming rapidity. Points to be recognized as indications that the child is outgrowing the braces or shoes must be called to the attention of the parents when correct application is demonstrated to them.

If elastic straps are attached to braces or shoes, inspection of the brace should include examination of this elastic for its resilience. These straps may go from the sole of the shoe to a point just below

the knee to form a sort of external dorsiflexor to relieve drop foot caused by paralysis of the anterior tibial muscle. Elastic is also used in many types of scoliosis braces.

Inspection of the skin when the brace is removed may reveal bruises, discolorations, skin abrasions, or dermatitis. Any deviation from the normal condition of the skin or underlying tissues should be reported. Suitable alterations can usually be made to overcome such friction.

Knee pads worn over the anterior aspect of the knee should tell the nurse of strong hamstring or flexor muscles around the joint combined with relatively weaker extensor muscles. Such pads are placed in front of the knee to prevent the child's feelings of insecurity and fear of jackknifing as he walks. A similar pad on the posterior aspect should tell her of strong quadriceps extensor muscles that tend to pull the knee into a hyperextended position (genu recurvatum). Frequently these knee pads get lost because the nurse and patient do not recognize them as an essential part of the brace.

The nurse in teaching parents and relatives must constantly emphasize the necessity of periodic checkups for all patients wearing apparatus of this nature.

SURGERY IN POLIOMYELITIS

The entire plan of reconstructive surgery in poliomyelitis (infantile paralysis) is based on the fact that joints are controlled by groups of coordinating but opposing muscles. In the ankle, for example, plantar flexion results from the action of the gastrocnemius (calf muscle group) and flexors of the toes. This is opposed and balanced by the extensor group of muscles—the tibialis anticus, the peroneus brevis, and the extensors of the toes. Inversion of the ankle is accomplished by action of the tibialis anticus and the tibialis posticus assisted by the flexors of the toes.

If the extensors of the toes are paralyzed, the foot will turn inward and there will be a dropfoot deformity. Likewise, weaknesses of various types will develop with paralysis of other groups of muscles.

Reconstruction surgery is based on the elimination of the joints that allow the deformity to occur by operative fixation, by the transplantation of certain selected tendons to replace the action of paralyzed ones, or by a combination of joint fixation and tendon transplantation.

There are a number of mechanical tricks learned through experience in operative surgery that may in some instances save part or all of the motion in certain joints and still eliminate the ability of the stronger group of muscles to create deformity.

Many operations are designed to correct various deformities and contractures that developed before the patient was first observed. These consist frequently in detaching the contracted muscle from its origin and allowing it to reattach to bone in a position that will accomplish straightening of the joint or limb.

Some special operations. When there is a permanent paralysis of the deltoid muscle with a frail and useless shoulder, the shoulder may be stiffened in a position of abduction (60 degrees for children and 65 degrees for adults), provided there is good power in the muscles about the shoulder blade and reasonably good power in the hand. Following the operation, the entire upper extremity and the upper half of the body (shoulder spica) are placed in a cast until bony union within the joint is present. Joint fusions are usually accomplished by the complete removal of all cartilage from the component surfaces. Frequently, a bone graft is used to transfix the joint, stabilize it, and speed the fusion time. Complete fusion usually takes place in from 3 to 6 months.

One of the commonest deformities in the hand consists in the paralysis of the opposing muscles of the thumb. This causes the loss of grasping and holding power. The condition may be improved or corrected by tendon transplantation. One method consists in transplanting one half of the long extensor tendon of the thumb to the posterior surface of the proximal phalanx of the thumb near its articulation with the metacarpal bone (Steindler). The method of Bunnell utilizes the flexor carpi ulnaris or the palmaris longus tendons, attaching them by a transplantation to the flexor tendon of the thumb through a loop around the carpal bones of the outer side of the hand.

Spine. Many of the worst cases of curvature of the spine are the result of spinal or abdominal muscle paralysis.

These curvatures should be prevented as much as possible during convalescence, but when they do occur they must be corrected.

The first step in the correction of paralytic curvature of the spine is through the use of corrective casts, such as the Risser cast. When the spine has been straightened, it is fused by surgery on the affected area and becomes rigid where the curve is most severe. The operation is frequently performed through a window that is cut in the back of the cast. The cast usually includes the head, the body, and one leg. It is worn for 4 to 6 months. This cast is replaced by another cast extending from the armpits to and including the pelvis thereby allowing the patient to become ambulatory.

In patients in whom curvature is the result of abdominal weakness, transplants of the strong ligamentous material from the outer side of the thigh (fascia lata) are made, replacing the paralyzed muscles (Lowman and Mayer). These bands usually are stitched to the brim of the pelvis and to the ribs to form inelastic stabilizing sinews beneath the skin that prevent rotation of the body and curvature. There are a number of applications of this method of stabilization.

Hip. When there is a flexion contracture of the hip, the muscle attachments, including a shell of bone, can be freed from the anterior and lateral portions of the iliac crest (Speed), thereby releasing the contracted muscles and giving correction of the deformity. A plaster hip spica is used to maintain correction for 6 to 10 weeks.

Knee. There are a number of operations designed to stabilize the knee. If both the knee and ankle are severely paralyzed, however, a long leg brace extending from the ischium to the shoe frequently constitutes the best form of

treatment. If stabilization of the knee is desired, it may be done by a bone block operation to limit flexion of the knee joint, a bone block operation to prevent hyperextension of the knee joint (backknee), or by complete ankylosis or fusion of the joint in a position of the greatest usefulness as far as the occupation of the particular person is concerned.

Before operative fusion is performed, it is well to test the probability of success and satisfaction to the patient by applying a plaster of paris cast over the thigh and leg and allowing him to get about for a few weeks with the leg in a fixed position.

Knock-knee and outward rotation of the tibia and foot are common deformities in patients with poliomyelitis. They can be corrected by an ostectomy of the bone just below the knee with inward rotation of the tibia. Immobilization in plaster for 8 to 10 weeks is required for healing.

Ankle. At the ankle, operations are designed to correct the most common deformities. Drop foot with inversion of the ankle and foot (equinovarus) is best treated by a modified Hoke operation that consists in the removal of a wedge-shaped portion of bone from the under-surface of the astragalus. The base of the wedge is forward and outward so that both deformities are corrected at the same time. The bone surface is freshened on both sides, and all cartilage is removed so that prompt ankylosis takes place. A plaster of paris cast from the toes to the groin maintains the corrected position during healing. The portion of the cast above the knee may be removed about 2 months after operation, but complete ankylosis rarely occurs in less than 4 to 6 months.

When the drop foot is uncomplicated by associated deformities, a posterior bone block in the astragalus will hold

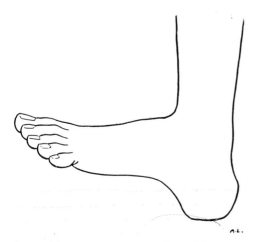

Fig. 202. Paralytic calcaneovalgus deformity.

the foot at a right angle. When the arch is abnormally high as a result of a contracture of the plantar muscles, the detachment of these muscles from the os calcis (Steindler) followed by manipulation and stretching will give correction in the more mildly affected patients. In the more severely affected patients the removal of a wedge-shaped piece of bone from the tarsal region (dorsal surface) may be necessary to supplement this procedure.

There are comparatively few tendon transplantations that are permanently successful in the lower extremities, but there is one that gives quite satisfactory results. In patients with clawfoot (retraction of the toes), successful results are obtained by the transplantation of the extensors of the toes into the metatarsal bones near the heads. It is usually necessary to fasten these tendons through drill holes in the metatarsal bones so that anchorage will be secure.

Epiphyseal arrest. Unequal growth of the legs may be an aftermath of poliomyelitis contracted in early childhood. To correct this condition by equalizing the length of the legs is an important consideration in orthopedic surgery.

Phemister and others a number of years ago showed that arrest of epiphyseal growth could be effected by forms of localized epiphyseal destruction or disturbance. Their plan was based on the fact that equalization of leg length could be obtained by such disturbance and retardation of growth at the epiphyseal line could be accomplished by a block osteotomy over the line with a 90-degree rotation of the fragment (a square plug). When this is rotated, it causes a fusion or elimination of the growth line, resulting in the stoppage of growth of the limb. The state of the epiphysis as shown by roentgenography and a family history of height statistics give a clue as to the time that epiphyseal growth should be stopped.

Walter Blount has shown clinically that the principle of epiphyseal arrest can be applied to many more problems. By the use of stainless steel staples, it can be applied not only to the equalization of leg length but also to the calculated control of knock-knees and bowlegs. Moreover, this process may be stopped and controlled by the timely removal of the staples. Blount has found that one staple on each side may break as a result of epiphyseal growth strain. About three staples are necessary to stop the growth. Strangely enough, however, if the staples are removed before complete closure of the epiphyses, growth is restored. These findings open up a new field of leg equalization as well as the correction of bowleg and knock-knee deformities at a calculated time before puberty or the closure of the epiphyseal lines.

In addition, deformities such as a flexed knee or a hyperextended knee can be corrected by staple fixation. The staples can be discontinued at the proper time. (See Fig. 203.)

Nursing care. As has been stated, surgery may be performed after poliomyelitis to correct deformities, to secure

Knock-knee

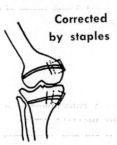

Corrected
by staples

Leg shortening

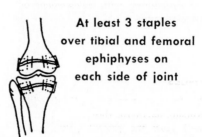

At least 3 staples
over tibial and femoral
ephiphyses on
each side of joint

Fig. 203. Drawings showing epiphyseal arrest used in knock-knee and for leg shortening.

stability of the joints, and to improve function. Some surgery is necessary because of neglect in early treatment or because of carelessness in following instructions given for home treatment. Nurses, therefore, should be very earnest in their attempts to see that instructions for home care are followed to the letter.

Surgery for stabilization of the joints may frequently be performed to permit the patient to walk without braces or crutches, and, even though it may accomplish this satisfactorily, some disappointment is often felt by the patient or his parents because the cosmetic effect has not been all that they had expected it to be. Time should always be taken before surgery to explain all the factors involved in the surgery and its probable outcome in order that disappointment may be avoided. Stories in newspapers and magazines during the past years have spoken so lavishly of miracle surgery that many persons expect an almost impossible result from orthopedic surgery and are disappointed when the outcome falls short of what they have expected.

The immediate aftercare is the same as that given to any orthopedic surgical patient, and it is an extremely important factor in the eventual outcome. Because most operations performed on patients with poliomyelitis are classified as clean surgery, the greatest care should be taken to eliminate the possibility of wound infection during dressings. Casts or other immobilizing apparatus must receive continued intelligent care both in the hospital and at home in order to accomplish the purpose for which they are intended. A great deal of the ultimate success of muscle transplants will depend upon prolonged and skillful physical therapy treatments, and nurses should make every effort to see that follow-up treatments are continued until the maximum recovery of function has been obtained.

STUDY QUESTIONS

1. Describe the early symptoms of poliomyelitis.
2. What are some of the common findings in the spinal fluid of a patient with early poliomyelitis?
3. Discuss some of the problems of the patient with residual paralysis following poliomyelitis.
4. What are the symptoms of bulbar involvement in poliomyelitis?

5. Describe desirable bed positions for the poliomyelitic patient with involvement of the lower extremities; with involvement of the upper extremities.

6. What position would be most comfortable for the patient with spasm of the gastrocnemius muscle? with spasm of the hamstring muscles?

REFERENCES

Ager, E. A.: Immunization as practiced today, Am. J. Nursing 62:74-79, 1962.

Boyd, T. E.: How the present poliomyelitis vaccine was discovered, Am. J. Nursing 57:722-725, 1957.

Dargan, F. P.: Occupational therapy for the poliomyelitic, Am. J. Occup. Therap. 9:272-277, 1955.

Dublin, T. D.: 1954 Poliomyelitis vaccine field trial, J.A.M.A. 158:1258-1270, 1955.

Hamil, E. M.: What is nursing in a respiratory center? Am. J. Nursing 57:42-44, 1957.

Knocke, L. S.: Some common types of braces, Am. J. Nursing 52:868-869, 1952.

Leprow, M., Serfling, R., Sherman, I., and Robbins, F.: A survey of immunization levels after an oral poliovaccine program in Cleveland, J.A.M.A. 187:749-757, 1964.

McCluskey, A.: The patient in a chest respirator, Am. J. Nursing 51:260-261, 1951.

Neu, H. N., and Ladwig, H. A.: The problem of the long-term respirator patient, Arch. Phys. Med. 37:351-357, 1956.

Nicholson, H. F.: The use and care of braces, Nursing World, pp. 36-38, October, 1952.

Paul, J. R.: Poliovirus vaccines—killed and alive, Am. J. Nursing 60:60-62, 1960.

Pfeiffer, E., and Stevens, M.: Weaning the respirator patient, Am. J. Nursing 56:454-457, 1956.

Rooney, A.: A Polio epidemic is averted, Am. J. Nursing 62:71-73, 1962.

Saunders, J. H., and Wendland, L. V.: Some emotional needs of patients with bulbospinal poliomyelitis, Nursing Outlook 3:374-376, 1955.

Saunders, J.: Inservice education at a respiratory center, Am. J. Nursing 57:44-45, 1957.

Scheele, L. A.: Control of poliomyelitis through vaccination, J.A.M.A. 158:1271-1281, 1955.

Siffert, R. S., and Losty, M.: Unequal leg lengths, Am. J. Nursing 55:294-295, 1955.

Spencer, W. A.: Treatment of acute poliomyelitis, ed. 2, Springfield, Ill., 1954, Charles C Thomas, Publisher.

Trott, A. W., and Kerr, M. L.: Tendon transplantation, Am. J. Nursing 54:1210-1214, 1954.

Van Riper, H. E.: The present status of the Salk vaccine for the control of paralytic poliomyelitis, New York J. Med. 56:2229-2237, 1956.

Wilson, J. L., and Dickinson, D. G.: Prevention of long-time dependence of poliomyelitis patients on tank respirator, J.A.M.A. 158:551, 1955.

Wright, J.: The Resper-aid rocking bed in poliomyelitis, Am. J. Nursing 47:454-456, 1947.

Wright, J.: Early treatment of poliomyelitis, Am. J. Dis. Child. 87:354-360, 1954.

Chapter 9

Cerebral palsy, including nursing care

DEFINITION

Cerebral palsy is the term applied to those conditions that are characterized by impaired functional muscular control as a result of abnormality in cerebral areas that affect neuromuscular functions. Spasticity is a type of cerebral palsy, although frequently the terms are used erroneously in a synonymous manner.

PREDISPOSING FACTORS

Certain factors that are essentially uncontrollable increase the likelihood of a child's having cerebral palsy during the period immediately surrounding birth.

First-born. This factor applies until the mother's fourth or fifth pregnancy occurs. If one of these first births results in cerebral palsy, there is an increasing likelihood that later children may suffer the disorder. The incidence in subsequent children, however, is not as great as in the first-born.

Premature birth. Approximately 40% of all persons with cerebral palsy have a history of prematurity. As might be expected in premature infants, the greater the prematurity the greater the likelihood of brain damage.

Abnormalities of labor. A prolonged period of labor or an unusually rapid labor is more likely to produce cerebral palsy.

Abnormalities of delivery. Unusual fetal presentation, major manipulative procedures, or cesarean section is more prone to be productive of the disorder.

Multiple births. One of twins, usually the second one delivered, has a greater likelihood of being afflicted than if the product of conception had terminated in a single birth.

Heavy birth weight. Babies with heavier than average birth weights are more likely to suffer brain damage. This apparently is caused by increased probabilities of cerebral trauma resulting from increased head size.

Race. Cerebral palsy reportedly is somewhat more common in Caucasians than in persons of dark-skinned races.

Sex. Males are slightly more prone to be afflicted than females, although a great difference does not exist.

INCIDENCE

Phelps reported that the frequency of babies being born with cerebral palsy as the result of prenatal or natal causes was 7 for each 100,000 general population per year. Morbidity figures according to live births vary among observers from 1:200 to 1:568. The total number of patients with cerebral palsy of all ages has been estimated to be between 400 and 600 per 100,000 general population.

CAUSE

Conditions that produce cerebral anoxia and hemorrhage or trauma, either singly or combined, are the most common etiologic agents. These factors, if of sufficient intensity or duration, may operate during the prenatal, natal, or postnatal periods of life and produce an irreversible brain abnormality resulting in cerebral palsy.

Prenatal conditions. The more common of the prenatal conditions include infectious illnesses in the mother early in pregnancy, particularly mild viral infections; abnormal placental attachments; toxemia in the mother; maternal hypotension; anemia; radiation, particularly early in gestation and if therapy is directed to the mother's pelvic organs; isoimmunization, such as Rh incompatibility between mother and fetus; and any condition in which the mother suffers intense or prolonged anoxia. The hereditary element per se is a very uncommon cause for cerebral palsy. Recent investigations have suggested that maternal nutritional deficits preceding and during pregnancy may bear an important relationship to the presence of brain abnormality and cerebral palsy in the offspring.

Natal conditions. The natal period refers to that period of pregnancy from the onset of labor to the birth of a viable child. Incidents that may produce brain damage during this time are primarily anoxia and trauma, either singly or combined. Some of the more common situations producing these damaging cerebral onslaughts are as follows: depressing maternal anesthesia that in turn temporarily enfeebles the vital centers of the baby, thus delaying the onset and effectiveness of natural respirations; placenta praevia or abruptio placentae, thus removing a source of oxygen to the baby before the infant's normal respiratory mechanism can operate; delaying birth unduly by force against the presenting part pending the accomplishment of desired preparations for delivery; prolapsed cord with delay in delivery of the head; difficult instrumental delivery; acute hypotension in the mother as a result of spinal anesthesia; precipitate birth resulting in cerebral damage as a result of sudden change in pressure from intrauterine to extrauterine life; breech presentation with delay in delivery of the aftercoming head; and vigorous manipulative procedures.

Postnatal conditions. Most situations occurring after birth that may lead to brain abnormality are more apparent. The more important of these circumstances include the following: kernicterus, often the result of erythroblastosis; brain infections, such as meningitis, encephalitis, and abscesses; cerebral trauma, often resulting from falls or other accidents; intense or prolonged anoxia resulting from any cause; brain tumors; and cerebral circulatory anomalies, often leading to rupture.

Certain systemic diseases may cause brain damage as a result of secondary effects. For example, cerebral thrombosis may be a complication of nephritis, nephrosis, or other disease; cerebral embolus may result from subacute bacterial endocarditis occurring as a complication of rheumatic fever, congenital heart disease, or other conditions; and rupture of minute cerebral blood vessels may occur with severe paroxysms of coughing in an infant with pertussis.

CLASSIFICATION

The most useful classification of cerebral palsy at this time is one based on

Table 1. Basic clinical types and characteristics in cerebral palsy

Type	Basic clinical characteristics
1. Spasticity	Increased resistance to manipulation; stretch reflex; hyperactive deep tendon reflexes; clonus; tendency toward contracture deformities; lower extremities often more involved than upper extremities
2. Athetosis	Involuntary and incoordinated motions without conscious control; normal reflexes when in relaxed state; upper extremities often more involved than lower extremities
3. Ataxia	Disturbance of autonomic balance; nystagmus; adiadochokinesis; difficulty in concentrating vision on a fixed field; normal tendon reflexes
4. Rigidity	"Lead pipe" resiliency of involved member; tendency to maintain position of extension; absent stretch reflex; near normal tendon reflexes
5. Tremor	Intention-tremor contractions occur only with attempted motions; nonintention-tremor contractions are present constantly; no hyperactivity of tendon reflexes

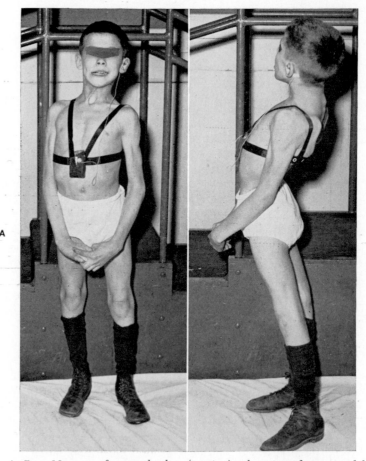

Fig. 204. A, Boy, 12 years of age, who has (tension) athetosis and associated hearing loss partially compensated for by a hearing aid. Note generalized hypertrophy of muscles, more involvement of the right shoulder than the left, pronated feet, and voluntary attempt to stabilize purposeless movements of the right upper extremity by clasping with the left hand. **B,** Lateral view of the same boy showing marked lordosis and genu recurvatum as a result of increased tension in an attempt to maintain standing balance as his center of gravity shifts.

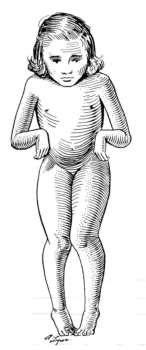

Fig. 205. Cerebral palsy with spastic quadriplegia. Flexion at all joints except the ankles. Adduction and internal rotation of the thighs. Scissors gait.

clinical findings. Autopsy material correlated with careful clinical observations in the same person has been insufficient to permit an authentic pathologic categorization according to types.

Table 1 lists the basic clinical types in decreasing order of frequency of occurrence as recognized by most physicians particularly interested in patients with cerebral palsy.

A mixture of more than one type may be present in the same person but probably is not found in more than approximately 1% of all patients.

The high spinal spastic type has been described in addition to those types as presented in Table 1. The site of damage in this type of cerebral palsy is at the level of the juncture between skull and atlas. The manifestation expected with this lesion is spasticity of the lower extremities.

Table 2. Extent of involvement

Descriptive term	Extent of involvement
Quadriplegia or tetraplegia	All four limbs
Hemiplegia	One side of body
Triplegia	Hemiplegia plus one limb of opposite side
Diplegia	Like parts on each side of body
Paraplegia	Both legs
Monoplegia	A single limb or part of body

The extent of involvement is variable from patient to patient. Table 2 indicates the descriptive terms used to denote parts of the body affected.

The degree of involvement is perhaps more important than the type of cerebral palsy when considering possibilities for physical rehabilitation. A mild degree of involvement suggests that extensive treatment measures are not necessary and can usually be accomplished by the parents in their home. One who is affected to a moderate degree needs special therapy measures that often include the use of braces and sometimes surgical procedures. One with a severe degree of involvement has only limited possibilities for physical rehabilitation even with the use of all special therapeutic measures available.

ASSOCIATED DEFECTS

The presence of one or more associated disabilities in the person with cerebral palsy is more often present than not. These disabilities are usually the direct result of the primary brain abnormality. Table 3 enumerates the more common associated defects that are found in the cerebral palsy population.

SOCIAL INFLUENCES

Very few diseases have social factors complicating the condition as extensively as does cerebral palsy. Formerly it was

Table 3. Associated defects frequently present in persons with cerebral palsy

Defect	Approximate frequency of occurrence
Mental defectiveness	25 to 40%
Educational retardation	Frequency is correlated with degree of severity; very common in patients other than mildly affected
Speech involvement	70 to 80%
Hearing defects	30 to 40%
Oculomotor abnormality	30 to 40%
Convulsive disorder	40%
Perceptual defects	Frequency undetermined; more common in those with athetosis
Symbolic language disability*	Frequency undetermined; probably fairly common
Physical growth retardation	Frequency is often related to the degree and extent of involvement; in part due to feeding difficulties
Emotional disturbances	Fairly common to varying degree

*Includes dysphasia, aphasia, reading disabilities, and allied abnormalities.

considered that all persons with cerebral palsy were feebleminded; thus institutional placement was the course to follow. Unfortunately, this attitude still exists in the minds of a segment of the population, and it has been conducive to the social isolation of afflicted persons in their homes. In addition, many other factors currently exist to the detriment of a healthful emotional state in one with cerebral palsy. Some of these are enumerated.

Parental guilt feelings and martyr complex. Studies have indicated that over two-thirds of all parents of children with cerebral palsy have feelings of personal guilt and consider that this handicapped child is theirs as a cross to bear. One would expect that such attitudes might be conveyed readily by the parents to the child in ways other than verbal expression. Parents who have these feelings to a strong degree are loathe to discuss their problems with others and tend toward voluntary introversion or extroversion and over-solicitousness as a compensatory device.

Family disagreements. Approximately one-half of the parents of children with cerebral palsy in one study admitted serious family disagreements regarding problems presented by their afflicted children.

Parental lack of information. The majority of parents have little or no authentic knowledge of etiologic factors, possibilities for successful rehabilitation, realistic aims, or even a basic understanding of what the term cerebral palsy means. Perhaps, as might be expected, the majority of parents exaggerate both the severity of involvement and the mental acuity of their child because of lack of knowledge or failure to accept the facts. Approximately one-half of the parents of these children make little or no use of literature available on the subject, and most of those who have attempted self-education in this manner have found the reading to be confusing or of no help. It is not unusual to find parents who are accomplishing no rehabilitation program at home because they are uninformed as to how they should proceed.

Professional help sought. The common response of parents of children with cerebral palsy is (1) rejection of the initial examiner and the information he gives when it is unfavorable, (2) the seeking of more favorable information from other sources, and finally, (3) the realistic acceptance of the child's condition. Thus, in one study of 200 parents of children with cerebral palsy having an average age near 8 years, the average amount of help sought per child was from nine medical physicians, two chiropractors, and one osteopath. Obviously, such shifting parental allegiance is detrimental to the possibility of any helpful approach to the child.

Oversolicitousness. Approximately 40% of parents admit to oversolicitousness toward their child. Experience suggests that this is a conservative estimate. School teachers, playmates, and other associates of the child with cerebral palsy are prone to manifest this same attitude and thus enhance the impact of this factor.

Limitations in socialization. Socialization experiences of the handicapped child are usually curtailed proportionately according to the severity of his physical handicap or associated defects. Approximately three-fourths of all children with cerebral palsy who are not in school have few if any playmates outside their home. In addition, it is not uncommon to find a child with cerebral palsy of 5 or 6 years of age who has never been inside a supermarket or five-and-ten cent store, seen an airport, or had similar experiences that are fairly commonplace for a nonhandicapped child.

THERAPY

An effective therapeutic program may require the services of an organized group of professional people in view of (1) the physical handicap itself, (2) the associated defects, some of which are usually present in one with cerebral palsy as mentioned previously, and (3) the social influences encountered by the child with cerebral palsy.

The broad aims of therapy should be to establish locomotion, communication, and self-help; to work toward an appearance of normality in all motor functions; to correct associated defects as effectively as possible; and to provide educational opportunities adapted to the given child's needs.

This plan of therapy may be accomplished in the home or in a hospital, or it may require special and prolonged facilities as provided in a hospital-school. In any eventuality, continued home therapy becomes essential for those patients who may have had their therapy initiated in a hospital or hospital-school. The needs of the patient and the home facilities available become most important in deciding which of these facilities is most advantageous for a given patient.

Obviously, to enable one to establish more specific aims in therapy, a thorough evaluation of the entire person becomes a necessity at the beginning of his management and must be effected recurrently as his needs demand. Usually, the scope of this evaluation goes beyond the capabilities of a single person and often requires the services of a physician, psychologist, speech pathologist, social worker, nursing personnel, and other professional persons.

The services of special therapists in physical therapy, occupational therapy, and speech pathology frequently are necessary to accomplish corrective exercises in a given patient or to instruct and demonstrate to parents sufficiently so that recommended procedures may be accomplished in the home. Parents can accomplish many of these exercises if they are instructed adequately in measures to be accomplished.

Medical help is required in several ways. Of importance is one physician who may act as a coordinator of the rehabilitation program for a given patient because of his particular interest in this condition. He may be a general practitioner or specialist in any one field. It is he to whom the parents may turn for counseling when questions arise. The consultation of other medical specialists frequently is necessary for purposes of correcting associated defects as well as aiding in the basic rehabilitation program.

Appliances such as braces or splints are used frequently for purposes of correcting or preventing deformities, reducing incoordinated and purposeless movements of the limbs, or affording increased stability.

Special equipment often becomes necessary as a means of effecting therapy procedures. Kneeling benches, stand-up tables, parallel bars, relaxation chairs, and special adaptations of feeding utensils are most commonly used.

Surgical procedures on tendons, nerves, or joints become necessary in a certain number of these patients. Neurosurgery has afforded very limited benefits thus far and is seldom used therapeutically.

Medications have extremely limited usefulness. Some products are of limited value for their relaxant properties; however, they are only adjuncts to other forms of therapy. Some medications are used to reduce salivary action and drooling. Preparations advocated earlier for improving mental acuity have since been found to have such limited value that they are unimportant. The drugs ordinarily used for control of seizures have similar usefulness in the patient with cerebral palsy.

Parent counseling is of great importance in making a program of therapy effective. The parents must be given basic information regarding cerebral palsy in general and facts pertaining to the condition as it relates to their own child. Realistic planning for rehabilitation (both physical and educational) and eventually for vocational anticipations should be accomplished. The counselor may be the physician who is coordinating the program or some other professional person if he has competent knowledge, adequate interest, and sufficient adeptness.

• • •

A person who has cerebral palsy is likely to have numerous and variable problems related directly or indirectly to his condition. Early recognition and attention to his problems, intelligent planning and accomplishment of a coordinated program of rehabilitation, and wise counseling are measures whereby satisfactory restoration may be effected in the majority of those so afflicted.

NURSING CARE

Cerebral palsy is one of the common causes of crippling in children. Yet it is not unusual for student nurses to complete their entire course of training without caring for such a patient on the hospital wards. Indeed, nurses often tell their instructors that their most impressive introduction to the patient with cerebral palsy is frequently outside the hospital entirely, on the street or in the home of some friend or neighbor.

Poliomyelitis (infantile paralysis) has received much attention during the past decade, and much has been done to eliminate this condition. One could hope that a similar amount of public interest might be evinced by this other comparable problem. However, cerebral palsy is a disability that does not strike spectacularly in epidemic form, and the results of it, although quite disastrous, are sometimes not appealingly dramatic. People are not instinctively drawn toward the unfortunate victim of this condition. They tend to be somewhat appalled and repelled by him, even when their sympathy for him is most manifest. Each nurse, as an individual in her own private world, may sometimes make the lot of the person with cerebral palsy more bearable because she has been able to interpret his situation sensibly and realistically to her friends or to her community. It can be admitted truthfully at the outset that this service may be a more important one than the relatively small amount of nursing care she will have the opportunity to give these patients in the hospital.

In ward classes student nurses discussing this condition frequently make the opinions of the public at large very graphic by their own reports of past experience. One student told how, as a child, she would cross the street to keep from passing a certain young boy. He jerked and twisted in all directions, and she was afraid of him. Furthermore, she had overheard some neighbors make the statement that his mother was frightened by a snake before he was born and that this accounted for his wiggling motions! She knows now that the boy was an athetoid, and she remembers that he always seemed to try to smile in a friendly fashion at the people who passed him. Another student told of a girl friend of hers in high school whose younger sister wasn't quite

right. The child was kept for years in an upstairs room. She was allowed to play only in a fenced-in backyard. One day the student saw the child in the backyard and noticed that she walked on her toes with her knees crossed and that she drooled and laughed raucously. The student remembers that she shuddered while watching the child and that she felt a great repulsion as though she were looking upon something not quite human. Now, however, she wonders why someone did not tell the parents of that child that perhaps something could be done for her.

Importance of early recognition and treatment

Early recognition is an important factor in the treatment of the condition. This is not always as easy as it might seem, particularly in the case of the mildly affected child. The more severely affected ones are not likely to be overlooked. With the history of a difficult labor, correlation between certain symptoms in the baby and his obstetric background makes the attending doctor and nurse particularly observant. Cyanosis,

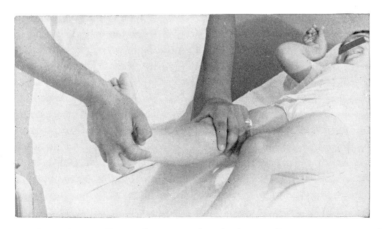

Fig. 206. Stretching the Achilles tendon. Note that the knee is kept in extension and that the entire sole of the foot bears the pressure (not simply the forefoot). (From Kenney, William C., and Larson, Carroll B.: Orthopedics for the general practitioner, St. Louis, 1957, The C. V. Mosby Co.)

convulsions, dyspnea, apnea, and twitching indicate an advanced degree of involvement. Increased crying, vomiting, hiccoughs, rigidity, or tenseness may be present in less severely affected babies. All symptoms of this nature should be faithfully recorded on the infant's chart and in considerable detail. Many such babies are also intractably difficult feeders, and this may be a significant factor in diagnosis.

In the infant with very mild involvement none of the above symptoms may be present. As the infant grows older, however, certain features make their appearance which should not escape the nurse's attention. Unless, however, the nurse knows at least the elements of normal child development, she will not be prepared to recognize departures from the normal in these children.

It is not at all uncommon for this condition to escape detection until the child begins to walk, although delay in walking may be significant. Sometimes a tendency to walk on the toes (contracture of the Achilles tendon) accompanied by adduction of the thighs and knees may be the only symptoms that are noted at this time.

It has been interesting to note that babies of a year or under are frequently brought to doctors' offices for some slowness in development, such as being unable to sit up or to lift the head, and the story is told that the baby was normal until he had an attack of stomach flu or a cold, or perhaps a fall, when he was about 6 months old. These incidents in the baby's short history could be the cause of the obvious existing cerebral palsy, but in many cases doctors feel that parents have simply not noticed or admitted that symptoms existed until the child reached 6 months of age, and it was no longer possible to ignore certain retardations in development. There is a definite resistance even among well-educated people to accept a diagnosis of spastic paralysis. It is still inherent in the public's understanding that these children are degenerate. There seems to be a stigma attached to them, and families tend to be ashamed, as they would never be ashamed of a child with poliomyelitis or, for that matter, with tuberculosis, though the latter might honestly be considered to present more aspects of blame and censure for the family than cerebral palsy.

It is very important that treatment be begun early. As far as possible the training of the child with cerebral palsy should follow the development of the normal child. If the condition is not diagnosed until the child is 3 years of age or older, a great deal of valuable time will have been lost. Nurses will remember that the average child tends to sit at 6 months of age, attempts to creep at about 10 months, and tries to stand alone at 15 months. In the mildly affected child this sequence might have been approximated with but little delay had training been instituted early enough.

Frequently parents are tempted to follow advice secured from unreliable sources, particularly about taking the child to unqualified practitioners. This tendency is expensive and dangerous, and the nurse must marshal her best (but unhysteric) arguments against it.

Probably no parents ever need help as badly as those with a child with cerebral palsy. Nurses need to know all community resource possibilities for the care and education of such children as well as those available in the state and nation. Cerebral palsy is an exceedingly complex problem, and the needs of the child for special types of treatment may be very great. Specially trained physical therapists, occupational therapists, speech therapists, and teachers may be required. The state society for crippled children and adults can usually give the nurse much valuable help on this problem and will be able to refer her to other agencies for additional help. Intelligent, sympathetic information given the family by the nurse sometimes prevents a great outlay of expense and energy in traveling from one healer to another in search of a miraculous, quick recovery for the child.

The nurse and the emotional aspects of this disease

What should be the attitude of the nurse toward these children? As far as possible it should be the attitude one has with a normal child. It has been repeatedly emphasized that workers in this field must remember the patient is first of all a child and only secondarily a victim of cerebral palsy. Friendliness, interest, affection, and dependability should be manifest in the nurse's actions, for the child needs these things and they add to his feeling of security and personal importance. It should be realized that patients with cerebral palsy are quicker than many other children to detect an unsympathetic presence. They are equally sure to sense a friendly one. It is essential to secure their confidence and friendship, for upon these things much of the success in treatment may depend. Furthermore, the nurse is urged to learn all she can about the child she is caring for, concerning both background and personal history as well as the improvement that the doctor believes possible. Has the child come from a home where family life has revolved around him as though he were a pivot? Has he been shoved in the background and treated with great negligence? The nurse's attitude toward the child may need to be altered somewhat by what she learns of his background. We know that the education of the parents is a very important part of

the treatment of these children. Treatment must carry on far into the future life of the child; otherwise, its value is questionable from the start. All treatment for these children is premised on this concept. Probably the two features indispensable to the treatment of the patient with cerebral palsy are these: mental capacity to make treatment of permanent value and the understanding and cooperation of the parents.

Too often the afflicted child has been utterly spoiled by the time he comes to the hospital. It may be because of a parent who has decided, with almost a religious fervor, to devote her whole life to the child to compensate him for being crippled. No responsibility of any kind has ever been given him, and he has never had to take the consequences for his misdeeds. Hospital experience will not be easy for such children, but if the situation is directed by an intelligent and understanding nurse it can be of great benefit. The child's moments of rebellion and temper will occur less frequently as he sees his unbecoming behavior duplicated in others like himself in the ward. The nurse's manner—quiet, firm, understanding, but unwavering where principle is concerned—will play a great part in the child's emotional development. This is so important that the nurse should never underestimate her share in the treatment of these children. Too often a complaint is made by the nurse that the physical therapist, the occupational therapist, and the teacher are the ones who really contribute toward the rehabilitation of these children, and we as nurses have little to do with it. This attitude is quite false. The child spends more time with the nursing group than with any other while he is in the hospital. The nurse's attitude and her teaching, by precept, example, and practice, can do much toward the emotional development of the child, and this service to him is not to be minimized.

Intelligence in cerebral palsy is not measurable by appearance. Facial contortions, a raucous voice, emotional instability, gutteral speech, apparent inability to understand what is being said, laziness, and lack of desire to do things for himself do not always signify low mentality. Opinions as to the mental capacity of persons afflicted with cerebral palsy vary considerably. Estimations of mentality based on mental tests that require some type of motor response are not considered reliable in giving an accurate measurement of the child's mental endowment. As better instruments for measurement are devised, however, and as knowledge of the various types of cerebral palsy increases, a more adequate estimation of the child's educability is becoming possible. Whereas too much optimism is always to be avoided until the child has been given the benefit of an examination by a specialist, to recommend custodial care for a badly affected child without such an examination is exceedingly unwise.

Defects of speech, hearing, sight, and sensation may be present in cerebral palsy. It can easily be seen that any of these defects might make the child seem less alert than he actually is. The athetoid is particularly likely to be slow to differentiate between sounds, and his ability to distinguish words may be greatly impaired. Defects of sight vary from lack of control of eye muscles and squinting to strabismus and nystagmus.

Cerebral palsy types are classified as spastic, athetoid, ataxias, rigidities, tremors, and others. The list grows as the knowledge of the disease progresses. The most frequent in occurrence are the spastic and the athetoid, and discussion of nursing care will be confined largely to these.

There is considerable variation in the treatment given to the two most common types of cerebral palsy patients. The child who presents the uncomplicated cortical involvement, the true spastic, has a set of symptoms that make efforts toward muscle reeducation the most important consideration. These children, confronted by a blocking of their voluntary efforts to perform an action, frequently tend to show signs of gradually developing frustration and apathy. There is reason enough to explain this, for each time the rigid spastic child attempts a movement, a sort of tug of war goes on between opposing muscles. Normal activity demands relaxation of one set of muscles while the other set contracts, but in the spastic child this does not happen. Constantly repeated blocking of his efforts may finally convince the child that the trial is not worth the effort, and he becomes harder to motivate than the person not so afflicted. Reeducation of muscles forms the basis of treatment, and muscle-checking to ascertain which muscles are strong, which are weak, and which are normal is essential to the program. But the emotional manifestations that characterize these children need some concurrent attention. They are not as a rule gregarious or outgoing in their attitude toward others. They tend to be fearful of new situations and of unknown experiences. They dread sharp, unexpected noises and are very much afraid of falling. Their fear of falling is based on experience, for a fall in an unrelaxed position is indeed an unpleasant occurrence.

The athetoid patient, on the other hand, can make normal movements without the block in the antagonist muscle that confronts the spastic patient, but he is deluged with a flood of involuntary purposeless movements that are beyond his control. He develops muscular tensions very early in life in an attempt to overcome this. Relaxation is the basis of treatment with the athetoid patient. Surgery and braces are seldom used because permanent fixed deformity does not occur in uncomplicated cases. These children are subject to spells of emotional instability approaching rages, but they are, on the whole, more out-going and affectionate. They like people and are less self-conscious than the rigid spastic patient.

In the third type of cerebral palsy, ataxia, the chief difficulty may be main-tenance of equilibrium. Because it is hard for these patients to balance them-selves, walking may be exceedingly difficult. These patients otherwise seem to be less severely involved than those with the two major types of the disease.

Certain principles apply to all types of cerebral palsy, and to avoid repetition these will be set down together. Such treatment as applies to one type or the

other is usually ordered by the physician who makes the diagnosis.

Relaxation, although paramount in athetosis, is important to all types of cerebral palsy. Too much stimulation of any nature is inadvisable. Surgical wards, wards used as centers of play for a noisy group of children, and loud radio programs of syncopated music are not good for these children. The environ-ment should be particularly quiet before meals, before the physical therapy treat-ments, and before retiring. The need for a controlled environment in the home is also to be emphasized. The atmosphere of the ward at all times for these chil-dren should be one of fairly even tenor. Fatigue comes quickly with even small effort. It must be watched for and its symptoms recognized. The child tends to want to go on beyond his fatigue level. Rest periods need to be a little longer for these children because they go to sleep only after a considerable

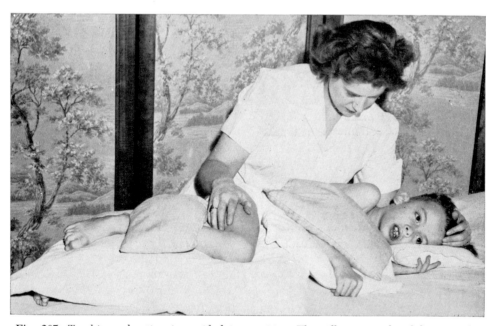

Fig. 207. Teaching relaxation in a side-lying position. The pillows are placed between the legs, under the upper arm, under the head, and the body is flexed. Here the control of athetosis is aided by the use of sandbags. (From Egel, Paula: Technique of treatment for the cerebral palsy child, St. Louis, 1948, The C. V. Mosby Co.)

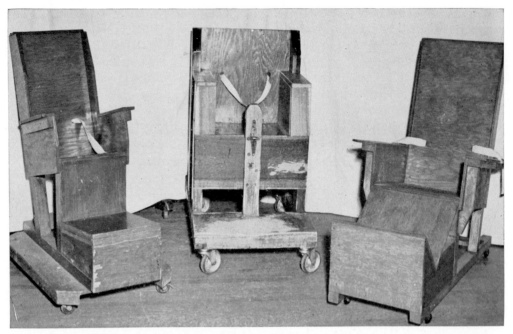

Fig. 208. Specially constructed chairs to promote relaxation in the patient with cerebral palsy. (From Egel, Paula: Technique of treatment for the cerebral palsy child, St. Louis, 1948, The C. V. Mosby Co.)

period of lying in a quiet room. In observing them after they have relaxed and gone to sleep, one will note that their exhaustion is sometimes out of all proportion to the activity they have engaged in. One of the chief lessons the patient wtih cerebral palsy must learn is how to relax voluntarily. In order to help the child to do this, nurses should be familiar with the methods used by physical therapists in teaching relaxation. Sometimes it is possible to help the child by reference to some familiar relaxing incident, experience, or sensation. For example, the child might be asked to try to imitate a soft and cuddly kitten, or a handful of sand, or a feather or leaf floating in the wind.

Nursing responsibilities in speech training

It is now generally conceded that the ability to talk is a primary need in cerebral palsy patients and that it is much more important, for instance, than learning to walk. Speech is bound up closely with every other type of learning, and every experience might be said to have its speech component. Nurses should attempt to follow up the child's periods with the speech therapist by paralleling each experience the child has during the day with conversation appropriate to that experience—that is, talk about clothes as the child dresses and talk about food as he eats.

Speech training for the patient with cerebral palsy should be given by qualified speech therapists. To be most effective it should be begun early, preferably between 2 and 5 years of age. By beginning this training early it will not be necessary for the child to unlearn the poor habits of communication that children with speech difficulties usually have. Parents may help prepare the child for speech training by having regular periods each day devoted to talking to the child. If the child is very young, talking should be accompanied by looking at pictures or handling the objects about which the parent is talking. This simple beginning in speech training will aid considerably in the child's development. It is a natural tendency for the child to try to imitate and echo the sounds he hears, and the child with cerebral palsy should not be deprived of this experience.

A factor that must be remembered by

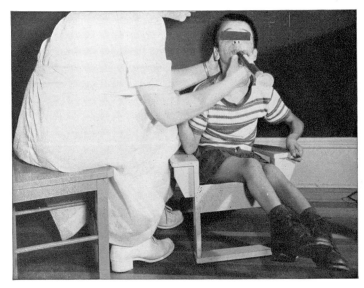

Fig. 209. Speech therapist developing the ability in a patient with cerebral palsy to exhale by blowing on a horn. (From Kenney, William C., and Larson, Carroll B.: Orthopedics for the general practitioner, St. Louis, 1957, The C. V. Mosby Co.)

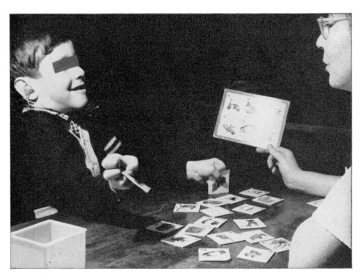

Fig. 210. Speech therapist using a combination of pictures and lipreading to aid speech in a deaf athetoid child. (From Kenney, William C., and Larson, Carroll B.: Orthopedics for the general practitioner, St. Louis, 1957, The C. V. Mosby Co.)

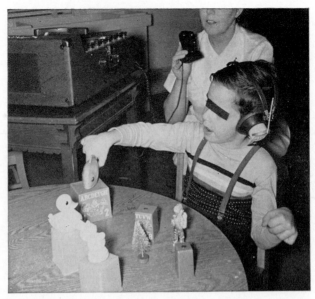

Fig. 211. Speech therapist using a Trainear portable amplifier to give instructions to a child with cerebral palsy. (From Kenney, William C., and Larson, Carroll B.: Orthopedics for the general practitioner, St. Louis, 1957, The C. V. Mosby Co.)

both nurses and parents is that the child must be urged to ask for the things he wants. If he can get what he wants without asking for it, he will try to do so. Speech therapists emphasize the fact that it is not wise to interpret the child's speech by satisfying his wants too easily. Much of the motivation to speak more accurately may thereby be lost.

Although poor habits of speech should, of course, be discouraged on the wards when the nurse knows the patient is capable of doing better, it is unwise to constantly call attention to the child's speech, particularly in a nagging manner. An emotional block toward the whole speech problem may be induced by nagging. Encouragement and assistance rather than correction should characterize the nurse's approach to this matter.

Teaching the child
to feed himself

Ability to feed himself is an important accomplishment for the child with cere-

bral palsy. Equipment for eating therefore should be optimal. Consultation with the occupational therapist will frequently reveal to the nurse ways of adapting existing hospital equipment to fit the needs of the child for handling his own food. Spoons can be built up with sponge rubber that can be wound around the handle to make a bulky object easy for the child to grasp. If this is covered with plastic material and secured at the base with waterproof tape, it can be washed and dried with the other hospital silver. A specially constructed chair with a slight backward tilt and a table with a space hollowed out for the child's body are especially useful. If the table can be constructed with depressions to receive a bowl, a glass, or cup so that things will not slide away from the child as he reaches for them, it will be particularly suitable for his use. Lacking this feature, however, it has been found that small rubber mats, frequently used under tumblers, and bowls equipped with suction cups

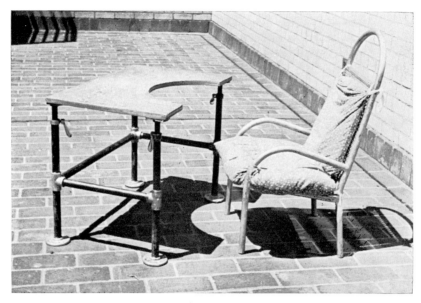

Fig. 212. Adjustable table and chair for patient with cerebral palsy. Made by hospital carpenter.

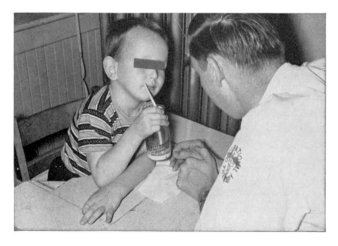

Fig. 213. Therapist teaching a patient with cerebral palsy to drink through a straw. (From Kenney, William C., and Larson, Carroll B.: Orthopedics for the general practitioner, St. Louis, 1957, The C. V. Mosby Co.)

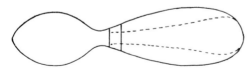

Fig. 214. Spoon built up with sponge rubber and covered with plastic material to make a good grasping handle for the child with cerebral palsy.

will help to keep the dishes from slipping about on the table. It is advisable to have the child's elbows supported by the table as he eats, since much greater relaxation will be obtained in that way. The feet should rest on a solid surface and not dangle in mid-air. A large waterproof bib will give the child freedom

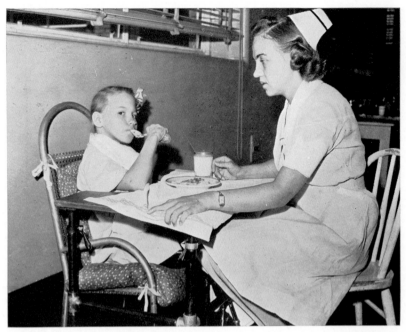

Fig. 215. Patient with cerebral palsy and equipment for assisting her to feed herself. Depressions in the table for holding dishes and cups are advisable for the badly affected child.

from fear of spilling food on his clothes. Many other details for making mealtime a more comfortable experience for the child can be worked out so that the period is less an ordeal for both the nurse and the patient than it sometimes is when no special equipment is provided.

Because much of the muscular coordination needed for chewing and swallowing is also necessary in speech, it is advisable that as soon as possible the child be given food that requires chewing. Chewing will aid considerably in developing control of the jaw and throat muscles. Some speech therapists advise that the child's training in swallowing can be aided materially by use of a lollipop. In sucking a lollipop the child will learn many of the tongue motions that are necessary in swallowing. A drinking straw is useful in teaching the child to narrow his mouth motion.

Most workers with cerebral palsy pa-

tients, however, advise that training for eating should not be done at mealtime. To avoid an emotional block, it is better for the child to learn these things at a time when his nutrition is not involved. Training in many of the details that concern eating are often incorporated in the physical and occupational therapy programs. Such skills are accomplished very gradually, and the child learns to master one motion thoroughly before he is advanced to another. If he can learn to raise an empty glass to his mouth, first by being guided by the therapist's hand and then by his own effort, he has advanced considerably toward being able to feed himself. After he has mastered the empty glass, a very small amount of liquid is added to it, and this is continued until he can lift a glass containing the usual portion of liquid.

Drooling is almost always a matter of great concern to the parents of the child with cerebral palsy. Training to overcome this habit is usually begun concurrently with speech therapy because it is considered to be the result, at least in part, of an inactive tongue. Speech clinicians tell us that something can be done for drooling in almost every instance. As the child learns to chew, suck, and swallow, he will automatically develop these reflexes that will aid in the control of drooling. It is also possible to aid the child in learning to swallow by having certain periods of the day when he practices swallowing rhythmically. For instance, in one exercise the mother or nurse counts to five and the child is instructed to swallow on the fifth count. Repeated faithful efforts in this will show results in the child's gradual ability to control drooling.

The child should have the benefit of quiet surroundings and suitable equipment when he is eating. In the hospital, where distractions are numerous, this is sometimes hard to provide without depriving the child of the companionship of his own age group. Consultation between nurse, physical therapist, and occupational therapist will frequently result in a flexible plan for the child that may be altered as his ability to feed himself and cope with distraction develops.

It must always be remembered that the child may need help, particularly with the last part of his meal. The severely affected patient cannot be deserted and expected to accomplish even minor tasks for himself. He may need help in adjusting his equipment. When he shows obvious symptoms of fatigue, he needs assistance. If he becomes disheartened by being given too much to do or too difficult tasks to perform, he tends to lose interest and courage. The nurse should keep this in mind even when she leaves him to perform a simple function of dressing or eating. Her encouragement and assistance will do much to promote in the child a feeling of accomplishment without tiring or discouraging him. There is a delicate difference in the matter of creating in the child's mind the ability and desire to do things for himself and confusing him by the assignment of impossible tasks that are beyond his capacity.

It is essential to teach the child to watch what he is doing. Once his concentration span is gone, he learns little by his fumbling efforts. The nurse must not be fooled, however, by the child's little tricks of feigning fatigue with a long-drawn-out sigh or a look of helplessness. He is likely to make tentative trials in this direction for the benefit of new nurses. (This is human nature and not peculiar to cerebral palsy.) Patience, understanding of the child's personality, and considerable firmness are necessary in combating these episodes. Back of this must be the continued interest in the child's welfare, for he quickly detects when this is absent.

Nursing care for the child with cerebral palsy in the hospital

Sometimes the child with cerebral palsy is kept in the nursery wards of the orthopedic division long after his age would permit him to be moved. This is done so that he may remain in a crib. A child 8 years of age with fairly normal intelligence does not respond to this kind of treatment. He resents it. It does something to his spirit. If the child can be moved into a ward with children of his own age group, some provision for this must be made.

A great effort should be put forth to speak to these children very distinctly. It is not considered wise to repeat oneself because it seems that the child has not understood. If there is some type of hearing defect, it may take him several seconds or more to understand and carry out the order or answer the question given him. Consideration must be given the problem he has with the mere task of motor response. If words are repeated his ability to respond is interrupted by deluging him with more stimuli. Facial expression should be carefully controlled, or he will detect impatience and be discouraged at the outset. He must be spoken to clearly, simply, and directly, and sufficient time must be allowed for him to comprehend and organize his response. Repetition is in order only when he has asked for it.

It should be recognized from the outset that it is an injustice for the nurse to rush through the care of the patient with cerebral palsy. These children do not progress at the hands of hurried, overwrought nurses. Their response to this haste is unmistakable—a tightening of all muscles, rigidity, and increased tenseness—the very things the child has been brought to the hospital to overcome. If it is at all possible, the nurse should postpone care of these patients until last in order to be able to give them more time to attempt to do things for themselves. This is sometimes impossible because of early morning assignments to physical or occupational therapy, but when it can be managed, the opportunity should not be neglected. Allowing the child to wash and dry his own face and hands or to brush his teeth may take what seems an unjustifiable amount of the nurse's time, but the reward attendant upon these efforts seems so great that no nurse should overlook it.

Toilet habits are not usually difficult to establish in the mentally unaffected patient with cerebral palsy and should be begun as early as with normal children. Specially constructed low toilet seats with armrests are desirable so that the child may be left alone. Continued use of the bedpan long after the child is progressing toward a considerable degree of independence is not wise. For the child who spends most of his time in bed, some arrangement should be made to place him securely and comfortably on the pan and leave him alone rather than to stand at his side holding him—a feature not conducive to good toilet training.

Very early in his training should come an appeal to the child to develop proper habits of cleanliness, such as clean hands, brushed teeth, and neatly combed hair. This may seem a small matter, but it will go far toward giving him a feeling of personal worth, without which no other training is of much avail.

The nurse's responsibility in teaching the patient

While the patient with cerebral palsy is in the hospital, coordination of all the services affecting him must be worked for constantly. Methods of relaxation followed by careful muscle reeducation in physical therapy and hours of urging toward self-help in occupational therapy and in the schoolroom can be undone by the solicitous nurse on the ward if she does not realize that the ultimate aim of treatment is to enable the patient to care for himself to the limits of his ability. It is far easier at mealtime to feed the child than to sit beside him guiding, urging, and, if need be, assisting him to eat. But if he is allowed to feed himself only on days when the wards are not busy, he will lose the desire to do it at all. It has been observed over and over again that the child loses the will to feed himself if there are days when the nurse does it for him. He likes her presence, and it is not necessary for him to put forth any effort. Another factor that inevitably leads to his caring less about doing things for himself is the fact that he frequently realizes it is such a nuisance to the nurse to wait for him. These children are observing. They soon recognize signs of irritation or bother on their nurses' faces. It is not uncommon for a child with athetosis to break into fits of uncontrolled weeping in the middle of a meal for no greater reason than that he feels himself a nuisance. Probably it must be admitted from the outset that because of this necessity to

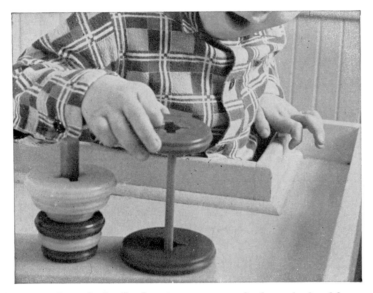

Fig. 216. Patient with cerebral palsy learning to grasp and release the hand by use of a large toy. Later, smaller objects will be used. Note also that the patient is in a standing table to help develop his ability to stand erect. (From Kenney, William C., and Larson, Carroll B.: Orthopedics for the general practitioner, St. Louis, 1957, The C. V. Mosby Co.)

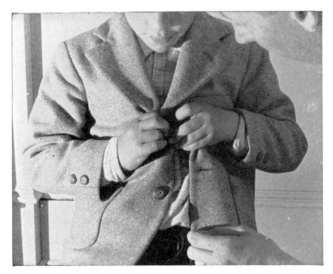

Fig. 217. Therapist teaching a patient with cerebral palsy to button and unbutton clothing. (From Kenney, William C., and Larson, Carroll B.: Orthopedics for the general practitioner, St. Louis, 1957, The C. V. Mosby Co.)

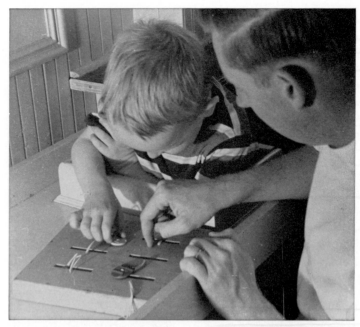

Fig. 218. Patient with cerebral palsy using a large model requiring, in general, the same type of movements needed to lace the shoes. (From Kenney, William C., and Larson, Carroll B.: Orthopedics for the general practitioner, St. Louis, 1957, The C. V. Mosby Co.)

hurry, hurry, hurry on the part of busy nurses on orthopedic surgical wards, the spastic child feels that he has no business being there.

The child's own wants in the matter of attempting new activities deserve consideration. The motive is strong at this time, and attention will be directed with greater success at something he really wants to do. Guidance is necessary to prevent frustrating disappointments.

Because one of the great aims of all treatment is to give the child as great a degree of independence as is compatible with his condition, considerable attention must be given toward assisting him to care for his own physical necessities. Teaching him to manage his own clothes is a point of great importance. This may be a very slow process in the badly affected child and may start with nothing more spectacular than an attempt to fold his garments as they are taken off. The less skilled movements naturally

come first, but some attempt can be made to prepare him to assume more of the task by allowing him to practice with a good-sized doll that has clothes fastened by a variety of gadgets, such as hooks and eyes, buttons, and zippers, as well as drawstrings and snaps.

When the child begins to walk on the ward, nurses should know exactly how he has been taught in the physical therapy department in order that consistency in instruction may be carried out. It is particularly important to note the child's habitual posture in walking and to discourage slumping attitudes or lazy methods of progression. It will help very little for the child to have 15 to 20 minutes' careful instruction in the physical therapy department once a day if he is allowed to form careless habits of walking the rest of the time on the ward.

Nurses learn from physical therapists of the use of mirrors in the physical training of the child with cerebral palsy.

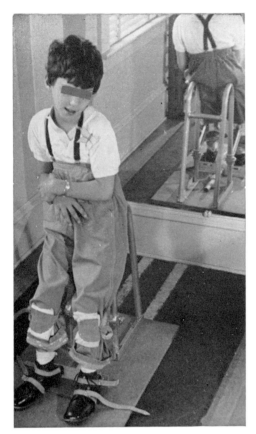

Fig. 219. Patient with cerebral palsy in stabilizer to achieve standing balance. (From Kenney, William C., and Larson, Carroll B.: Orthopedics for the general practitioner, St. Louis, 1957, The C. V. Mosby Co.)

It is often a remarkable fact that such a child learning to walk by the aid of lines drawn in front of a mirror will straighten his body almost as though by reflex when he comes within the range of vision of the mirror. He does not like the look of the stoop-shouldered youngster he sees ahead of him, and he will do his best to alter that appearance. Physical therapists frequently advise parents to use a weighted doll carriage in assisting the child to walk. Walkers are thought by some authorities to be inadvisable because the child, unless closely supervised, tends to push himself along without lifting his feet from the ground

and thereby develops undesirable habits of progression. Parallel bars, which furnish a sort of stabilized canelike support for the child, are considered more useful. Frequently, some type of support for the child's feet can be constructed to give a wider base for standing and walking. "Duck shoes" or "ski shoes" have been used for this purpose, and these are firmly fastened to the child's everyday shoes during his walking exercises. They are dispensed with as soon as possible, and the child is urged to attempt walking in the normal fashion.

The nurse caring for the patient with cerebral palsy over a considerable period of time will soon learn that there are certain conditions and occasions under

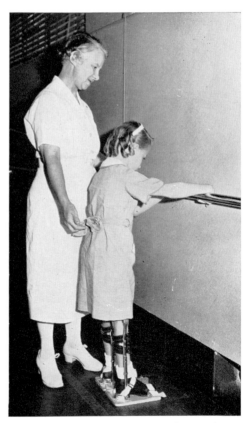

Fig. 220. "Duck shoes" strapped to ordinary shoes for balancing exercises preceding walking attempts.

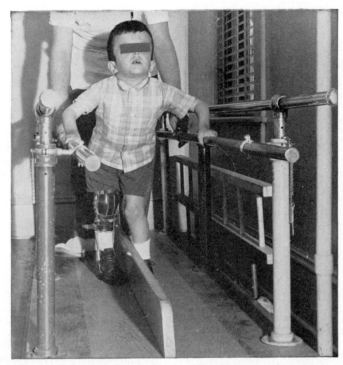

Fig. 221. Patient with cerebral palsy learning reciprocal gait in the parallel bars. Note the center piece to prevent scissoring. (From Kenney, William C., and Larson, Carroll B.: Orthopedics for the general practitioner, St. Louis, 1957, The C. V. Mosby Co.)

which the child relaxes best. Soothing music, gentle rhythmic movements of the limbs, warmth, light massage, and submersion in warm pools frequently are efficacious in assisting the child to relax. Since she knows that a great deal of the patient's progress depends directly upon his ability to meet new situations and environments successfully, the nurse will seek to increase the child's ability to relax in other less optimal circumstances. This will require time and thought and will be accompanied by many backsets, but the carry-over is possible if the child's mentality is normal.

POSTENCEPHALITIC CEREBRAL PALSY

The postencephalitic cerebral palsies that follow some virus-induced disease that has affected the cortex of the brain are usually severe in nature. Loss of motor function occurs, and varying de-

grees of impairment in speech and intelligence sometimes are so severe in nature that any return of these functions is despaired of. Until a trial is made, however, pessimistic predictions are hardly justified, for considerable return of function has been possible in a number of the most severely affected patients of this type. These children, struck down suddenly, usually from a healthy normal childhood, present a most tragic spectacle because of the abruptness and devastation of the disease. A hopeless attitude is all too easy for the nurse and parents in dealing with these children, and often the best treatment that can be visualized by them is complete and conscientious care of the child with a view to his physical comfort and cleanliness. A more far-sighted attitude would be displayed in an effort to utilize the child's unaffected faculties as soon as the acute illness is over. Frequently, more is left from the wreckage than is at first apparent. One very bright boy, 14 years of age, with extremely severe involvement after encephalitis initiated by measles, was distressed immeasurably by not being able to make known his wants. A perplexed but sympathetic student nurse set herself to work out the problem with a piece of white poster paper. She divided her paper into six sections and made a crude drawing in each section: in one a bedpan, in another a urinal, in another a glass of water, and so on. By standing at the patient's bedside and pointing to the articles one after another, the boy could move his head sufficiently to let her know what he needed at the moment.

Nursing care after surgical treatment

Student nurses frequently see patients with cerebral palsy only when they are admitted to orthopedic wards for surgery. This is by no means the best time to make the child's acquaintance because he is likely to be more tense and emotional than at any other time. From the nurse's standpoint at least, it would be desirable to have him admitted long enough before surgery for her to establish some measure of rapport with him and to assure him of her friendliness, interest, and desire to help him. Only in this way can his great burden of apprehension and insecurity be alleviated. Fortunately, most surgeons feel that it is very unwise to operate on such children until they have become adjusted to their surroundings. Their hyperexcitability is likely to lead to acidosis if surgery follows too soon upon admission to the hospital. Furthermore, operations on rigid spastic patients are usually performed after a period of muscle training. If this interval devoted to muscle reeducation is spent in the hospital, the nurse can

help the patient make his adjustment to the ward situation more satisfactorily than is possible if he enters immediately preceding surgery.

Many operations have been made necessary in these patients because of failure to prevent secondary contractures that come about from constant positions of creeping, crawling, and sitting. These positions are the ones maintained by the child a great portion of the time if he is unable to walk. Parents should be instructed to have the child alternate these positions with periods of prone-lying. This tends to stretch the contracted flex-

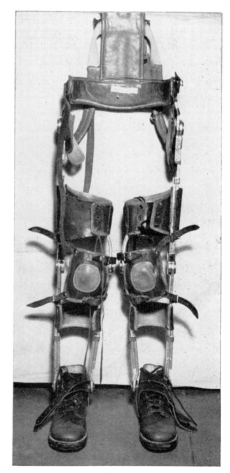

Fig. 222. Long leg braces with pelvic girdle worn by patient with cerebral palsy to prevent flexion contractures and to increase stability.

ors of the hip and to overcome the forward position of the shoulders. Another variation can be obtained in the back-lying position with a small pillow beneath the dorsal spine. At such times elevation of the bed or crib on boxes at the head will permit the child to see what goes on around him and not give him a feeling of isolation from ward or home activities.

The incidence of acidosis after surgery is rather high with these children, and considerable attention is given to pre-operative feeding of stick candy and orange juice. Intravenous glucose is occasionally administered to fortify the particularly excitable child against acidosis.

Postoperatively, these children sometimes display great apathy and prostration, greater than the mild surgical procedure they have been subjected to would seem to warrant. The nurse is urged to respect the child's desire to be let alone as much as is compatible with good care. If he is in casts (long leg or hip spica) after surgery on nerves or tendons, every alteration of his position tends to cause agonizing muscle spasm in the extremities. Even without such movement, his face will be contorted with expressions of pain at very frequent intervals as a result of spasm in the muscles at the site of surgery. Often, these spasms make him very resistant to any type of nursing care, and only the most skillful handling on the part of the nurse will be tolerated willingly. The patient must be turned very gently. No portion of the trunk must be allowed to change position during the turning process. Steady support along the body and cast is essential during any change of position.

The spastic child's postoperative nausea seems unduly prolonged. The intake of such children must be watched carefully because acidosis comes on with great rapidity in these cases. The doctor must be informed of the total 24-hour intake so that he may administer intravenous glucose if he thinks it necessary.

The skin of these children tends to break down easily when subjected to constant pressure. Attention to the child's every complaint regarding sensations of pressure is extremely important. Loss of some degree of sensation, however, is not uncommon in these children, and pressure areas may form beneath casts without any complaint from the child. Scrupulous care of the patient's skin, accompanied by frequent inspection of the cast for odor, rough edges, and the like, is indispensable.

If an adductor tenotomy has been performed, the site of incision in the groin is a frequent cause of concern to the nurse, particularly if the child is very young or is one who cannot be depended upon to call for the bedpan. Sometimes collodion dressings are applied, or waterproofing may be put on over the dressings and the edges may be sealed with waterproof adhesive tape. The nurse is occasionally given permission to change these dressings when the necessity arises. Although careful aseptic technique must be carried out, it is a recognized fact that these tissues seem to be resistant to urine-induced infections.

When the order is given to bivalve the casts and to remove the child from them for certain periods during the day, it has been observed that the child cries bitterly when the splints are put on again. Acute muscle spasm and tenseness sometimes make it almost impossible to reapply these splints, and, if force is used, the child frequently has a miserable night. It is advisable to try to bring about relaxation of the child's muscles rather than to use force in this circumstance. A prolonged bath in warm water sometimes helps to relax muscles and makes the application of these splints less painful for the child. The nurse's humane urge to leave off the splints after an unsuccessful attempt to apply them must be tempered by her realization that the tendency toward recurrence of deformity in these patients is very great, and much of the improvement made by the operation may be sacrificed if splinting is not carried out faithfully.

This difficulty is not so pronounced in the application of the braces that may be ordered later for the postoperative spastic patient. By the time braces are ready his postoperative tenderness has subsided. It has been found convenient to have the shoes that are attached to such braces cut open to the toes and eyelets made over the dorsum of the foot, since much easier manipulation of the foot is possible in this way. Grasping the sock over the instep and thereby guiding the foot into the shoe serves to overcome the tendency of the child's foot to go into plantar flexion as the shoe is applied.

Central nervous system operations, such as cordotomy and ramisection, are performed much less frequently than formerly. The nursing care for these patients is the same as combining the care of a patient who has had a laminectomy with that of a patient with hyperirritability and neuromuscular tension. Noticeable lessening of spasticity is sometimes observed, but it has been noted that this tends to be transitory. Changes in this regard must be carefully observed and recorded by the nurse throughout the postoperative period. The risk attending these operations is not inconsiderable, and the child will be seriously ill for some time.

Teaching parents home care of these children

Instruction for follow-up home care is so vital that the success of all hospital treatment may be said to be based upon it. Demonstrations of treatments and imparting information about the child are far from sufficient. If possible, the parents should spend several days in preparation for taking the child home. The mother should be allowed to see the treatments and nursing care on several occasions and to observe certain emergencies that arise in connection with the child's daily routine so that she will see how these have been dealt with in the hospital. It is particularly important for the parents to realize how serious an error it is to break down or interfere with the patient's nascent sense of his own independence and worth. On the other hand, although parents should be urged to encourage the child in his activities, some warning may be needed if they seem to be overly ambitious for the child's progress. Sometimes the parents' enthusiasm and desire for the child constantly to do better serve only to increase his tension, and he may be totally unable to relax in their presence. Furthermore, parents should understand that the child will occasionally go through a period when no improvement whatever seems to occur. These plateaus are part of the natural cycle of the patient with cerebral palsy, and too much concern should not be caused by their occasional appearance.

In giving instructions for home care to the parents of these children, the nurse may help them see the advantages of enlarging the child's horizon by means of friendships with other handicapped children as well as with normal children. The orthopedic public health nurse may be of considerable help to the parents in finding these friends. Assisting the child to forget himself is believed by some to be the major objective of treatment, since loss of agonizing self-consciousness is one of the surest ways to improve motor skill. Developing such objectivity may be a lifelong job, but the child should be brought to understand that the human race as a whole has the same fight before it. The obstacles are greater for those with cerebral palsy, but the rewards are greater, too, in the realization of the immense obstacles overcome.

Some attempt to educate the child's friends and associates in their approach and relationship with him may be advisable. Only friends who are by nature considerate of others should be encouraged. Outright rudeness or thoughtless remarks made to the handicapped person often discourage him from further attempts of a social nature. To help the child in meeting the inescapable crises, some explanation needs to be given to him about human nature and its variable response to the handicapped person. He should be brought to realize very early how children and grown-up people will frequently display unintelligent, ignorant attitudes toward him that are unthinkingly cruel on some occasions and foolishly sentimental on others. Perhaps the child old enough to comprehend these things can be made to realize that he himself must develop attitudes of tolerance and forbearance toward persons of limited abilities. His own limitations, after all, are largely physical. He should therefore be able to make allowances for errors in others who are even less well equipped than himself.

There are many crafts adaptable for the home use of the child with cerebral palsy. Finger painting is excellent for the child whose hand grasp is poor. Work with clay and embroidery on burlap with yarn and large blunt needles provide training toward muscular coordination. Looms and basketry are also excellent. Occupational therapists advise us that whatever craft the cerebral palsied child undertakes should be within his mental and physical capacity. The materials chosen for work should not be difficult to handle. In addition, the work should be the child's own, not that of the parents, nurses, or therapist. Motivation can too easily be destroyed if many alien hands interfere with the child's progress in making something that he would like to think of as entirely his own.

Community projects for the assistance of patients with cerebral palsy are numerous, and the alert public health nurse can help to interest local groups in the subject. One particularly good idea that has been worked out in a community is a so-called lending library of equipment for these patients—for example, reclining chairs, specially constructed tables with adjustable legs, dishes, etc. This, of course, entails having a carpenter available who can alter the equipment to suit the needs of the current borrower. As a family finishes using the particular item, it is sent back to the library where the carpenter makes the adjustments for the next borrower. Another example of community cooperation is a manual training class in a high school that has taken as a special project the construction of equipment recommended by a local orthopedist for use by persons with cerebral palsy.

The public health nurse can be of inestimable help to the parents of these children in many ways. She needs to know definitely what instructions were given the parents before taking the child home. She is entitled to know also the treatment and success of treatment that the child had in the hospital. If these details are made available to her before the child returns home she is fortified to assist the parents and the child in carrying out recommended treatment. It is essential that she have this information before the child goes home so that there will be no intermission or backsliding. Even a week of this can undo much of the effect of the hospital experience.

STUDY QUESTIONS

1. Study and list the possible causes of cerebral palsy.
2. What early symptoms might indicate the presence of this condition?
3. Discuss briefly the differences in treatment of the two main types of cerebral palsy.
4. Discuss the nurse's part in habit training in cerebral palsy.
5. What are some of the problems that might be encountered in the postoperative care of the patient with cerebral palsy?
6. Does the child's physical disability influence his mental and emotional development? Explain.
7. Can you visualize the problems parents and family are confronted with when a child is born with cerebral palsy? What assistance can the nurse give the parent?

REFERENCES

Abel, M.: Feeding the child with cerebral palsy, Am. J. Nursing **50**:558-560, 1950.

Bare, C., and others: Self-help clothing for handicapped children, National Society for Crippled Children and Adults, Chicago, Ill., 1962.

Cardwell, V. E.: Cerebral palsy: advances in understanding and care, Association for the Aid of Crippled Children, 1956, 345 East 46th St., New York 17, N. Y.

Carlson, E. R.: Born that way, New York, 1941, John Day Co.

Corner, G. W.: Fetal and neonatal anoxia and cerebral palsy, Cerebral Palsy Rev. **16**:4-6, 1955.

Deaver, G. G.: Cerebral palsy: methods of treating the neuromuscular disabilities, Arch. Phys. Med. **37**:363-367, 1956.

Denhoff, E., and Holden, R. H.: Understanding parents: one need in cerebral palsy, Cerebral Palsy Rev. **16**:9-11, 1955.

Gardner, E. D.: Fundamentals of neurology, ed. 4, Philadelphia, 1963, W. B. Saunders Co.

Glick, S. J.: Vocational, educational, and recreational needs of the cerebral palsy adult, New York, 1954, United Cerebral Palsy of New York.

Glick, S. J., and Donnell, C.: Nonmedical problems of the child with cerebral palsy, Nursing Outlook **1**:101-103, 1953.

Glick, S. J., and Donnell, C.: Nonmedical problems of the adult with cerebral palsy, Nursing Outlook **1**:277-279, 1953.

Hanna, R.: The function of a cerebral palsy treatment center, Cerebral Palsy Rev. **16**:5-8, 1955.

Lesser, A. J.: Progress in service for children with cerebral palsy, Cerebral Palsy Rev. **16**:8-9, 1955.

Mercer, Sir Walter, and Duthie, R.: Orthopedic surgery, ed. 6, Baltimore, 1964, Williams & Wilkins Co.

Pendleton, T.: Trainable cerebral palsied children, Phys. Ther. Rev. **41**:582-585, 1961.

Pendleton, T., and Simonson, J.: Training children with cerebral palsy, Am. J. Nursing **64**:126-129, 1964.

Rusalem, H.: Vocational adjustment of the handicapped child, Cerebral Palsy Rev. **15**:11-13, 1954.

Stewart, M.: The child with cerebral palsy and the nurse, Am. J. Nursing **52**:1228-1230, 1952.

Chapter 10

Common painful affections in adults

Low back pain, including nursing care

In recent years there has been an increasing number of patients complaining of pain in the lower portion of the back; hence much attention is paid to this disability in an attempt to determine precisely the origin of pain in each case.

With a detailed history, complete examination of the back, and adequate roentgenography, it is usually possible to determine whether the cause is likely to be infection, tumor, arthritis, or mechanical in nature. Any disease, injury, or affliction known to involve bones or joints throughout the body is capable of choosing the bones and joints of the lower part of the back. By far the majority of backaches are the result of mechanical stresses, and it is this type of backache that will be discussed.

ANATOMY OF THE LOW BACK

The anatomy of the lower part of the back should be reviewed for an understanding of the nature of mechanical causes of backache. The entire spine is composed of vertebral bodies that are separated by disks. These disks are resilient and capable of absorbing shock much the same as shock absorbers on automobiles. This shock-absorbing mech-

anism is nature's way of protecting the brain from impact shock, such as might occur in a jump from a height or a fall on the ice in a sitting position. When the disks are injured or chronically strained by repeated heavy lifting, they undergo changes so that they lose their resilience and become narrowed. This is called degeneration and is commonly painful.

The facets are small joints, one on either side of each vertebral segment, that form the fulcrum for motion when the spine is flexed, extended, rotated, or bent sideward. These facets are covered with smooth articular cartilage that allows easy, gliding, symmetric motion when they are normally placed. Frequently the facets are asymmetric or anomalous in their position as a result of congenital malformation. When this is the case, the cartilage wears out prematurely and can be the cause of pain in the lower back. The pain often begins as "catches" in the back and is referred to as the facet syndrome.

Asymmetry of the facets is only one of the many anatomic variations that can occur in the lumbosacral area. The most frequent anomaly is an incomplete fusion of the lamina of the first sacral segment. Another common variation is sacralization of the fifth lumbar segment, which means that the fifth lumbar segment takes on characteristics of the sacral rather than the lumbar spine.

SPONDYLOLISTHESIS

Spondylolisthesis, or the slipping forward of one vertebral segment on another, constitutes the congenital anomaly most likely to produce a backache. The presence of spondylolisthesis does not always mean a backache, but perhaps 60% do eventuate in symptoms.

POSTURAL STRAINS

Postural strains comprise a group of backaches that are mechanical in nature and occur in normal spines in the absence of predisposing causes such as anomalies. As the term implies, the strain is the resultant effect upon supporting ligaments that resist any poor posture for long periods.

The entire group of mechanical back-

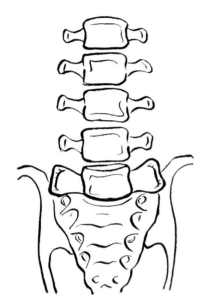

Fig. 223. Anomaly of the fifth lumbar vertebra. Note that in this particular case there is sacralization on both sides of the vertebral body. (From Kenney, William C., and Larson, Carroll B.: Orthopedics for the general practitioner, St. Louis, 1957, The C. V. Mosby Co.)

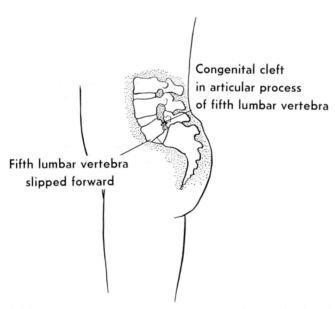

Congenital cleft in articular process of fifth lumbar vertebra

Fifth lumbar vertebra slipped forward

Fig. 224. Spondylolisthesis (Type II).

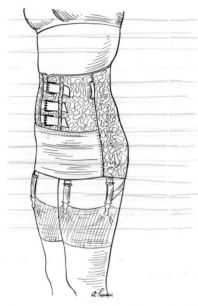

Fig. 225. Sacrolumbar support. It is made of brocade, elastic, and straps. It has a keystone pad over the sacrum and is heavily reinforced with corset stays.

aches has a similar pattern of treatment. An attempt should be made in all cases to detect the predisposing cause, be it a congenital anomaly or a faulty postural habit. By eliminating the abnormal stresses the symptoms can be controlled.

Elimination of abnormal stresses is accomplished by teaching the patient the correct positional use of the spine—that is, proper standing position, proper lifting habits, proper sitting positions, and the avoidance of twisting motions. Frequently this can be supplemented by a support such as a low back brace or corset that will act as a reminder rather than a true support for the back. Weak musculature should be built up to proper strength by exercises.

RUPTURED DISK

Perhaps 10% of the backaches that are brought to a physician's attention will be caused by a ruptured disk. As the name implies, a portion of the nucleus pulposus, which is the central portion of an intervertebral disk, herniates through the posterior ligament that invests it. This herniated fragment of disk comes to lie within the spinal canal, and by occupying space it crowds or actually causes pressure on the nerve roots within the spinal canal. Nerve roots when irritated become painful, and the pain is radiated along the entire course of the nerve; hence it is likely that ruptured disks will cause pain radiating into the leg and foot. This has commonly been called sciatica, but the term is not correct because only one of the many nerve roots that make up the sciatic nerve is affected.

Lifting from a stooped position is the most common cause of rupture of the intervertebral disk. Whenever back pain is associated with radiating leg pain, a ruptured disk should be suspected. Weakness of muscle groups, changes in sensation, and loss of ankle or knee jerk are helpful signs to localize the particular nerve root that is irritated. Another way to determine the exact level of the ruptured disk is by the use of contrast media intrathecally. Radiopaque material introduced by spinal puncture technique will be visible in the fluoroscope and reveal a filling defect at the site of the ruptured fragment. This procedure is known as intraspinal myelography.

The treatment for a ruptured disk is likely to be operative, since removal of the protruded fragment of disk will relieve the radiation pain. Operative treatment is imperative only when there is evidence of increasing nerve root pressure. In milder protrusions nonoperative treatment, namely bed rest, will often relieve the acute symptoms.

In all types of backaches so far discussed, spinal fusion can be done to relieve pain when conservative measures have failed. The pain will be eliminated when there is no longer motion through

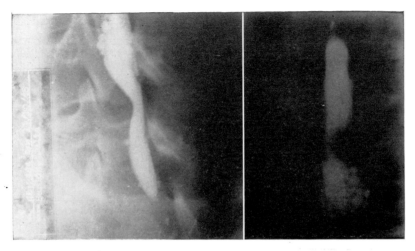

Fig. 226. Ruptured nucleus pulposus protruding into a column of radiopaque contrast media during myelography. (From Kenney, William C., and Larson, Carroll B.: Orthopedics for the general practitioner, St. Louis, 1957, The C. V. Mosby Co.)

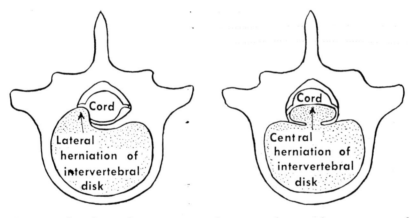

Fig. 227. Ruptured nucleus pulposus. Diagram showing mechanism of pressure on cord.

the affected segments. Fusion is frequently carried out after removal of a ruptured disk in order to stabilize the degenerated level in which the rupture occurred. For details of spinal fusion, see pp. 327-328.

NURSING CARE

Early mild back strain is usually treated by recumbency and heat. Adequate recumbency for this condition requires a hard bed and supports under the lumbar spine and knees. The support under the lumbar spine should be a hair pillow or folded sheet. It should be a firm support, and a sheet folded lengthwise is preferable to a feather pillow. If the patient prefers to lie prone, he will usually be most comfortable with a pillow under the lower abdomen and another supporting the feet so that the knees are mildly flexed. Radiant heat may be ordered, or moist hot packs similar to those used in poliomyelitis may be used. Prolonged heat, however, will increase congestion, which is extremely undesirable in low back pain. Hot paraffin is sometimes used to supply heat in these cases, and it is put on by brush in repeated applications until a thick coating is obtained. It will maintain heat in the part for as long as 40 minutes. Massage is not usually a part of the physical therapy for these patients, particularly in the acute stage, since muscle spasm is somewhat exaggerated by it. Deep massage in the less severely affected patient is sometimes of considerable comfort, but it must be used with caution. Medications usually consist of aspirin or some other type of salicylate given at 3- to 4-hour periods. Muscle-relaxant drugs are occasionally ordered for relief of muscle spasm.

Back-strapping with adhesive tape frequently provides temporary relief in mild cases. This procedure is performed by the orthopedist, but there are sometimes emergencies in which the orthopedic nurse may be called upon to do this at the request and under the direction of the physician. Adhesive strips 3 to 4 inches in width are used and should be long enough to extend from the anterior iliac spine on one side across the back and beyond the anterior iliac spine of the other side. Considerable traction is exerted on each strip as it is applied, and a lumbar pad of felt to supply pressure over the sacral region may be used under the tape. From three to four strips of adhesive tape are necessary, and these extend from the trochanter level to above the iliac crests. The patient may be standing or may be lying in bed while these are applied. It has been found that when standing the patient can provide assistance if he is allowed to stand in a corner and brace himself with his hands against the walls. Strapping gives only temporary relief, but occasionally symptoms may subside and the patient will be able to return to his work. Occasionally, strapping is used in conjunction with recumbency or traction. The main contraindication here

is that the use of heat is restricted because of the presence of the tape.

In using such large amounts of adhesive tape, skin irritation is not infrequent. Tincture of benzoin is sometimes used to paint the skin before application of the tape.

Bed rest is usually ordered for severe pain in the lower portion of the back. The patient is most comfortable in a semi-Fowler position. In this position, with the backrest elevated approximately 20 degrees and the knees flexed slightly, there is less tension of the back muscles and of the hamstrings. At times the attending physician will find it necessary to apply traction to relieve spasm of the thigh and back muscles. Simple Buck's extension can be used intermittently to relieve back pain. In the acute stage of this condition, however, the patient is likely to be uncomfortable in any position, and, for this reason, he is allowed to assume whatever attitude he can find to give him relief. Morphine may be necessary to control pain that is sometimes so severe that the patient is in continuous agony. Nurses tend to minimize low back pain as one of the minor afflictions until they have cared for a patient with an acute case and watched the intense suffering that he endures from it.

When the acute pain has subsided, exercises may be ordered for the purpose of improving the patient's body mechanics and thereby building up a resistance against further back strains as the result of postural deviations. Nurses should make an attempt to watch these exercises as they are taught in the physical therapy department. Usually, such exercises begin with teaching the patient —first in the lying position and then standing—to flatten the lumbar spine by active contraction of the abdominal and gluteal muscles. Diaphragmatic breathing is also emphasized. Sometimes the

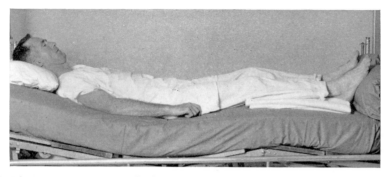

Fig. 228. The patient with acute back pain is usually more comfortable with the backrest elevated 20 to 30 degrees and the knees flexed slightly.

exercises are done by the patient in bed as often as every hour during the day. He may be taught to contract the gluteal muscles five or ten times, using a steady, slow rhythmic contraction. A second important bed exercise for this condition is one in which the patient lies on his back and raises his head and shoulders a short distance from the bed without using his elbows to brace himself. This also may be done five to ten times an hour until he is doing the exercise 100 times daily.

Use of the therapeutic corset. Practically all physical therapy after treatment for these patients is designed to create a set of corset muscles sufficiently strong to serve as an internal splint for the low back. Until this can be accomplished, some kind of corset or brace is customarily prescribed. Nurses should understand that a corset for this condition should be prescribed by the physician. Patients who attempt to purchase corsets for low back pain without the advice of an orthopedist frequently spend a great deal of money on garments that are absolutely inefficient and may even exacerbate their condition. Corsets for low back pain have a dual purpose. In the first place they should provide a type of immobilization for the painful back, and secondly they should assist in maintaining the trunk in good posture. The therapeutic corset is often a some-

what perplexing problem to the student who has relatively little chance to obtain experience in its application. Students should be given the opportunity to watch the prescription corsetière as she does the final fitting to observe points of special importance in the construction and application of the garment.

The corset is made to fit the curves of the back so that no loose or gapping spaces occur anywhere. Its length must be sufficient to assist in the control of the buttock muscles, and it should be high enough to approximate the lower portion of the shoulder blades. The front of the corset must be long enough to support the abdomen adequately. Ober states that the fit of the garment over the iliac crests is the most important consideration. He recommends that the iliac crests fit into the cloth of this part of the corset as into a pocket so that the garment cannot roll up whatever the activity of the patient.

Perineal straps are sometimes used to prevent the corset from rolling up, but these are not considered essential if the fit of the garment is adequate. (Sacroiliac belts, however, may frequently have this feature attached.) Pads made of flannelette sewed into place over the sacrolumbar region of the corset are not uncommon, but again these are considered superfluous if the corset is carefully constructed to fit the curves of the

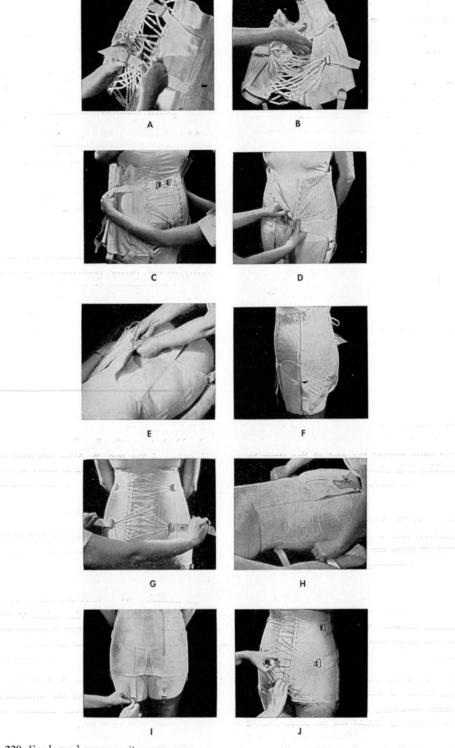

Fig. 229. For legend see opposite page.

back. Back-lacing is considered desirable for proper fitting in therapeutic corsets.

The patient should be observed in a sitting position after the corset is applied to see that it does not slip from its original position. A garment that fits loosely or that rolls up is of no value. The front stays should not press down on the pubic bone because this will cause the patient considerable discomfort. The garters are an important part of any therapeutic corset and should be kept in good condition. The posterior and lateral garters are particularly important for the correct fitting and placement of the corset. Nurses should observe that they are not fastened in such a way that they go off at an angle when attached to the hose. The front garters must be attached to the hose without undue tension, for tension may make it impossible for the patient to stand erect.

Nursing care of the patient with a herniated disk

Conservative treatment. Rupture of an intervertebral disk is a well-recognized cause of pain in the low back. Conservative treatment for this condition may be the same as for any type of low back pain, namely, recumbency, heat, support, and exercise. A semisitting position is sometimes found to be efficacious for the comfort of these patients. The backrest is elevated about 20 degrees, and the legs and thighs are elevated on pillows along their entire length. Forward flexion of the lumbar spine is thereby encouraged. Physicians who prescribe this position do not permit lying in the prone position (hyperextension of the spine) at any time.

Muscle spasms frequently cause great discomfort for these persons. The application of heat by means of a hot water bottle, hot moist packs, or in some in-

---

Fig. 229. Application of a corset for conditions of the low back. **A,** Release the buckles by turning them backward on the straps, holding the buckle between the first finger and thumb, and slide toward the end of the strap to within 2 inches of the end. **B,** After releasing the buckles it is advisable to bend the bones in the top and bottom in the back in order to conform to the curves of the body. **C,** Standing position: Place the support on the body with the center back well down under the gluteus muscles (as shown). The bottom of the front should curve down to the pubic bone; the bones of the support, if any, should not press on the pubic bone. **D,** Hooking the support in the standing position: If the top hook of the support is fastened first, it will hold the support on the body while the fitter is hooking the rest of the support from the bottom upward. **E,** Reclining position: Same procedure as in standing position. **F,** Fastening side hose supporters: In both standing and reclining positions, fasten side hose supporters in such a manner that the front portion will draw straight down on the side as shown. **G,** Pulling the adjustment straps in the standing position: Draw, slightly, the top strap or lacer sufficiently to settle the support at the waistline. Then hold the lower straps, one in each hand, and give a steady pull, thus laying a foundation about the pelvis. **H,** Reclining position: The patient must raise her body to enable the fitter to obtain a proper grip on the straps and to give a firm, steady, outward pull. Procedure is the same as for standing position. Caution: Always tighten the opposite straps at the same time, one in each hand, and not first one and then the other. **I,** Fasten front hose supporters: Fasten front hose supporters straight down without tension. **J,** Inspection of fitting: See that there is no slack in any of the lacers; if slack is present, retrace lacers with the fingers. Tuck ends of the adjustment straps backward through the loops designed to receive them. When correctly adjusted, the back opening should not be more than 2 or 3 inches wide; if it is, a larger size should be chosen. Have the patient sit down to make sure that the support is comfortable and that it does not slip from its proper position on the body. (Courtesy S. H. Camp and Co.)

stances a heating pad may give relief. Pelvic traction or Buck's extension may be applied and muscle relaxant drugs prescribed. In some instances, however, narcotics will be necessary before relief is gained. When this patient is turned, it is important that the shoulders and hips be moved in one plane. Twisting of the spine is avoided by teaching the patient to turn log fashion. A wide drawsheet that extends from the shoulders to below the hips may be used. A pillow is placed between the patient's thighs. The nurse, reaching across the patient, grasps the rolled drawsheet and gently turns him toward her onto his side. The patient's hips will need to be pulled back toward the center of the bed, and the uppermost limb adjusted on the pillow previously placed between the thighs. Another method of turning this kind of patient is described in the nursing care of the patient with a spinal fusion. The use of a child's bedpan or a bedpan with a tapering back will cause the patient with back pain less discomfort than the ordinary adult bedpan. To place the patient on the pan, he is rolled onto his side, and the pan and a small pillow or roll to support the lumbar region are placed in position. The patient is then rolled back on the pan. Having him use the trapeze should be avoided. A foot support to hold the covers off the feet and to prevent drop foot adds to his comfort and is a necessity if there has been motor or sensory changes in the limbs.

Prior to ambulation the patient is fitted with a corset or brace that provides support and immobilization of the back. The purpose of the support is to prevent recurrence of the condition. It should be worn when the patient is not in bed. Also, a pair of good walking shoes should be worn when the patient is permitted to begin activity. Another important aspect in preventing recurrence of this condition is instructing the patient in correct body mechanics. Proper methods of lifting and stooping must be practiced if recurrence is to be avoided.

Conservative treatment usually consists of several weeks of bed rest. Frequently these patients become quite discouraged and feel that little progress is being made. They may fear being operated upon or question whether they will be able to return to their usual activities without recurrence of the condition.

Nursing care following laminectomy. Laminectomy is sometimes necessary for patients with lesions of the intervertebral disk. The surgical procedure provides for removal of the portion of the nucleus pulposus that is protruding or ruptured from the intervertebral disk. To do this a portion of the lamina of one or more vertebrae is removed. The nursing care of a patient after a laminectomy without fusion is a relatively simple problem, quite different from the nursing problem encountered in laminectomy for fractured spines or cord tumors. When spinal fusion is not done simultaneously with the laminectomy, the patient is usually permitted to move about in bed at liberty and is encouraged to exercise his feet and legs at frequent intervals. Nurses are instructed to observe the patient's ability to do this after the operation and to record this carefully during the early postoperative period. Blood pressure readings are taken postoperatively at frequent intervals. The patient should be placed on a firm mattress. Maintenance of the supine position may be ordered for the first 24 hours postoperatively. Pressure on the operative area helps prevent formation of a hematoma. The usual precautions in turning patients with conditions of the spine are observed in the care of these patients. The body is turned in one piece, and twisting at the hips is carefully avoided. Face-lying and side-lying positions are often permitted. When the patient lies on his side, a pillow between the legs will prevent strain on back muscles. A pillow to support the upper arm will prevent sagging of the shoulder. Early ambulation is frequently prescribed for the patient who has had a laminectomy. This in itself helps to prevent many postoperative complications, such as retention, distension, phlebitis, and hypostatic pneumonia.

Postoperative care of the patient with spinal fusion. The postoperative care of the patient with spinal fusion will vary somewhat in different clinics, but a general outline will be given.

Shock blocks, a warm bed with rubber-covered pillows, and a firm mattress should be at hand when the postoperative bed is being prepared. Some doctors require their patients with spinal fusion to lie prone for the first few days and be turned only for voiding. This is usually because they fear pressure and necrosis at the operative site. Others prefer that the patient lie flat on his back without being turned for several days. These patients are usually most comfortable if pillows are used to support the legs along their entire length. Some relaxation of the back muscles is obtained by this slight elevation. Furthermore, it is thought by many surgeons to be a means of overcoming a threat of thrombophlebitis in the femoral vessels. When the pillows are arranged, they should not be placed in such a fashion that flexion of the knee is exaggerated. The first pillow should be placed high enough under the thigh to support the limb along the full length of the hamstring muscles. The lower pillows support the knee and lower leg on a slight incline without undue knee flexion.

When a plaster bed is to be used after surgery, allowance should be made for the dressing that the patient will be wearing. This dressing, consisting of gauze sponges and combination pads, is sometimes quite generous, and, if no allowance is made, pressure upon the incision is inevitable. The plaster bed must be well prepared for the patient. Wrinkles and ridges should be eliminated. The doctor preparing the bed will have padding inserted at the proper points. The stockinet must be pulled out to cover all the raw edges and taped down securely. Straps are often added to the bed, and its final finishing is done by a bracemaker. If this is not done, the nurse is responsible for drying the plaster and for having straps with buckles in readiness. The entire shell may be covered with stockinet sewed on neatly. The area around the buttocks must be protected with a waterproof material. All this should be done before surgery because the patient can seldom spare either section of the shell long enough for repair afterward. The advisability of having the patient lie in the plaster bed for a time before surgery is great. Any points of discomfort incidental to the shell can thus be discovered before the patient is compelled to lie in it permanently.

When a good plaster bed has been made preoperatively, orders will usually be given to turn the patient for morning and evening care. This turning may be done the first evening if the patient's condition permits. A patient in severe shock, however, will often benefit by being allowed to lie quietly until the next morning. If the patient lies on his back, careful check of the pulse and blood pressure will be necessary to detect hemorrhage since the dressings are not visible.

There may be a mild and temporary decrease in the tone of the genitourinary and gastrointestinal tract as a result of the inevitable shock to the sympathetic nervous system. Considerable liberty is allowed the nurse in giving fluids to these patients. Fluids are usually encouraged as soon as nausea is past. Diet is increased as the patient tolerates it.

If the patient is an adult, it is advisable to have sufficient help so that the initial turnings may be accomplished with as little discomfort as possible. He is naturally apprehensive at this time, and everything should be done to give him a sense of security. Later turnings will be accomplished much more easily if this is done. The patient in a well-fitting plaster bed can be turned with relatively little pain to his back. If the graft has been taken from the tibia, slight changes of position in the knee joint will cause muscular pull on the tibia, which causes the patient considerable pain. It is important that all who are assisting with the turning of the patient recognize the fact that the knee should not be flexed or extended in the turning during the first few days. The nurse handling the leg from one side of the bed should very carefully transfer it to the nurse receiving it on the other side without changing its position. Pillows must be ready to receive it before the leg is lowered to the bed. The patient may be turned on the leg if this seems to be more comfortable for him. As a general rule, however, the plaster bed is made with some abduction of the legs, and it is easier to turn the patient with the leg operated on uppermost. After a week or so the pain and muscle spasm in this leg will have subsided, but during the early days it is very acute and is a source of great concern to the patient. At present, however, many surgeons are taking the graft from the crest of the ilium instead of the tibia. Thus, the difficulty in turning and the pain experienced by the patient are somewhat lessened.

The patient is moved all in one plane to the side of the bed. The undersheet is then changed by a nurse on the opposite side of the bed. Pillows are arranged to receive the leg from which the graft has been taken, and a support is made ready for the feet. The plaster shell should be securely fastened at the axillary level and around the hips. If the cast has been applied after surgery and is still soft and compressible, the bed should be covered with rubber-covered pillows where the cast will rest. If possible, the arm toward which the patient is to be turned should be placed above the head. For operations on the dorsal spine, however, it is sometimes better to have the arm on which the patient is to be turned stretched downward along the side of the cast. The nurse standing at the side of the bed toward which the patient has been pulled must take responsibility for seeing that this arm is freed immediately after turning is done. Otherwise, the pressure of the heavy plaster bed on the arm may cause considerable bruising. The patient is turned toward the clean side of the bed as a unit, without twisting at the hips or knees. One nurse can accomplish this if the patient is not too large. For a large adult, however, two nurses are advisable. One nurse places her hands on the patient's shoulders and hips, and the other assumes responsibility for the leg operated on, with some assistance from the nurse who stands on the opposite side of the bed.

Once turned, the patient should be made as comfortable as possible. The feet should be supported on a pillow placed under the ankles so that the toes do not dig into the bed. The posterior shell of the cast is removed, the dressings are carefully inspected for signs of hemorrhage or drainage, and the surrounding skin is washed and then rubbed gently with alcohol. The circulation of the back, head, and neck is important for the well-being of patients who have had spinal surgery and should be given frequent attention. Back rubs should include the scalp, neck, and thighs. The patient should be urged to lie prone for as long as he can do so in order to re-establish circulation in the dependent areas of the back and thighs. He may ask to be turned back almost immediately, but a little explanation of the purpose of the position will often help in prolonging the period.

Turning the patient with spinal fusion who is not immobilized. Patients with spinal fusions frequently are not immobilized in plaster. Extreme care and gentleness in turning are essential for these patients to avoid motion of the spine that will be accompanied by excruciating pain. To maintain good alignment some doctors request that these patients be kept flat and that they lie either on their abdomens or on their backs. In other instances patients are permitted to move and turn as they wish.

When a patient is being turned from his back to his abdomen after spinal fusion, without benefit of cast or brace, the nurse will apply the same technique used with the patient in a plaster cast. First, the patient is moved to one side of the bed. If the bed is made with a wide drawsheet, the sheet

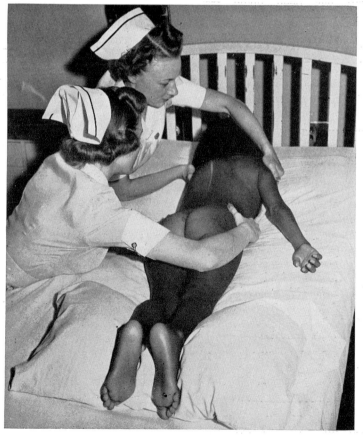

Fig. 230. Method of turning patient after spinal operation when no supportive apparatus is used. A pillow placed between the legs to prevent sagging of the hip would be used if patient were to lie on the side. Upper arm also should be supported in side-lying position.

may be used as a slide for the patient. This helps to avoid twisting movements of the spine. Clean linen is placed on the opposite half of the bed. Two nurses stand at the side of the bed toward which the patient is to be turned. The patient's arms are kept close to his side, and he is instructed to make his body rigid. The first nurse places her hands on the patient's far shoulder and arm, and the second nurse grasps the patient's hip and thigh. Slowly and gently, they turn the patient onto his abdomen toward themselves. Following this, it is necessary to move the patient back to the center of the bed. This again can be accomplished with the drawsheet. When the patient lies in the prone position, the dorsum of his feet need to be supported by a pillow. His arms may be placed in any comfortable position.

If the patient is turned on his side, the nurse will remember what constitutes a good side-lying position. The pillow between the legs to prevent adduction of the uppermost limb will avoid added strain on sore back muscles.

Frequently patients with spinal fusion are placed on the Foster frame. Adult patients can be turned more easily and with less pain when immobilized with the frame. For care of the patient on a frame, see pp. 401-404.

During the early days after surgery carelessness in turning seldom takes place. The patient is so apprehensive that it is necessary to guard one's every movement lest unnecessary pain be caused him. After 10 days or 2 weeks, however, when the patient's general condition is on the upgrade and the acute pain in the leg and back is much diminished, haste and carelessness sometimes do occur, for nurses on busy wards tend to try to turn such patients with insufficient help. Healing in spinal grafts takes place slowly, as does all bone healing, and gentle handling must continue for many weeks. The so-called critical time after spinal operations is given as 4 to 5 weeks. Particular care in handling the patient during these times should be observed. Spinal pseudarthrosis can occur because of careless postoperative handling of the patient with spinal fusion. The patient will learn to help the nurse in turning. Fewer persons can accomplish the same effect for which many persons were needed during the first postoperative days. Such things, however, as twisting or piecemeal turning, arching, or sagging of the buttocks and shoulders during the procedure should never be tolerated.

Edema of the face sometimes occurs in patients after spinal fusion, particularly if maintenance of shock position is necessary. This can be remedied by removing the shock blocks or lowering the bed as early as seems compatible with the patient's general condition. A temporary impairment of bowel function is often encountered. Enemas are usually ordered between the fourth and sixth days, but they may not be efficacious unless they are preceded by very mild laxatives. Rectal impaction must not be allowed to occur before a cathartic is given. Occasionally, oil enemas will be more successful than large volume enemas. The establishment of regular habits of elimination will soon help to overcome the need for enemas or laxatives and should be part of the patient's routine. The back and legs of the patient must be supported while he is on the bedpan so that all sections of the body are in the same plane. These patients will have less discomfort if a bedpan with a tapering back is used in place of the regular bedpan. Attention to such details will sometimes pay surprising dividends in helping the patient to resume normal habits of elimination.

Patients who must lie prone are in

danger of pressure areas over the iliac crests. This is particularly true of the thin patient in a bivalved cast. Reddened or bluish areas around the bony crests should receive immediate attention as skin breakdown in that area is extremely rapid. The areas must be massaged frequently, and crescent-shaped pieces of white felt may be lightly taped around the crests and will often serve to overcome the hazard of lying prone. Circular doughnuts or pieces of felt with circles cut out of the center are not advisable, for they frequently serve to cut off circulation to the part still further.

The patient's progress and his resumption of normal activities—such as sitting, standing, and walking—will depend upon the diagnosis that made the spinal fusion necessary. Fusions in patients with disabilities of the low back usually progress more rapidly than those in patients who have had tuberculosis or similar infections of the vertebrae. It is urgent that patients who are to remain in bed for a prolonged period have constant intelligent care to parts of the musculoskeletal system not primarily affected but so important to them when they become ambulatory. The physician may prescribe deep-breathing exercises, exercises for maintaining muscle tone in the feet, quadriceps setting, and, later, flexion and extension of the knees. The feet should be provided for by a support to keep the covers from pressing on the toes and to maintain the normal physiologic position of the feet in standing. Knee hyperextension should be eliminated by a small rolled towel placed under the head of the tibia just below the popliteal space. Outward rotation of the hip, if not controlled by a cast or plaster bed, should be prevented by sandbags or a trochanter roll. Unless contraindicated, the patient should be provided with occupations that will ensure normal varied use of the arms and shoulders.

The patient will usually be provided with a brace before he is allowed out of bed. It is essential that the nurse know how to apply the brace correctly and that she recognize its importance to the patient's ultimate recovery. The

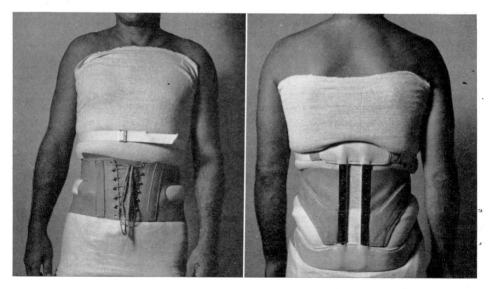

Fig. 231. Anterior and posterior views of a low back brace.

physician will usually order the patient to wear the brace at all times, in bed or out, until permission to omit it for short periods is given.

Applying back braces. Nurses should remember that low back braces and spring back braces may ride up considerably, particularly on heavy women. Perineal straps to prevent this are sometimes used but are never very comfortable for the wearer. If the brace has a well-fitting pelvic band, this will often overcome the tendency of the brace to ride up. A safe rule to remember is that in every back brace the pelvic band should fit low enough to hold the upper part of the buttocks adequately. When the brace is applied, the abdominal leather apron must be laced very snugly at the lower portion, diminishing in snugness as the lacing ascends. It is important in applying back braces to observe that the spinal uprights are far enough apart not to press on the vertebral prominences, but also close enough together to fit well between the scapulae.

Another important point to remember is that it is essential that a back brace allow the patient to sit with the hips at right angles, with no impingement of the metal or the leather on the groin. The patient must be able to sit without having the brace pushed up by the chair.

Spinal braces, such as the Taylor back brace, are not infrequently used for postoperative immobilization after fusions of the low back (sacroiliac fusion, sacrolumbar fusion, or combinations of the two). These supports are often applied in the operating room, and the patient wears them continuously for a period of several months. For back care he is carefully turned in the brace. The metal and leather part of the apparatus is then lifted off the back, but the canvas apron that supports the abdomen is left under the patient as he lies prone, making it easy to reapply the brace once the back is cared for. A thin cotton vest of some knitted material is usually worn beneath the brace.

Bursitis

LOCATION

Throughout the body there are a number of places where bony prominences are exposed to irritation, either from outward pressure or from the friction effect of tendons, ligaments, and even the skin over these bony prominences. These prominences are protected by small sacs or compartments that are filled with a lubricating synovial fluid produced from the walls of the sac. This allows the gliding of the various structures over bony prominences without friction. A bursa may develop in an area where none normally exists if persistent irritation continues. The ordinary location of these bursae is as follows:

1. Shoulder
   (a) Over the acromial process
   (b) Tuberosity of the humerus (subdeltoid)
   (c) Under the coracoid process
2. Elbow
   (a) Olecranon
   (b) Epitrochlear (tennis elbow)
3. Hip
   (a) Gluteal (under attachment of gluteus maximus)

(b) Trochanteric (greater trochanter and lesser trochanter)

(c) Ischial (Weaver's bottom)

4. Knee

(a) Prepatellar (housemaid's knee)

(b) Pretibial (under patella tendon)

(c) Superficial pretibial (over tibial tubercle)

(d) Popliteal

(e) Bicipital

5. Foot

(a) Achilles (under attachment of Achilles tendon)

(b) Retrocalcaneal (anterior to the Achilles tendon)

(c) Inferior calcaneal (under the attachment of the plantar fascia to the heel—policeman's heel)

(d) Bunion (may develop on either the inner or the outer side of the foot when there is bony prominence of the metatarsal head as seen in hallux valgus)

SYMPTOMS

Inflammation of a bursa may develop gradually as the result of a repeated strain or injury or may develop acutely as the result of more severe damage. There are pain, swelling, and marked tenderness. When active motions involve the function of the bursa, pain is greatly aggravated. Passive motions, however, are usually not as painful as they would

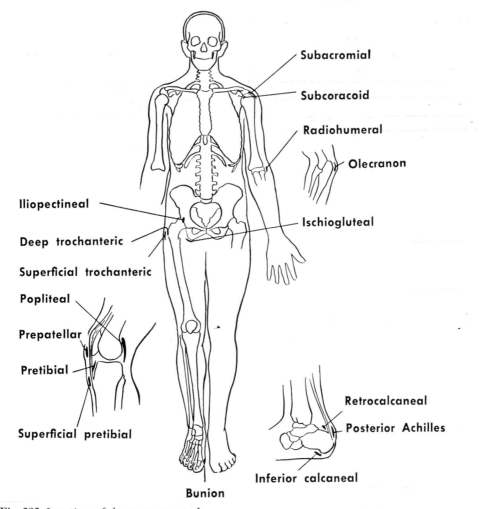

Fig. 232. Locations of the most common bursae.

be if there were joint involvement. Acute inflammation of a bursa may develop when bacteria or toxins from remote focal infection settle there.

TREATMENT

The causes of bursitis, such as irritation and infection, should be removed.

In the noninfectious types of bursitis complete rest and the application of heat are important. A plaster of paris cast or a flannel spica applied to the extremities often is effective in giving relief. The bursa should be locally protected by the use of a doughnut pad of cotton or felt.

Subdeltoid bursitis. Subdeltoid bursitis is one of the commonest forms and may need special treatment. The subdeltoid bursa is situated between the deltoid muscle and the rotator cuff of the shoulder. The inflammation arises in this bursa secondary to degeneration in one of the tendons of the rotator cuff, usually the supraspinatus. Calcium is deposited into the degenerated area so that it is often possible to see a calcific deposit in a roentgenogram of the shoulder, which is painful as a result of bursitis. Pain is the outstanding symptom and frequently radiates down the arm. Restriction of motion in the shoulder may be so severe that this condition has been referred to as frozen shoulder.

Treatment of subdeltoid bursitis will depend on whether it is in the acute or chronic stage. In acute bursitis the treatment is aimed at relief of pain. The simplest way to release the calcium that is under tension and is responsible for the active pain is to insert a needle and wash it out. This can be done with Novocaine. At times the calcium is inspissated (dried out to form a hard pebble) and may require surgical excision. Many times the acute attack will cure itself by absorption of the calcium; however, this may require a period of a few days during which time the patient must be well medicated for pain and the shoulder must be immobilized in a sling.

Chronic bursitis does not demand immediate treatment to relieve pain, although pain is present. The main consideration is to stop irritation of the degenerated rotator cuff so that it may heal. Avoidance of extreme motion and lifting, plus local heat, may control the symptoms and allow the process to subside. Many physicians prescribe radiation therapy, but the beneficial effect is variable. Pendulum exercises to regain lost motion are perhaps the most important treatment. Local injection of hydrocortisone into tender areas often helps to relieve pain.

Disabilities of the feet

ANATOMY OF THE FOOT

The feet, small or large, must take the burden of weight bearing for various sizes and shapes of bodies. They bear the weight of the body when walking or standing and serve as levers in raising and propelling the body forward. The bony structure consists of seven tarsal bones, five metatarsal bones, and fourteen phalanges. At birth much of this structure is soft tissue (cartilage), and for this reason the foot of the newborn infant (when deformity exists) lends itself to corrective measures much better than the foot of an older child. There are two main arches, the longitudinal and the transverse (metatarsal). These arches are present at birth. The baby's foot, however, may appear quite flat because of a fat pad that fills the longitudinal arch space. The medial aspect of the longitudinal arch extends from the os calcis to the head of the first metatarsal. The lateral aspect extends from the os calcis to the head of the fourth and fifth metatarsals. This arch is supported by two groups of muscles: (1) those on the inner and (2) those on the outer side of the ankle. The inner group of muscles consist of the tibialis anticus, normally attached below the internal cuneiform, the posterior tibial muscle, normally attached to the scaphoid, and the flexors of the toes, whose tendons act by leverage under the astragalus (sustentaculum tali) to support the arch. All these muscles work in coordination and are assisted to some extent by the intrinsic muscles of the foot. The outer side of the foot is supported by the peroneal muscles—longus, brevis, and tertius. These muscles tend to balance the arch-elevating effect of the muscles of the inner side of the foot and at the same time work in unison to support the arches of the foot.

The metatarsal arch extends medially from the base of the fifth metatarsal to the base of the first metatarsal. This arch is supported by the balanced action between the flexors and the extensors of the toes combined with the intrinsic muscles of the foot.

When muscle action fails from disuse or disease, the strain is transmitted to ligamentous structures, such as the plantar fascia, and to other ligaments

about the joints. Strain is often accompanied by inflammatory change. Thus, it can be readily understood that the patient who has been at bed rest needs adequate support for his arches when ambulation is permitted. This patient needs a well-fitted shoe and not paper slippers.

MOVEMENTS OF THE FOOT

When caring for the bed patient, it is essential to know the normal movements of the foot and ankle. If these motions are not contraindicated and are performed passively or actively, joint contractures can be prevented and muscle tone maintained. Plantar flexion (equinus position) and dorsiflexion of the foot take place at the ankle joint. Inversion (supination) and eversion (pronation) movements of the foot are made possible by the subastragalar joint. Adduction and abduction motions take place in the midtarsal joints. Flexion and extension of the toes take place at the metatarsophalangeal and the interphalangeal joints.

SHOES

Characteristics of a well-fitted shoe. Properly fitted shoes are an important factor in the prevention of foot deformities. If pain and foot discomfort are to be prevented, the shoe size and shape need to conform to the foot. The foot must not be forced into an ill-fitted shoe. The shoe length, with weight bearing, should extend approximately ¼ to ½ inch beyond the end of the great toe. A shoe that is too short will cause crowding of the toes, and the great toe will be forced into a hallux valgus position. A straight inner last is desirable. Continuous wearing of pointed shoes will result in a hallux valgus deformity and the formation of a bunion. A properly fitted shoe must have a sufficiently wide sole at the ball of the foot to permit

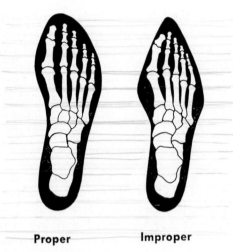

Proper   **Improper**

Fig. 233. Note that the shoe with a pointed toe forces the great toe into a hallux valgus position.

free movement of foot muscles. The length should be proportioned so that the ball of the foot is accommodated at the widest part of the shoe. This part of the shoe needs to be flexible to permit bending of the toes. The shank should give fairly good support. The heavy person or the person who stands for long hours may need a stronger shoe and a more rigid shank than the person who sits for long periods. The shank of a child's shoe, unless ordered otherwise by his physician, should be flexible. The heel needs to fit the heel of the foot. Sling-strap slippers give little or no support, do not hold the heel in position, and tend to cause blisters and calluses. The height of the heel depends upon the purpose of the shoe. A shoe that is to be worn when working or walking should have a heel of reasonable height. It is difficult for the person who walks or stands in high heels to attain good posture and to practice good body mechanics. The weight of the body is thrown forward on the ball of the foot. This results in calluses and strain on the metatarsal arch.

Children's shoes. The baby who has

not started to walk needs covering for his feet only to keep them warm. These shoes need to have soft soles that permit motion of the feet and use of foot muscles. When he learns to walk, his shoe should have a thin leather sole sufficient to protect his foot but flexible enough to permit normal motion and use of the muscles, particularly at the ball of the foot. The best shoe for a growing infant, especially if there is any abnormality, is of the high-topped variety with a firm sole, narrow heel, and broad toe.

PREDISPOSING CAUSES OF FOOT STRAIN

Foot strain caused by inherently weak muscles can begin with the first steps that a child takes. This weakness may persist and cause foot strain throughout life.

A second common cause of foot strain is ill-fitted shoes. There has been a tendency in the past to conform to style rather than to the shape of the foot, and the result has been high heels, narrow wedging toes, and a narrow sole. Fortunately this is at present being partly overcome, and there is an attempt to make shoes to conform to the shape of the average foot, but such correct shoes are still none too popular. Although ample width is essential in the metatarsal region, a shoe should not be sloppy or ill-fitted about the instep and heel. One of the common causes of foot trouble, particularly in women, is the tendency of the manufacturers to make

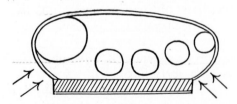

Fig. 234. Pressure exerted to cause metatarsal arch strain when shoe is improperly built. Such a shoe may have plenty of room.

shoes that are sufficiently large in circular dimension, but the sole of the shoe is narrower than the ball of the foot. This is likely to cause strain on the metatarsal arch, because pressure is exerted upward along the lateral borders of the foot, and, in spite of the fact that the person has ample room within the confines of the shoe itself, there is no freedom of muscle action. A frequent statement is: "If my shoes were any bigger I couldn't keep them on my feet."

A third cause of foot strain is inadequate muscular and ligamentous support. (The arches of the foot are supported by ligaments, tendons, and muscles.) The child that is growing very rapidly may complain of some foot discomfort. Muscular strength is not keeping up with the growth of the body. Prolonged inactivity will result in weakness and atrophy of the soft tissues supporting the arches of the foot. If weight bearing is permitted in soft bedroom slippers, the patient may develop painful feet. Excessive body weight puts an additional strain on the foot. The muscular and ligamentous support of the arches may become inadequate, and the inevitable is painful, flattened arches. Excessive exercise in soft rubber-soled shoes, when the individual is not accustomed to such activity, may result in foot strain and pain.

BUNIONS

There are two types of bunions, the acquired and the hereditary. Acquired bunions are definitely caused by wearing shoes that are too pointed and too narrow or too short.

Hereditary bunions are caused at least in part by a congenital abnormality. The space between the first and second metatarsals is increased so that bunion development in almost any type of shoe is unavoidable.

There is a distinct difference between

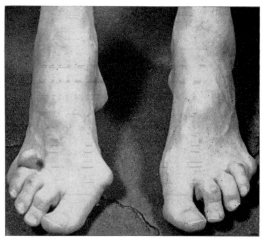

Fig. 235. Hallux valgus deformity with bunion, overlapping fifth toe (right), hammer toes, and corns.

hallux valgus and bunions. The first deformity is of bone, and the second is the result of an overgrowth of the soft tissue (bursa formation) over the bony prominence developing even in a normally shaped foot.

The pain and discomfort from bunions can in most instances be relieved by properly fitted shoes and by support of the metatarsal arch by means of arch supports and metatarsal bars and by sufficiently wide shoes. Sometimes the sufferers from these deformities are not willing to accept the type of shoe necessary for relief. Sometimes bunions may be so severe that bony correction is required.

In this severe type of bunion, operative removal of the bony overgrowth with about two-thirds of the outer side of the distal end of the first metatarsal head is necessary.

In the congenital type, osteotomy at the base of the first metatarsal may be combined with tendon transplantation according to the method of McBride. An osteotomy at the distal end of the metatarsal may also be necessary to restore the alignment.

Congenital bunion   **Acquired bunion**

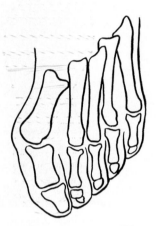   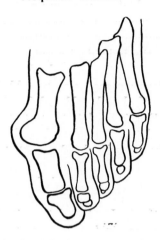

Fig. 236. Note difference in angle between first and second metatarsals.

LONGITUDINAL ARCH STRAIN

The pain in longitudinal arch strain both in children and in adults is usually felt in the arch of the foot and in the muscles of the legs. As a rule the pain that is caused by arch strain is present only after exertion and fatigue. If there is an inflammatory condition accompanying such a strain, it is usually characterized by aggravation of the pain on first arising in the morning or upon sudden activity after short periods of rest. Pain that is present only after activity is usually the result of muscle and ligamentous strain rather than inflammation of the joints and ligaments.

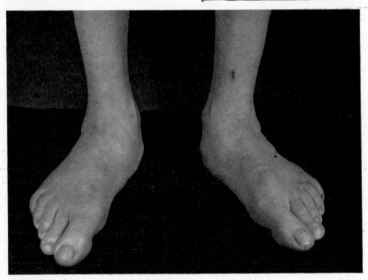

Fig. 237. Pronation of the foot. A common postural disturbance. Note flattened or depressed position of the longitudinal arch. If the foot is observed from the back, the Achilles tendon curves toward the midline. Frequently, the patient with pronated feet will complain of backache and pain in the calves of the legs.

Treatment is designed to relieve the strain on the tibialis anticus and posticus muscles by means of temporary arch supports made of felt and leather and designed to the individual requirement. A Thomas or orthopedic heel with an inner elevation may also be added, particularly if knock-ankle deformity is present. Felt is used instead of steel because the latter is rigid and tends to decrease the muscle development for correction.

A distinction should be made between acute arch strain and permanent or chronic flatfoot. In the latter it is justifiable to use rigid arch supports of stainless steel or Monel Metal. In acute arch strain exercises with temporary lifts and supports may be of distinct value in restoring muscle power after the strain has been relieved. In chronic flatfoot, however, exercises are of little value. It may be necessary at times to use a high-topped shoe to offset the demands on the muscles that also control the ankle.

METATARSAL ARCH STRAIN— METATARSALGIA

The metatarsal arch is supported primarily by muscles, and, when the muscular action fails because of abuse or disuse, strain is placed upon the ligamentous structure and upon the arch. If strain is severe enough, there is a flattening of the arch and weight is taken on the heads of the second, third, and fourth metatarsals. The person with this condition will develop a callus over the ball of the foot, and walking will become quite painful. To relieve this pain felt or rubber pads covered with leather may be placed just posterior to the heads of the second, third, and fourth metatarsals. The pad gives support to the arch and relieves pressure. The physician may also request that a metatarsal bar (anterior heel) be attached to the

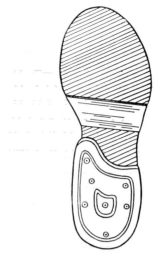

Fig. 238. Thomas (or orthopedic) heel used often in combination with a metatarsal bar.

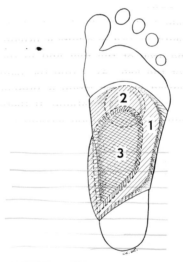

Fig. 239. Design for arch support based on the normal weight-bearing surface. The pads are of felt or rubber and covered with leather. Pad 3 fills the normal arch space. Pad 1 distributes pressure evenly over a larger area, and pad 2 increases pressure under the metatarsal arch at any desired point.

shoe (Fig. 238). This, again, gives the arch support and relieves pressure on the metatarsal heads.

In strains of either longitudinal or metatarsal arches, a support of felt and leather may be designed from the pedo-graph or outline of the weight-bearing surface of the foot (Fig. 239). It is the object of supports not only to relieve pressure in the area of the foot that does not come in contact during weight bear-ing but also to distribute the pressure evenly through the nonweight-bearing area and a small portion of the weight-bearing area.

One of the main requirements in strain of the metatarsal arch is to give sufficient room for action of the muscles that support the metatarsal arch. There-fore, adequate width of the shoe in the metatarsal region is necessary. Many broad short feet need EE or EEE shoes, which are difficult yet possible to obtain.

EXERCISES

The treatment described is aimed at relieving the symptoms and enabling the person to get about without discom-fort. If the condition is to be corrected, however, the strength of the muscles that normally support the arch must be restored. This may be accomplished by active exercises. The following exercises are frequently prescribed to relieve arch strain.

For the metatarsal arch. One exercise prescribed to strengthen the metatarsal

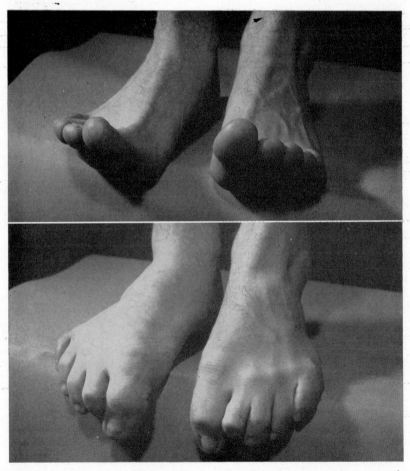

Fig. 240. Contracting the toes rhythmically over the edge of a stair step to strengthen foot muscles.

arch is the towel exercise. A towel is placed on the floor, and the feet are placed parallel to each other about an inch apart with the heels just over the posterior border. The toes are then contracted alternately one foot with the other so that the towel is gradually accumulated under the arch. Another exercise for the metatarsal arch is the marble exercise. Ten to twelve marbles are placed on the floor, and by action of the flexor tendon they are picked up, moved, and released rhythmically. A pencil may also be used. The toes may also be contracted rhythmically over the edge of a large book upon which the subject is standing.

For the longitudinal arch. In the standing position the feet and toes are inverted so that the weight is borne on the outer border of the feet. This exercise should be repeated thirty times. Another exercise for the longitudinal arch is performed by rising on the balls of the feet, raising the heels, and everting the ankles. This is to be repeated twenty to thirty times.

For contracted heel cords. Two exercises for contracted heel cords are performed as follows: (1) Stand on the heel, raising and inverting the forefoot, and (2) stand with the ball of the foot on the edge of a stair and drop the weight downward, stretching the heel cords. These exercises should be done at lease twice daily and should be repeated, starting about twenty times each, and increasing to about fifty.

OTHER DISABILITIES OF THE FEET

There are other causes for disabilities in the foot as a result of disease, trauma, and disturbances in circulation.

Apophysitis. Apophysitis is a disease of the heels of growing children as a result of traumatic and metabolic disturbance. There is an irritation of the posterior epiphysis of the os calcis. Pain

and tenderness are characteristic. Treatment consists in removing the counter of the shoe and temporarily raising the heel ½ to ¾ inch. Calcium, phosphorus, and vitamin D should also be administered.

Koehler's disease. Koehler's disease is characterized by pain, tenderness, and slight swelling about the tarsal scaphoid. It is caused by trauma, direct or indirect, and by circulatory disturbances in the bone, causing degenerative changes and compression within the scaphoid. It is relieved by casts or by arch supports and a lift or wedge along the inner side of an elongated heel.

Freiberg's disease. Freiberg's disease is a condensation or infraction in the distal end of the second metatarsal, usually resulting from trauma and aseptic necrosis and characterized by shortening of the metatarsal, tenderness about the metatarsal head, and some strain of the metatarsal arch. It is treated by support of the metatarsal arch.

Clawfoot and hollow foot. Clawfoot and hollow foot consist in a contracture of the muscles and ligaments of the plantar arch as a result of relative overactivity of the extensors of the toe as compared to the flexor action. This may

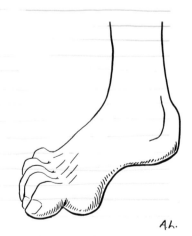

Fig. 241. Clawfoot deformity with retraction of the toes and high arch (cavus).

be influenced or instigated by continued metatarsal arch strain, arthritis, or spastic or infantile paralysis. The condition is frequently accompanied by calluses under the metatarsal heads and by corns on the dorsal surface of the interphalangeal joints of the toes. The treatment may require proper support of the metatarsal arch with arch supports and metatarsal bars, tenotomy of the extensor tendons to the toes, tendon transplantation of the extensor tendons to the metatarsal heads, or, in severe cases, resection of the metatarsal heads or proximal portions of the phalanges.

Hammer toes. Hammer toes may be either congenital or acquired as a result of spasmodic contracture of the extensors of the toes. The first interphalangeal joint is usually prominent and flexed. A corn usually develops on top and on the end of the toe. Correction can easily be obtained by resection of a portion of the proximal phalanx so that the toe is shortened and the muscle contracture released.

Knock-ankle and flatfoot deformities. Knock-ankle and flatfoot deformities in children are common and are frequently accompanied by bowlegs or knock-knees and internal rotation of the tibiae so that the child walks with a pigeon-toe and knock-ankle gait. It is difficult to tell whether or not there is a true flatfoot deformity in young children when they are beginning to walk because of the frequent existence of a fat pad under the arch. Arch supports are not often indicated, and the correction can usually be accomplished by lifts and elongated heels. When the internal rotation and pigeon-toe deformity is not severe and the principal deformity is knock-ankle, an elongated heel with an inner lift of ⅛ to ¼ inch will usually correct the deformity within a few months. If a pigeon-toe condition is present, it may be necessary to add to the shoe alterations ⅛ inch or more outer elevation of the soles.

When the pigeon-toe deformity is severe with marked internal rotation of the ankle on the knee, it is best to use elastic rotators attached to the outside or the inner side of the shoe. They spiral the leg and are fastened to a belt at the waist. (Fig. 243.) The adjustment of these rotators may exert the necessary tension to maintain correct alignment. In

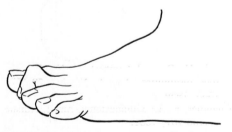

Fig. 242. Hammer toe. A corn usually forms on the top and the end of the toe.

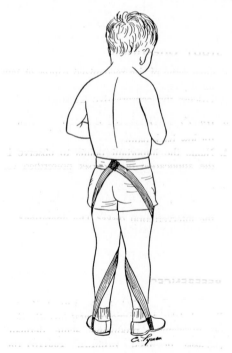

Fig. 243. Elastic rotators attached to shoe below and belt above for the correction of pigeon toes. When the child sits, the rotators relax.

6 to 18 months the alignment becomes fixed and the deformity disappears.

Bowlegs in children are not uncommon up to the second year and probably compensate for foot deformity, or vice versa. After the bowleg deformity has subsided, a reversion to the knock-knee status may take place and persist to the seventh or eighth year. During this time frequent changes in shoe elevations may be necessary to meet the current requirements of balance.

GOOD HYGIENIC CARE OF THE FEET

Good hygienic care of the feet, daily bathing, and massage will help to relieve tired, aching feet. Contrast baths improve circulation and tone of the foot muscles. The person who spends many hours on his feet may secure relief from aching feet by changing shoes during the working hours. Proper length hose and care in trimming of the nails will help to prevent painful ingrown toenails and dangerous infection. The nails should be trimmed straight across. Irritation and pressure caused by ill-fitted shoes will result in corns and calluses. A corn is an overgrowth of the outer layer of skin and is nature's way of protecting the soft tissue. Pads may be used to relieve the pressure. To secure permanent relief, however, it is necessary that the shoe fit properly and that pressure on the area be relieved. Maintaining clean healthy skin will help greatly in preventing athlete's foot (dermatophytosis). Wearing clean hose and permitting shoes to air and sun is of considerable value. Blisters and abrasions of the skin should have proper care. This is particularly important for the older person who has poor circulation or the person with diabetes whose tissues heal slowly.

STUDY QUESTIONS

1. Give some of the recognized causes of low back pain.
2. Discuss the conservative treatment of low back pain.
3. What type of exercise is usually prescribed for low back pain?
4. Name the important points to observe in the application of a corset prescribed for low back pain.
5. What is the conservative treatment used for low back pain caused by affections of the intervertebral disks? The operation?

6. What are some of the points to observe in applying a back brace to the patient with low back pain?
7. List criteria to use in evaluating a properly fitted shoe.
8. Describe the bony structure of the foot.
9. Why is it important that the convalescent patient wear a well-fitted shoe instead of a bedroom slipper?
10. List causes of foot strain.
11. Of what value are the foot exercises frequently prescribed to correct foot strain?

REFERENCES

Baer, R. L., Rosenthal, S. A., Litt, J. Z., and Rogachefsky, H.: Experimental investigations on mechanism producing acute dermatophytosis of feet, J.A.M.A. **160**:184-190, 1956.

Bruck, H.: Nursing the laminectomy patient, Am. J. Nursing **51**:158-161, 1951.

Bruck, H. O., and Lambert, C. N.: Common foot disabilities, Am. J. Nursing **59**:1580-1583, 1959.

Chandler, F. A.: Laminectomy, Am. J. Nursing **51**:156-157, 1951.

Colonna, P. C.: Spondylolisthesis, J.A.M.A. **154**:398-402, 1954.

Howorth, B. M.: Low back pain, Am. J. Nursing **55**:40-43, 1955.

Howorth, B. M.: Your feet and your shoes, Am. J. Nursing **52**:1368-1372, 1952.

Janes, J. M., and Stifter, R.: Spinal fusion, Am. J. Nursing **55**:1062-1065, 1955.

Locke, R.: Foot care for diabetics, Am. J. Nursing **63**:107-110, 1963.

Mercer, Sir Walter, and Duthie, R.: Orthopedic surgery, ed. 6, Baltimore, 1964, Williams & Wilkins Co.

Pasternak, S.: The patient with a ruptured disk, Am. J. Nursing **62**:77-80, 1962.

Selke, O. O.: Foot strain, Orthopedics **2**:48-49, 1960.

Shands, A. R., Raney, R. B., and Brashear, H. R.: Handbook of orthopaedic surgery, ed. 6, St. Louis, 1963, The C. V. Mosby Co.

Stimson, B. B.: Backache, Am. J. Nursing **51**:672-674, 1951.

Tondra, J. M., and Carlin, G. A.: Plantar warts —their etiology and treatment, Am. J. Nursing **55**:828-829, 1955.

U. S. Children's Bureau: Your children's feet and footwear, Children's Bureau Folder No. 41-1954, Washington, D. C., 1954, U. S. Government Printing Office.

Chapter 11

Special operative procedures

Types of operative procedures

This chapter has been included to acquaint the student with the types of operative procedures carried out for disabilities of bones and joints. It is not meant to include all varieties of operation but rather to point out broad categories and to discuss a few in detail.

ARTHRODESIS

A number of operative techniques have been designed to fuse various joints that are disabling. The main purpose of any fusion is to eliminate motion from the joint. This is helpful in healing disease such as tuberculosis of the hip, knee, or spine. Fusion may also serve to eliminate instability of a paralyzed foot, or it may be useful to correct deformity such as might occur in the ankle following a severe injury.

Triple arthrodesis. Triple arthrodesis is a surgical procedure performed on the foot to increase stability. The poliomyelitic patient with a flail extremity or the older child with an untreated clubfoot may have this procedure performed to eliminate motion and to maintain a better position of the foot. It consists in fusing three joints of the foot, the subastragalar joint, the astragaloscaphoid joint, and the calcaneocuboid joint. The

fusion of these joints eliminates the movements of inversion and eversion of the foot and lessens the amount of abduction and adduction of the forefoot. Ankle motion is not changed. Fusion is accomplished by removing the articular cartilage of the joints involved.

Following this surgical procedure a short leg plaster cast is applied. The foot is immobilized in plaster until healing and fusion have taken place, approximately 8 to 12 weeks. Weight bearing is not permitted during this time. Postoperatively, a considerable amount of bleeding may be expected. The limb should be elevated for 3 to 5 days after surgery to minimize swelling and thus lessen the pain. Even so, narcotics usually must be given to provide comfort for this patient. Careful and frequent check of the circulation in the toes must be made. Often it is necessary that the cast be split and spread.

Spinal fusion. Spinal fusion warrants detailed discussion because it is so common and involves considerable nursing care. Fusion of the spine is accomplished by obtaining solidity between the posterior segments of the vertebrae. Usually, the solidity is achieved by the use of bone grafts

327

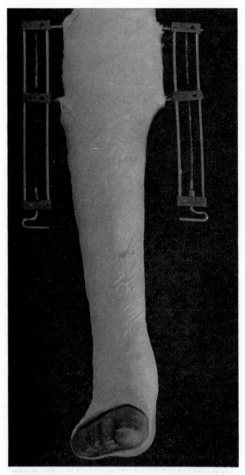

Fig. 244. A pin has been placed through the lower end of the femur and the upper end of the tibia to maintain compression apposition during the healing stage after an arthrodesis of the knee. The two hand screws allow for daily adjustment to bring the two bone wires closer together to maintain compression at the site of the fusion.

placed on the lamina of the area to be fused.

Refinements of technique are diverse and are determined by the type of graft, placement of the graft, and preparation of the graft bed. In addition, most surgeons fuse the facets at the proper levels to assure solidity of fusion.

It has been implied that spinal fusions are performed to relieve backache,

which is true, but there are other equally important indications. Scoliosis can be corrected in part, and the correction can be maintained by fusing the spine in the corrected position. Here as a rule many levels are fused, and the aftercare to ensure fusion must be closely supervised. The same is true when fusion has been performed to control active tuberculosis of the spine. The patient must remain for some months in recumbency with immobilization, and thereafter ambulation must be begun gradually with continued support to prevent motion of the spine.

ARTHROPLASTY

An arthroplasty is an operative procedure that attempts to re-create a joint as nearly like the original as possible. It has been applied to the elbow, hip, knee, shoulder, and small joints of the hand with varying degrees of success in the order listed.

The creation of a new joint is truly a reconstructive operation and requires skill by the surgeon as well as strong will by the the patient to achieve a good result. At best a surgically constructed joint will not equal a normal joint, but if well done technically it can approximate the normal if the patient will faithfully carry out a long program of exercises to maintain motion and to build muscle strength.

Hip arthroplasty. In arthroplasty of any joint some material must be superimposed between the newly shaped joint surfaces to prevent ankylosis of the joint. In the elbow, fascia lata has been found to be satisfactory interposition material. In the hip, where weight bearing is necessary, fascia lata is not so satisfactory; therefore, stronger material has been used, namely Vitallium, which is a metal that the body tolerates well. Vitallium cup arthroplasty has so far been used mainly for the hip in

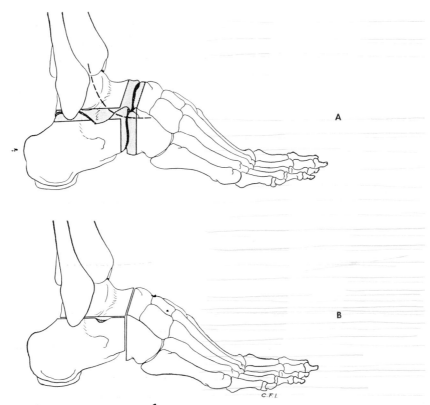

Fig. 245. Triple arthrodesis. **A,** Line of skin incision. Shaded area indicates amount of bone removed. **B,** Completion of operation. (From Speed, J. S., and Knight, R. A.: Campbell's operative orthopedics, ed. 3, St. Louis, 1956, The C. V. Mosby Co.)

adults and for the following conditions:

Indications for cup arthroplasty of the hip.

1. Malum coxae senilis (painful hypertrophic arthritis of the aged)
2. Traumatic arthritis (secondary arthritis that follows surgery)
3. Rheumatoid arthritis (arthroplasty indicated to relieve pain, correct deformity, and improve function)
4. Unreduced congenital dislocation of the hip
5. Old septic arthritis
6. Complications following fractures of neck of the femur
   (a) Aseptic necrosis of the head of the femur
   (b) Nonunions (calls for various types of reconstruction using the arthroplasty principle with Vitallium cup; reconstruction dependent on what remains of the original joint that can be utilized)

To illustrate what has already been mentioned regarding the importance of supervised convalescence, the following routine is frequently employed after cup arthroplasty.

Postoperatively this patient is placed in balanced suspension traction. The purposes of this traction are (1) to provide support for the limb, (2) to maintain the extremity in a position of abduction, (3) to provide increased comfort for the patient, and (4) to facilitate nursing care. Bed position and posture (Fig. 250) are extremely important for the patient with cup arthroplasty. The affected limb is maintained in a position of abduction and internal rotation. To help the patient maintain this position, the nurse will not only

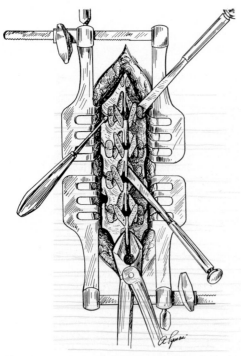

Fig. 246. Fusion of the spine. Hibbs method.
Upper chisel for obtaining bone chips from superficial surfaces of articular facets.
Curette for removing cartilage from articular facets.
Lower chisel for producing bone flaps from spinous processes in four directions.
Bone-cutting forceps for cutting chips from remaining portion of spinous processes to be laid down center. Muscles and ligamentous structure hold chips in place when wound is closed.

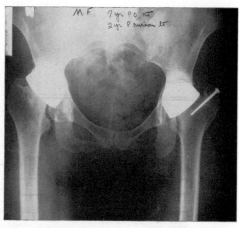

Fig. 247. Roentgenogram showing position of Smith-Petersen Vitallium cup after bilateral arthroplasty of the hip.

need to teach him what constitutes good position but also help him to attain it in many instances. A sandbag placed against the medial aspect of the unaffected limb will remind the patient that he must not recline so that his body lies diagonal of the bed. If this position is permitted, abduction of the extremity is lost. A sandbag placed against the chest wall on the unaffected side will help him to keep the iliac crests level. A footboard or bolster for the unaffected extremity will help maintain good position, and when the backrest is elevated, there will be flexion of the hip joints

and not flexion of the lumbar spine. A small pad placed beneath the lumbar region will add greatly to the patient's comfort. It must be remembered, however, that extension of the hip joint without increased lumbar lordosis is desirable. Several days after surgery the patient should be doing things for himself. He needs to be encouraged to use the trapeze for shifting his position and to assist with nursing care procedures. Exercise and use of the unaffected extremity will help maintain muscle strength and prevent generalized weakness.

On approximately the fourth postoperative day, muscle-setting exercises are begun. The patient is instructed by the doctor or the physical therapist pertaining to quadriceps and gluteal muscle-setting exercises. (Many times the patient is taught these exercises preoperatively.) In quadriceps-setting exercises the patient is instructed to press the popliteal space against the mattress and to lift the heel off the bed. With this exercise the kneecap can be felt to move as the quadriceps muscle tightens. As has been previously stated, it is important that the tone and strength of this

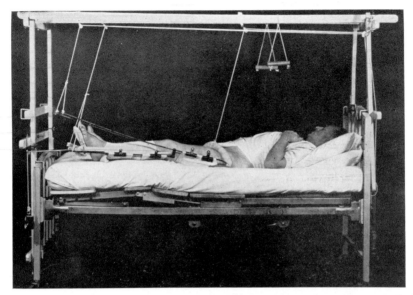

Fig. 248. Postoperatively, balanced suspension traction is applied to maintain the desired position of the extremity. The half-ring Thomas splint with the Pearson attachment provides support for the limb. Note the wooden Balkan frame attached to the bed.

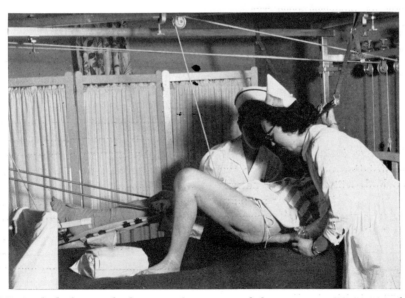

Fig. 249. Method of giving back care to the patient in balance traction. By grasping the trapeze and pushing with the normal extremity with the knee and hip flexed, the patient is able to lift the buttocks off the bed. Because of the balanced weights, the splint supporting the affected extremity elevates as the patient's body is lifted.

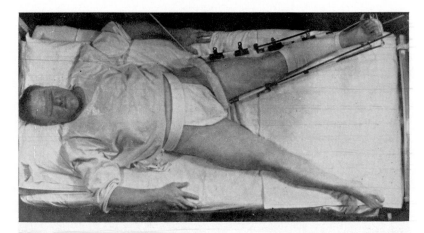

Fig. 250. The desired position for the patient with a cup arthroplasty in balance traction. Note that the patient is in the center of the bed and that the iliac crests are level. Both limbs are abducted. This position helps maintain the cup and head of the femur in the acetabulum. The affected limb is held either in a neutral position or in a position of slight internal rotation.

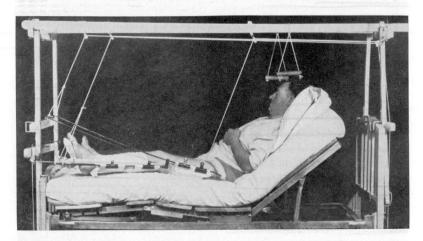

Fig. 251. Sitting position for the patient with cup arthroplasty with limb in balance traction. It is important that these patients be in the sitting position at intervals throughout the day and that their bed be flat at other times. The purpose of this is to provide flexion and extension of the hip joint. The nurse, however, must secure instructions from the surgeon for each patient pertaining to elevation of the bed. How soon postoperatively and how much the bed may be elevated will vary depending on the stability of the hip joint.

muscle (knee extensor) be maintained during the period of bed rest. If this exercise is practiced faithfully during the time spent in traction, the process of standing and walking will be much easier. With gluteal-setting exercises the patient is taught to pinch the buttocks together and to attempt to move the leg to the side of the bed. This tightens the abductors (gluteus medius muscle). In addition to these exercises, the patient is instructed to dorsiflex and plantar flex the ankle and to bring the foot into a position of inversion. The patient must actually dorsiflex the foot and not just move the toes. Several days postoperatively the surgeon will request that the backrest be elevated. The amount of

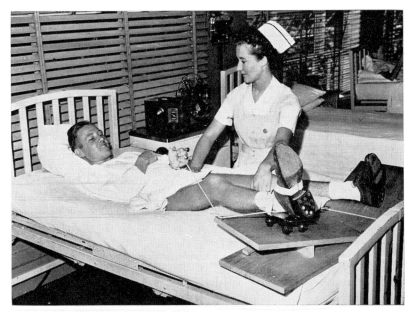

Fig. 252. Skate used with shoe. Nurse keeps hand on opposite side of pelvis to prevent further compensating adduction of the normal hip as the reconstructed hip is pulled into abduction by the patient.

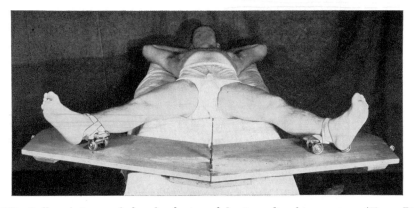

Fig. 253. Roller skates used for developing abduction after hip surgery. (From Pitman, Eleanor: Hip injuries and nursing care, Am. J. Nursing **40**:395-400, 1940.)

elevation and length of time will be increased gradually as the patient is able to tolerate increased flexion of the hip joints. When the patient becomes accustomed to this position, he may prefer having the backrest elevated and the hips flexed. It must be remembered, however, that a position that permits complete extension of the hip joints must be assumed at intervals.

Within approximately 3 weeks (depending on the surgeon's wishes) traction is removed. After the removal of the traction, roller-skating exercises are started. This exercise provides for abduction at the hip joint and strengthens the abductor muscles. With the bed flat a roller-skating board is placed under the patient's feet, and the skates are fastened to his ankles. The rope attached to the skates is threaded through the pulley at the outer edge of the board. The patient abducts the limb as far as possible with the hip muscles, and then by means of the rope he can passively increase the amount of abduction (within limits of pain). In the beginning, however, the nurse must be alert for signs of fatigue and muscle soreness. If muscle soreness develops, progress will be delayed. Later, this exercise may be ordered two or three times daily for 10-minute periods.

Usually about the twenty-eighth day postoperatively or earlier, the patient is permitted to stand. He is assisted to the sitting position and then to the standing position. He places both feet on the floor but does not place his full weight on the affected extremity. This is the beginning of a period of concentrated exercises, walking with crutches, and special exercises on the bicycle and skates. These exercises must be continued faithfully for many months if maximum hip motion is to be gained

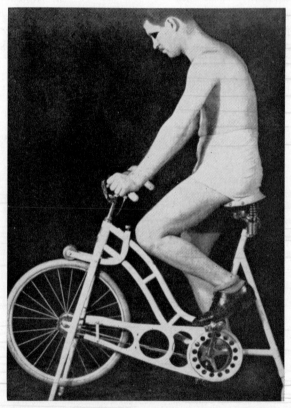

Fig. 254. The stationary bicycle provides flexion and extension exercises of the hip and knee joints. The patient must sit well back on the bicycle seat, and his foot is placed squarely on the pedal. He pushes down with his heel and pulls up against the foot strap placed across the dorsum of the foot. The first time he may not be able to make a complete turn with the pedal. The nurse must remember, however, that in the beginning all of these exercises are for short periods and are gradually increased to periods of 10 minutes or more and are performed several times daily. To promote development of the hip muscles resistance may be applied against the bicycle wheel. To increase flexion of the hip joint the bicycle seat may be lowered.

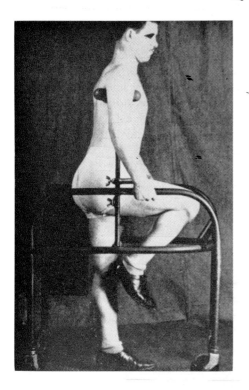

Fig. 255. Walking in the walker. Note extreme flexion of the affected extremity. When using the walker or crutches, the patient should be encouraged to use this type of step rather than a shuffling gait. With unilateral cup arthroplasty the patient is taught the three-point crutch gait. Both crutches are advanced with the affected extremity, and the patient takes approximately half his body weight on the affected extremity. With bilateral cup arthroplasty, the four-point gait is taught, left crutch, right foot, right crutch, left foot. The patient is also taught stair climbing. This is the same for the patient with a cup arthroplasty as for any patient with crutches. When going down the stairs, the crutches and affected extremity are placed on the lower step, preceding the normal leg. When going up the stairs, the patient's normal leg is placed on the next step and then followed by the crutches and the affected extremity.

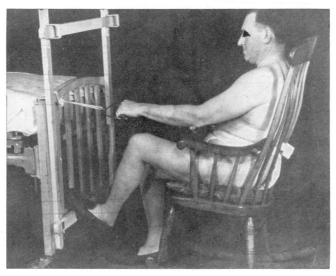

Fig. 256. Rocking chair exercises. Note that the patient sits with hips well back in the seat of the chair and that the foot of the affected extremity is placed on the bed. As he pulls himself forward in the rocker, flexion of the hip joint is increased. The same effect may be accomplished by placing a sandbag or footstool beneath the foot. Weights may be added to the arm of the chair to pull the patient and chair forward.

and maintained. Before discharging the patient, provision must be made to supply him with the apparatus needed for exercise in the home.

The exercises that promote flexion and extension of the hip joint and that increase muscular strength are illustrated. These exercises are a very important part of the treatment and care of the patient with a cup arthroplasty, and are ordered specifically by the surgeon for the individual patient. The patient undertakes gradually one exercise after another to keep motion and to build muscle until further gain cannot be made. After a year or more the new joint will have reached its optimum function, although small gains may still be made year after year.

OSTEOTOMIES

The shaft of any long bone may be malaligned as a result of congenital deformity, disease such as osteogenesis imperfecta, or a fracture that healed in malposition. Any such deformity may be corrected by operative means; this constitutes an osteotomy. When it is feasible, the osteotomy will be fixed by internal means, such as wire, metal screws and plates, bone grafts, or specially designed fixation material. The aftercare will be similar to the treatment of a fracture at a comparable site, for

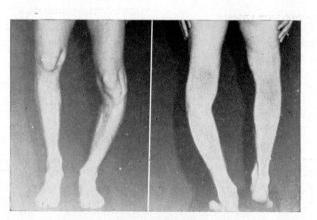

Fig. 257. Anterior and posterior views illustrating extreme bowing of left tibia.

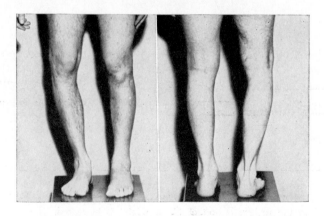

Fig. 258. Postoperative photographs showing correction gained by osteotomy of the proximal end of the tibia.

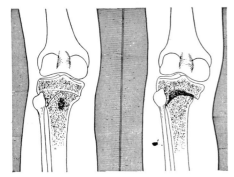

Fig. 259. Line drawing illustrating osteotomy of the tibia used in correction of genu valgum deformity.

in essence an osteotomy is a controlled fracture.

TENDON TRANSPLANTATION

Several principles of tendon transplantation might be of interest to nurses. It is well to know the reason in a given case for the tendon transplant.

Substitution. In patients with poliomyelitis there is frequently residual paralysis of certain muscle groups that can be easily determined. In any such circumstance if strong muscles exist in the same extremity, the strong muscle may be transplanted (1) to gain certain function, as in opponens pollicis transplant to the thumb, and (2) to eliminate bracing, as in anterior tibial substitution.

Replacement. In crushing hand injuries certain tendons may be damaged beyond repair. In such instances a tendon from a less important area may be surgically grafted to replace the damaged tendon, and this is known as a free graft.

Realignment. Uncorrected deformities are sometimes increased by the pull of normal muscles in an abnormal direction. Such muscle pull can be redirected by surgical transfer so that it tends to correct the deformity. An example is a shift of the anterior tibial tendon to a more lateral position in a patient with clubfoot.

ARTHROTOMY FOR INTERNAL DERANGEMENT OF THE KNEE

The knee, the elbow, and the phalangeal joints are the only true hinge joints in the body. The knee, being a weight-bearing joint, is the most susceptible to

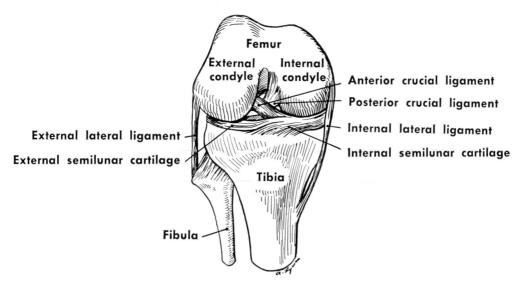

Fig. 260. Ligaments of the knee joint and semilunar cartilages shown with the knee in flexion.

strain and ligamentous injury. These commonly occur in athletes and industrial workers and usually are the result of twisting motions or lateral strain. When the knee is in complete extension, stabilization is accomplished by the internal and external lateral ligaments. These become taut in the extended position but relax somewhat in flexion (Fig. 260). The anterior crucial ligament also is tightened in extension and tends to stabilize the joint in complete extension.

The posterior crucial ligament prevents forward displacement of the tibia on the femur when the knee is in flexion.

Types of injury. Rupture of the anterior crucial ligament may occur when the knee is forced into a back-knee position. Rupture of the posterior crucial ligament may occur when the force is exerted on the lower leg from behind with the knee in flexion.

The most common athletic injury is tearing of the internal lateral ligament. It is caused by exerting pressure against the other side of the knee when the foot is anchored against the ground. This is often called football knee and requires a period of 3 to 6 weeks to heal. The first 3 to 4 weeks are spent in a walking cast that extends from the groin to above the ankle. To prevent the cast from sliding down by gravity, adhesive tape is usually applied over a coat of compound tincture of benzoin (to prevent skin irritation) and is turned upward at the lower end of the cast. After this a knee support is frequently used for a period of several weeks. The reenforced, laced, elastic type seems to be the most efficient. The knee-cage brace with a steel reenforcement and joint may be preferable in some cases.

Rupture of the crucial ligaments is usually caused by rather severe knee injuries. Fortunately, most of these rup-

tures will heal if cast immobilization is used for sufficient periods of time. If not, operations for the replacement of the ligaments with tendons or strips of fascia become necessary.

Rupture of the internal and external semilunar cartilages occurs frequently. Rupture of the internal cartilage is the more common. It occurs as a result of a twisting motion. The foot is anchored on the ground, and the body and thigh twist when the knee is flexed so as to cause rotation of the condyles of the tibia on the condyles of the femur. Rupture of the external semilunar cartilage occurs as a result of a reversal of this motion.

The rupture may occur as a detachment of the anterior attachment of the cartilage or the posterior attachment of the cartilage, or it may be the bucket handle type in which the cartilage is split, part of it entering the central compartment of the knee joint and part of it remaining in the normal position along the outer margin of the joint. Repeated locking is indicative of this type.

Treatment. Immediate operation is not always necessary in semilunar cartilage injury. Many patients will recover if closed reduction is accomplished with or without anesthesia and a walking leg cast is applied for a period of 3 to 4 weeks. If there is recurrence, then removal of the cartilage is usually indicated. Removal does not usually lead to any interference with the function of the joint. There are many active athletes who have had a cartilage removed.

After surgery no cast is used, but a compression bandage helps prevent postoperative hemorrhage. Motion is begun after 24 to 36 hours, stitches are removed in 8 to 10 days, and walking on crutches with tapping is started at 2 weeks. About 3 months are required for full recovery.

Amputation surgery and rehabilitation, including nursing care

Although amputation surgery is as old as surgery itself, the past 20 years has brought enormous progress to the field. With the help of antibiotics, vascular surgery, and effective control of diabetes, many limbs are now being saved that would have required amputation in the past. Since World War II intensive research in the development of artificial limbs, or prostheses, and an excellent education program have been sponsored by several federal agencies. Greatly improved care for the patient with a threatened or doomed limb is now generally available. The outlook for returning to a nearly normal life is much brighter today for the amputee as a result of these developments.

Amputation is far more common in civilians than in members of the armed services, even during wartime. Nurses will encounter patients with amputations on the general surgical wards as well as on the orthopedic wards. The ultimate goal in the care of each patient is maximum restoration of physical, economic, emotional, and social capacity. This means the amputee must learn to walk using his artificial limb, learn to care for his own toilet and dressing, and sometimes learn a new job in keeping with his new abilities. To accomplish this goal requires effective teamwork and meticulous nursing care. The nurse must have a fund of knowledge that will enable her to offer advice or assistance when the occasion arises. Besides the knowledge of the care required immediately after surgery, she must teach stump hygiene and know something of prosthesis construction, fit, and function.

The major causes for amputations are as follows:

1. Injury. Amputation sometimes becomes necessary as a result of severe crushing or extensive lacerations of arteries and nerves.
2. Disease. Vascular disease, especially arteriosclerosis, may result in gangrene of a limb caused by in-

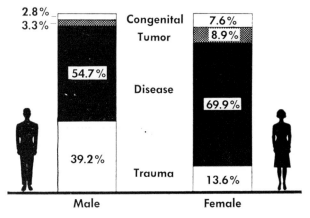

Fig. 261. In both men and women diseases such as arteriosclerosis are the major cause of amputation. (From Glattly, Harold W.: A preliminary report on the amputee census, Artificial Limbs 7:5-10, 1963.)

1-10
343
11-20
571
21-30
554
31-40
808
41-50
1127
51-60
1551
61-70
1885
71-80
863
81-90
153
91+
4

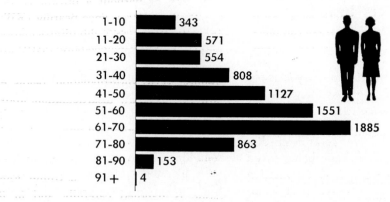

Fig. 262. Most amputations occur in the later years of life because diseases that lead to amputation are more common in this age group. (From Glattly, Harold W.: A preliminary report on the amputee census, Artificial Limbs 7:5-10, 1963.)

Male
77%
23%
Female

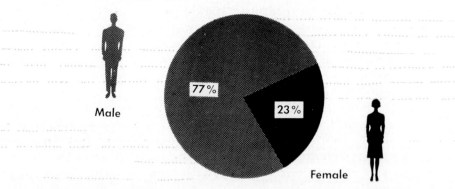

Fig. 263. More than three-fourths of the amputees fitted with artificial limbs are males. (From Glattly, Harold W.: A preliminary report on the amputee census, Artificial Limbs 7: 5-10, 1963.)

Site
Percentage
Shoulder disarticulation 1.1
Above elbow 3.7
Elbow .3
Below elbow 8.6
Wrist .8
Hip disarticulation 1.8
Above knee 44.1
Knee bearing 1.1
Below knee 36.8
Syme 1.7

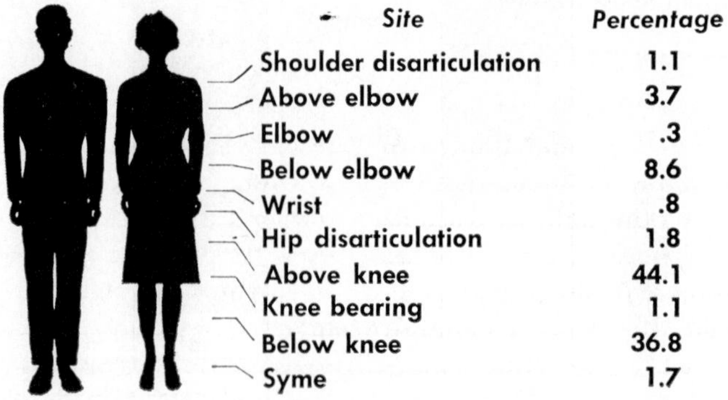

Fig. 264. Note that 85% of the prostheses delivered are for lower extremity amputations. (From Glattly, Harold W.: A preliminary report on the amputee census, Artificial Limbs 7: 5-10, 1963.)

adequate blood supply to the tissues. The elderly patient with an above-knee amputation as a result of arteriosclerosis is by far the most common amputee. Diabetes is often accompanied by severe vascular disease as well as loss of skin sensation and marked susceptibility to infections. Extensive osteomyelitis may so damage a limb that the patient prefers amputation and a prosthesis.

3. Tumors. Malignant bone tumors are most common in the second decade of life and in many cases are best treated by amputation.

4. Congenital. Absence of limbs (phocomelia) or severe malformations of a limb present at birth are the result of faulty embryonic development. Thalidomide, once a popular sedative in Europe, caused multiple severe limb malformations in the infants born of mothers who had taken the drug. Amputation may be necessary if the malformed limb will not respond to other corrective treatments.

In a recent survey of prostheses fitted it was found that more than three-fourths of the amputee patients were males. Of all amputations 85% were of the lower extremities and only 15% were of the upper extremities.

AMPUTATION SURGERY

As much as possible the surgeon attempts to perform the amputation with a standard technique at standard sites, saving as much of the limb as feasible. Each level of amputation, therefore, has certain characteristic features and problems with which the nurse should be familiar. For example, the Syme amputation is a removal of the foot at the ankle joint (disarticulation) and it is done in younger patients with good circulation. It provides an excellent weight-bearing stump that allows the patient to walk with or without a prosthesis. Below the knee (BK), knee bearing (KB), above the knee (AK), hip disarticulation (HD), and hemipelvectomy (HP) are other standard levels in the lower extremity. Wrist disarticulation, below elbow (BE), elbow disarticulation, above elbow (AE), and shoulder disarticulation (SD) are standard upper extremity amputation levels.

The surgeon designs neat skin flaps to cover what will be the new stump. Each tissue is handled carefully and in its own prescribed way to avoid unnecessary damage. The major vessels are doubly secured with suture ligatures before being divided. In closure of the wound only enough sutures are used to bring the tissues into approximation without undue tension. Drains placed deeply within the wound may be brought out through the skin incision line to allow escape of fluid and blood from beneath the skin flaps. Suction tubes to serve the same purpose may be brought out from the skin adjacent to the incision line.

Occasionally, a guillotine amputation is necessary because of uncontrolled infection. In this type of amputation the tissues and bone are severed at the same level without making skin flaps. The wound is not closed but usually can be approximated using skin traction postoperatively, or it may require secondary closure in the operating room some days later. A snug compression dressing is applied in the operating room. Some surgeons prefer skin traction that may be applied in the operating room or immediately after the patient is conscious. This is necessary in some cases to ensure proper conditions for healing. Methods of applying traction may vary somewhat. Stockinet and skin glue, moleskin straps, and rubber surface traction are in common usage.

If stockinet is used, the material is rolled doughnut fashion and applied over the dressing. The top of the stockinet is secured to the skin of the leg above the dressing by some kind of skin adherent.

The most commonly used type of traction is made by four strips of adhesive tape that are applied on each of the four aspects of the thigh above the dressing—medial, lateral, posterior, and anterior. A circle of heavy wire, stabilized by two crosspieces of wire, or a wooden hexagon may be used as a

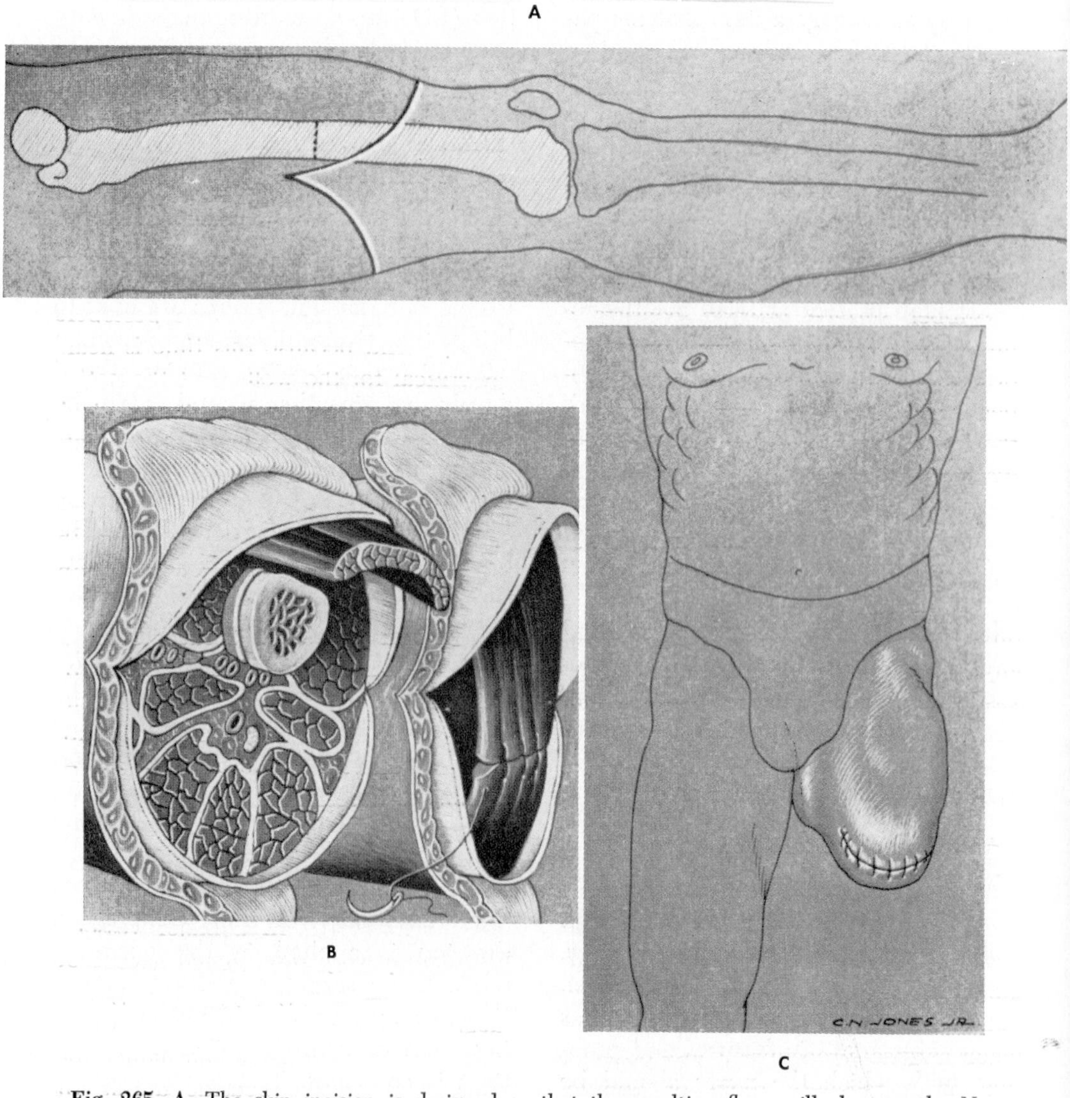

A

B

C

Fig. 265. A, The skin incision is designed so that the resulting flaps will close neatly. Notice that the anterior flap is slight longer than the posterior flap. B, Each tissue is gently and cleanly incised. Here the muscle and fascia are sutured in layers over the end of the bone. C, The completed amputation: The line of closure falls slightly on the posterior aspect of the stump. (From Slocum, Donald B.: An atlas of amputations, St. Louis, 1949, The C. V. Mosby Co.)

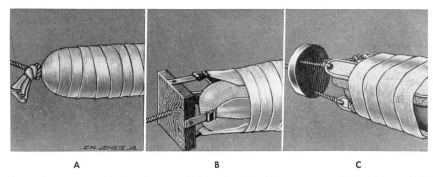

Fig. 266. Skin traction. **A**, Stockinet and skin glue. **B**, Adhesive tape. **C**, Rubber pad. (From Slocum, Donald B.: An atlas of amputations, St. Louis, 1949, The C. V. Mosby Co.)

spreader for the adhesive. Rope extends from this spreader to a pulley attached to the end of the bed. A 5-pound weight attached to the traction is usually considered adequate.

Rubber surface traction consists of lining the adhesive tape strips previously described with thin strips of sponge rubber. These strips are then bandaged to the skin above the stump, and the weights are applied as in most skin adhesive traction. The suction of the rubber on the skin maintains it in place. The advantage of this kind of traction is that it can be removed entirely for physical therapy treatments. Occasionally, a protective wire cage or plaster cast is applied to keep the fresh wound undisturbed, to keep the limb in the desired position, or to prevent contractures.

CARE OF THE PATIENT AFTER AMPUTATION

Immediately following surgery, patients who have had an amputation are subject to complications inherent in the administration of any anesthetic and major surgical procedure. Close observation in a recovery room or another facility where suction apparatus, oxygen, infusion packs, and other emergency equipment are at the bedside must be maintained for several hours following surgery. It is not enough to have these

facilities in the next room—they must be at the bedside for immediate use. The nurse who is in charge of the recovery area has this as her sole responsibility. Nothing whatsoever must distract her attention from the postoperative patient, because this time is nearly as critical for the welfare of the patient as is the actual operation. Frequent observations and recordings of the vital signs are necessary. Restraints may be necessary until the patient is fully alert to prevent disturbing the dressing, the intravenous infusions, and suction tube apparatus. The patient is encouraged to cough and take deep breaths every 15 minutes. The doctors may position the patient temporarily in the side-lying position to avoid aspiration of vomitus into the airway. If elevation of the extremity is necessary because of shock or hemorrhage, it is wiser to raise the end of the bed than to place pillows under the stump. Extensive bleeding from a loosened ligature on a major vessel is fortunately very rare. When it does occur it is an emergency of the gravest degree. To avert a possible catastrophe, many surgeons order a tourniquet routinely kept at the bedside during the postoperative period.

Curiously enough, the pain following amputation is almost always quite mild. Mild analgesics usually suffice, and often no analgesic at all is necessary after the first 24 hours. Pain of great severity may indicate a wound complication, and the doctor should be notified at once of the patient's discomfort.

The doctor will usually permit sips of fluids as soon as the patient is fully awake and free of nausea. The following day, a light diet is usually well tolerated. The insulin requirements of diabetic patients undergoing amputation may fluctuate in the postoperative period. This is especially true when infection is a complicating factor. When control is difficult, the doctor may order frequent small doses of regular insulin and may request frequent fractional urine determinations for urinary glucose.

Amputation is usually accompanied by a more or less profound degree of psychologic shock, which, of course, can be readily understood. This reaction is seen less frequently in patients who have been psychologically well prepared for their surgery. It is most profound in the patient who has an amputation as a result of an injury and has not had time to adjust to the loss. The nurse may note evidence of this psychologic shock in her patients by manifestations of depression, hostility, denial, and occasionally, feelings of futility. The elderly patient often demonstrates extreme confusion during the postoperative period, and young patients may have feelings of mutilation or emasculation. These reactions in general are seen less often in the patient

with a well-balanced, stable personality. The patient will need reassurance from the nurse starting even before surgery and continuing during the first few difficult days after surgery. The nurse is in an excellent position to supply reassurance that he is not to become a cripple, unable to walk or look after his own needs. The nurse, fully aware of the advances made in the past few years in regard to walking with artificial limbs, may be a source of great encouragement to the patient at this time. She should supply continual firm, affirmative support and constant reassurance. This type of support should be continued throughout the rehabilitation period.

Nurses should be alert from the outset to detect signs of flexion and abduction contractures at the hip. This is a natural position for the patient to assume in bed, partly because he feels he is protecting the fresh wound from any disturbance. The hip becomes contracted in this position quite insidiously. Strenuous measures must be taken to avoid this complication because it makes efficient walking with a prosthesis difficult, if not impossible. Even a slightly sagging bed can contribute to contractures, and bed boards may be necessary to provide a firm support. Pillows under the thigh are almost certain to result in some degree of flexion at the hip level. To prevent these complications the above-knee amputee should lie prone

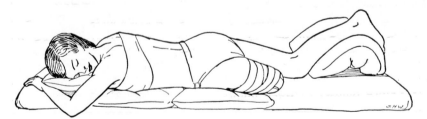

Fig. 267. Prone position. The pillow under the patient's lower trunk protects the wound from pressure on the bed and maintains the hip in extension. (From Moskopp, Mary-Elizabeth, and Sloan, Jane: Nursing care for the amputee, Am. J. Nursing **50:**550-555, 1950.)

for ½-hour intervals several times during the day. If the patient uses the backrest or a wheelchair for long periods during the day, he should be encouraged to spend a comparable period in a position of full extension to prevent contracture of the hip flexors. Bed exercises will be started after a day or two, not only to prevent contracture but to start building needed muscle strength.

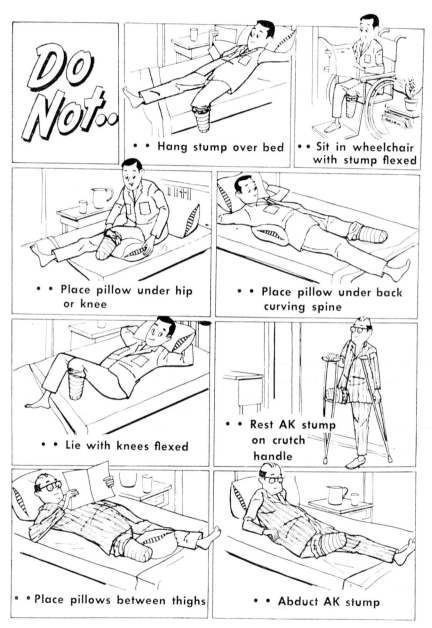

Fig. 268. To avoid contractures and to assure the best conditions for wound healing the patient should be cautioned to avoid the activities shown. (From Wilson, A. Bennett, Jr.: Limb prosthetics today, Artificial Limbs 7:1-42, 1963.)

A great deal of the patient's future ability to walk will depend on the remaining limb, and care should be taken to keep it in normal muscle tone. Supports should be provided to encourage good anatomic position in bed. A sensitive heel sometimes develops in the remaining foot because of the patient's inclination to push himself up in bed by digging his heel into the mattress. An overhead trapeze will help the patient to pull himself up in bed without using his heel.

The patient may be allowed out of bed as early as the day after amputation to reduce the danger of embolism. He should be fitted with a good shoe when he begins to bear any weight on the foot.

These things will not be difficult to encourage in the healthy adult, but the debilitated, elderly patient will need to be encouraged by frequent explanations as to the necessity of what he is doing. Otherwise, it tends to seem too much trouble to him to warrant the effort he must put forth.

PHYSICAL THERAPY

Two forms of treatment that are almost universally followed after amputation are bandaging and exercise. It is desirable, although sometimes not possible, that these be given under the direction of a physical therapist. If such service is not available, nurses must request demonstration from the physician. It is not enough in these circumstances that the demonstration be given to the patient alone because the nurse will need to encourage and guide the patient in the doctor's absence.

Bed exercises may be started on the first or second postoperative day. These help greatly in the prevention of contractures as well as in preserving and increasing muscle power for the training to come. While lying in the prone posi-

tion, the patient is instructed to bring the stump close to the normal leg, to lift it, and to contract the gluteal muscles as he does so. Nurses supervising this bed exercise should see to it that the patient lies with his foot over the edge of the mattress and keeps the normal leg on the mattress while he is extending the stump. Another exercise the surgeon may sometimes suggest is that of squeezing a pillow between the thighs. If the patient has a below-knee amputation, considerable attention may be given to strengthening the quadriceps muscle as well. One commonly used exercise is to have the patient tighten the kneecap, using the quadriceps muscle for 10 seconds and then relaxing for 10 seconds. The exercise is repeated four or more times, several times each day. Patients understand more quickly if they do this in unison with the normal leg and are taught to feel the medial portion contract during the final 10 degrees of full extension.

Heat and massage may also contribute a great deal toward preparing the stump for efficient weight bearing. These treatments should be done in accordance with the doctor's prescription by a person trained in physical therapy if at all possible. Otherwise, the nurse entrusted with the treatments should seek explicit instructions and demonstrations from the doctor.

Radiant heat may be provided by sunlight or an electric ultraviolet lamp. Infrared lamps may be helpful in improving local circulation and promoting scar healing but carry the danger of burning the stump. The stump should be kept dry at all times until healed, and it is not permissible to use hot packs or the whirlpool bath. Heat should be used with extreme care, particularly in patients with diabetes or diseases of the vascular system. For such patients the doctor may order a foot cradle and a lamp suspended over the limb area. This type of heat will increase the circulation of the limb without endangering the stump area itself.

When the patient can be out of bed, it is essential that he learn to balance himself properly as he stands on his remaining foot. Parallel bars or crutches will assist him in attaining this balance. In the patient with poor vision, poor balance, or tremors, a walker may be of great benefit. The body should be held straight and the stump should hang straight without flexion or abduction. There should be no distortion of the body because of the missing limb. Drawing in of the abdominal muscles and pinching the gluteal muscles together will give the patient a girdle sense that will enable him to avoid shifting

his weight to the side of the normal leg.

COMPRESSION OR SHRINKER BANDAGING OF STUMP

As soon as the wound is healing well, the doctor may order some type of shrinker or compression bandage to be applied to the stump. The preferred material for this bandage is usually cotton elastic. Bandages are worn at all times except during physical therapy treatments and until the patient is fitted with a prosthesis. With careful bandaging the stump can be molded into the desired shape for fitting with a prosthesis. Without bandaging the stump tends to remain boggy, swollen, and flabby—in this condition a prosthesis cannot be satisfactorily fitted. The chief cause of de-

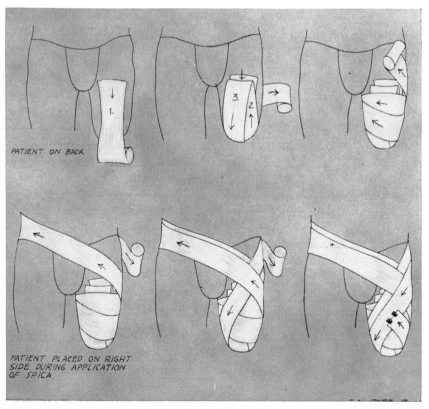

Fig. 269. Application of compression bandage. (From Slocum, Donald B.: An atlas of amputations, St. Louis, 1949, The C. V. Mosby Co.)

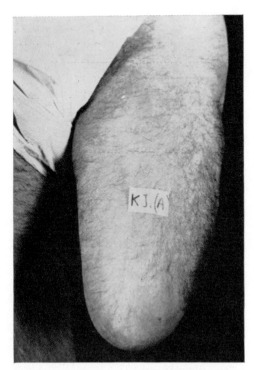

KJ.(A

Fig. 270. Proper compression bandaging will result in a well-molded stump that is ready for prosthetic fitting. (From Wilson, A. Bennett, Jr.: Limb prosthetics today, Artificial Limbs **7:** 1-42, 1963.)

lay in the fitting of the prosthesis and rehabilitation of the patient is an improperly molded stump as a result of inadequate or incorrect compression bandaging. A poorly applied bandage is probably worse than no bandage at all. If it is properly applied, however, a shrinker bandage may play a most important part in the ultimate rehabilitation of the amputee.

Because the bandage needs to be reapplied several times during the day to be most effective, nurses should be familiar with the correct application. Too often nurses are satisfied to leave this task to the physical therapist, but this is hardly a wise procedure since the bandage will frequently need to be reapplied when no physical therapist is available. Occasionally, in busy seasons, it has

been necessary to permit patients to apply their own bandages. Results from this, for the most part, have not proved satisfactory.

For the thigh of an average adult two or three 4- to 6-inch all-cotton elastic bandages will be necessary. For convenience and security they are sewed together end-to-end. The bandage is started on the front of the thigh at the groin level. It may be anchored in place by having the patient hold it with his thumbs, one on either side of the thigh. The bandage is then carried down the center front of the thigh, over the end of the stump, and up the back of the thigh to the gluteal fold, where the patient may secure it with his index fingers. (Unless the patient is very large, his hands should be able to encircle his thigh in this fashion.) Now the bandage is carried down the back of the thigh, going somewhat obliquely this time, over the end of the stump, back up to the groin level, and then down obliquely again, this time over the inner aspect of the stump. Each time the recurrents are held by the patient's fingers and thumbs and each time the end of the stump must be compressed securely. The maximum force of the bandage should always be at the stump end and should diminish as the bandage ascends. These recurrents (three) are then secured by one or two circular turns of bandage around the thigh at the groin level.

Two spiral turns of the bandage downward to the end of the stump are now made, and the patient is turned on his normal side. The bandage is then carried spirally upward around the thigh, compressing the soft tissues on the side of the stump in an upward and outward direction, and then over the outer side of the buttock near the ilia crest. It crosses the abdomen at the umbilicus line and then around the hip of the normal side across the back and around the amputated leg at the groin level. A spiral to the end of the stump is made and a second spiral is made as before, always working from within outward and always using the bandage to compress soft tissues at the stump end. The bandage is finally brought back to the stump and completed by a few spiral turns as the length of the bandage allows. It may be secured by safety pins or bandage clips.

The finished bandage should be observed to see that the spiral crossings to make the hip spica bandage do not lie on the front of the thigh, a condition that encourages hip flexion. Also, the bandage must cover the inner surface of the thigh as high as possible on the groin. If this is not done, a fleshy roll will be likely to occur at the top of the bandage that will be uncomfortable to the patient and will also cause the bandage to slip downward from that level. An unhealed stump must not be bandaged too snugly, and bandages for healed stumps should not be applied so snugly that actual discomfort occurs.

The below-knee bandage is applied in much the same manner as the one for the thigh stump, omitting, of course, the technique for the hip spica. If the bandage extends above the knee, the patella should remain uncovered and the leg should be held in extension. The popliteal area must not be compressed by too snug a bandage.

Because compression bandages must be reapplied several times during the day, it is advisable to have several sets on hand. They should be carefully washed between each wearing with mild soap and warm water and very thoroughly rinsed. They should be squeezed out and laid on a flat surface to dry because they tend to lose their elasticity if hung. When dry, they should be rolled snugly but without stretching.

As soon as the wound is well healed and the patient understands stump wrapping, exercises, and positioning, he will be discharged from the hospital. He is seen at frequent intervals by the doctor to supervise these activities. As soon as his stump is well molded and firm, he is ready for prescription of an artificial limb and rehabilitation.

PROSTHESIS PRESCRIPTION

When the stump is well healed and firmly molded (ordinarily 2 to 3 months after operation), the patient is ready for consideration of a prosthesis. In well-run amputee clinics experience has shown that the prescription and training in the use of the limb is best carried out jointly by a doctor familiar with amputees and prostheses, the prosthetist who will construct and fit the limb, and the physical therapist or occupational therapist who will train the patient in its use. Rehabilitation counselors and social workers usually are also involved. The interested nurse is in an excellent position to contribute to this team through her familiarity with the patient. Many factors must be considered in selecting the proper type of prosthesis and prosthetic component. Some of the more important considerations are the following:

1. Age. Special problems exist at the extremes of life. Children need simpler mechanical devices and their limited attention span makes special training techniques necessary. They outgrow their prosthesis every 2 to 3 years. The elderly amputee may need extra stability to prevent falls.
2. Occupation. Obviously, an active laborer will require heavy duty components and construction, whereas a weak, elderly nursing home patient will desire a lighter prosthesis.
3. Agility and intelligence. A feebleminded patient cannot be expected

to master a complicated upper extremity prosthesis. An obese, clumsy patient will require more safeguards and stability than the average patient.

4. Other health problems. Cardiac reserve is seldom an absolute limiting factor in training because the exertion required to walk with an artificial limb is less than that required for crutch walking. Poor vision, poor balance, paralysis, diminished skin sensation and tolerance are other health considerations.

5. Finances. Artificial limbs are very expensive. Recently developed components—for example, the commercially available hydraulic knee unit—add greatly to this expense. Charitable or governmental agencies furnish 70% to 80% of all prostheses today. Therefore cost must be kept as low as possible. Luxury components can rarely be used.

6. Motivation. The most important consideration of all is motivation, for without it the patient will not use the prosthesis and all rehabilitation efforts are doomed. The nurse, by her knowledge of the patient, can contribute greatly in this evaluation. In general, it is uncommon that the prosthetic prescription team decides that the patient is not a candidate for an artificial limb of any sort.

After prescription the prosthetist takes a mold and certain measurements of the stump to use in construction of the prosthesis. After the mold is taken shrinker bandaging should be discontinued because further shrinkage of the stump will result in an ill-fitting prosthetic socket. The construction of artificial limbs requires the highest standards of craftsmanship and technical skill. The prosthetist must have a thorough understanding of the intricate mechanics of body motion that he is attempting to replace. Socket construction is critical for a proper fit and distribution of weight. Sometimes it is hand carved in basswood or willow wood; otherwise a plastic laminate socket is constructed from a plaster mold. Only certain definite areas on the stump and buttocks are capable of withstanding the pressures of body weight, and the socket must distribute the weight accordingly. Alignment is equally critical, because the position of the prosthesis at all times must closely match that of a normal limb. Lastly, the prosthetist must finish the prosthesis so that it will be pleasing to the eye, carefully matching the patient's own coloring and contour, or else the patient may not wear the limb at all. The prosthetist must be exacting in each detail of construction—it is no mail order procedure.

PROSTHESIS COMPONENTS

Familiarity with prostheses can be gained only by seeing several of each type. The nurse should examine the workings and fit of each artificial limb she encounters. For the interested nurse whose duty requires working with large numbers of amputees, attendance at one of the three large prosthesis schools (Northwestern University, New York University, or University of California at Los Angeles) would be invaluable. The following brief account of the commonest prosthesis components can best be understood if actual prostheses can also be seen and investigated.

The Symes prosthesis is constructed to permit direct weight bearing on the end of the tibia. A small side or rear opening panel in the shank allows the bulbous stump to enter the prosthesis. The socket is made entirely of plastic laminate. A SACH (Solid Ankle, Cushion

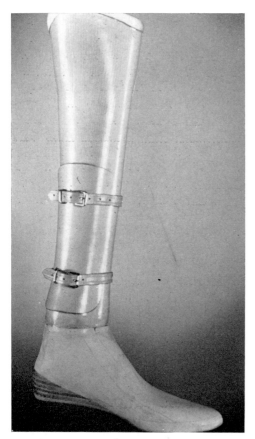

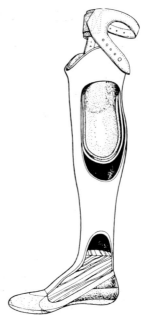

Fig. 272. Cut-away view of the patellar-tendon-bearing prosthesis for below-knee amputees. Usually, only a light strap above the knee is necessary for suspension. (From Wilson, A. Bennett, Jr.: Limb prosthetics today, Artificial Limbs **7**:1-42, 1963.)

Fig. 271. The Canadian Syme prosthesis. A panel on the medial side permits the bulbous stump to enter the prosthesis. A SACH foot is used in this prosthesis. (Courtesy Prosthetic and Sensory Aids Service of the Veterans Administration, Washington, D. C.)

Heel) foot is provided, and this has no actual moving ankle joint. Sponge rubber in the heel simulates the ankle function of absorbing the impact of heel strike with each step. With no moving parts, this foot combines a pleasing appearance with trouble-free wear.

For the below-knee amputee, the patellar-tendon-bearing (PTB) socket has become widely popular. This socket is constructed of plastic laminate with a thin leather and sponge-rubber liner. The bulk of the weight in this instance is distributed to the patellar tendon, which is admirably suited for the job. Usually a single cuff around the thigh just above the kneecap is sufficient for suspension. The SACH foot is generally used in combination with the PTB socket prosthesis. The older hand-carved wooden socket, or so-called soft socket, depends on hinged upright thigh bands and leather lacers to carry much of the weight. The lower end of the socket is left open and it is combined either with a SACH foot or a single axis ankle foot components. Although for years it has proved to be a satisfactory prosthesis, it has a few disadvantages and is being gradually replaced by the PTB socket.

The above-knee amputee faces additional problems because the prosthesis must have a knee articulation. Many types of knee units are in current use, but nearly all incorporate a design that promotes friction during the swing phase of walking. This is necessary to limit the height of the rise of the heel from the floor and to prevent a jarring impact as the knee is again extended just prior to the time the heel strikes the floor. The knee is so aligned that when standing with the knee fully extended, it is balanced against sudden flexion—a disaster that would send the wearer sprawling on the floor. An automatic knee brake (the Bock safety knee) is useful for elderly or infirm patients because it prevents the knee from buckling whenever weight is borne on the prosthesis, whether the knee is safely extended or not. For the especially active wearer, there are new hydraulic (Hydra-Cadence) knee units available that produce a marvelously smooth gait.

These are expensive and occasionally troublesome.

The quadrilateral socket, or Berkley socket, has virtually replaced the older, round socket or plug socket for the above-knee amputee. As the name implies, its rectangular shape does not conform to the shape of the stump, but it does make use of the remaining muscles of the stump. Weight is distributed principally on the ischial tuberosity and the tough origins of the hamstring muscles. The socket is carved from wood or molded in plastic. In some cases a total contact socket is used to alleviate or prevent certain stump skin problems. As the name implies, all portions of the stump are in contact with the socket wall. The suction socket has definite advantages for the active above-knee am-

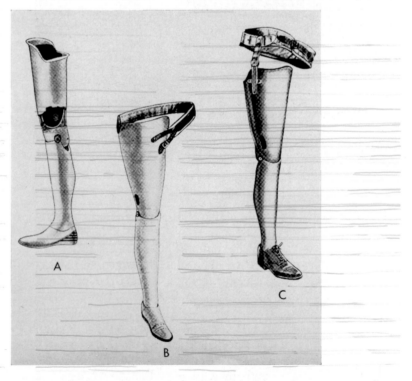

Fig. 273. Three means of suspension in above-knee artificial limbs. **A,** Cut-away view of suction socket. Note again the SACH foot. **B,** A Silesian bandage. Note the single axis ankle-foot component. **C,** Pelvic belt suspension. (From Wilson, A. Bennett, Jr.: Limb prosthetics today, Artificial Limbs **7:**1-42, 1963.)

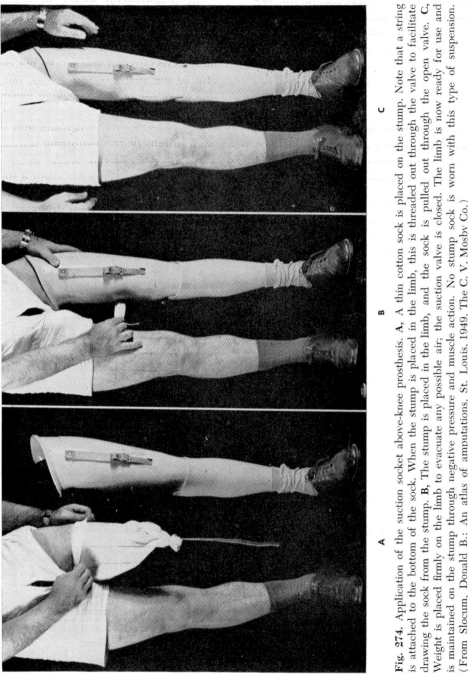

Fig. 274. Application of the suction socket above-knee prosthesis. **A,** A thin cotton sock is placed on the stump. Note that a string is attached to the bottom of the sock. When the stump is placed in the limb, this is threaded out through the valve to facilitate drawing the sock from the stump. **B,** The stump is placed in the limb, and the sock is pulled out through the open valve. **C,** Weight is placed firmly on the limb to evacuate any possible air; the suction valve is closed. The limb is now ready for use and is maintained on the stump through negative pressure and muscle action. No stump sock is worn with this type of suspension. (From Slocum, Donald B.: An atlas of amputations, St. Louis, 1949, The C. V. Mosby Co.)

putee. Not only does it reduce the need for harnessing but it gives improved perception of the movement and location of the prosthesis. The wearer feels that the prosthesis is more a part of his body. When once applied, the stump is pumped up and down to expel all air from the bottom of the socket. A valve is then closed that permits no air to enter, and a suction effect is created.

The Canadian hip disarticulation prosthesis is the current standard prescription for patients who have had a hemipelvectomy or hip disarticulation. The socket is a plastic laminate mold designed to distribute weight on the

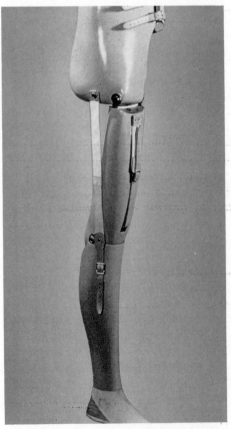

Fig. 275. The Canadian hip disarticulation prosthesis. (Courtesy Prosthetic and Sensory Aids Service of the Veterans Administration, Washington, D. C.)

ischium or other available structures. The hip joint hinge is located toward the front of the socket in a position ahead of the thigh. This alignment eliminates the need for a lock at the hip joint because it cannot buckle suddenly during standing or normal walking. This arrangement also facilitates sitting while wearing the prosthesis. The remaining components consist of a constant-friction knee and a SACH foot.

For the upper-extremity amputee prosthesis function and fitting presents some quite different problems. Replacing the prehensile human hand is clearly an impossibility, and prostheses can only provide a rough approximation of this function. In most cases the prosthetic hand provides only holding and assistive functions for the intact hand. Placing the hand at a desired position in space away from the body and holding it there becomes an intricate problem in levers, cables, and locks. Cosmetic appearance is of far more concern to the average upper extremity amputee. These many problems lead to a lower rate of success in the number of amputees who successfully wear upper extremity prostheses as compared to lower extremity prostheses.

For the wrist disarticulation or below-elbow (BE) amputee, the replacement consists of some type of terminal device that is powered by a cable arrangement from the shoulder. Many types of terminal devices are available, but these divide naturally into hooks and mechanical hands. The term hook is a misnomer that conjures ugly visions of pirate captains, but it is so entrenched in common usage that we are left little alternative except to refer to it nonspecifically as a terminal device. Actually, it is seldom used as a hook, and it would make a clumsy weapon in combat. Most hooks are of the voluntary opening variety, which means that the wearer actively opens the hook to grasp objects, but

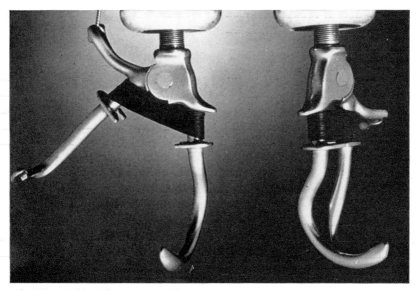

Fig. 276. A common type of voluntary opening hook. Opening is achieved when the wearer applies pull to the cable. Closure is powered by stout bands of elastic rubber. (Courtesy Prosthetic and Sensory Aids Service of the Veterans Administration, Washington, D. C.)

that closure is powered by stout bands of elastic rubber. Voluntary closing hooks remain open until the wearer activates the mechanism to close or pinch an object. This provides more delicate function, but it is inclined to malfunction more frequently. A simple voluntary opening hook is the more efficient, functional, and trouble-free terminal device. It is the logical choice for the new amputee.

Mechanical hands are complex pieces of apparatus that are made in answer to the demand for better cosmetic appearance. In this they do quite well, for they do simulate the form of a hand and a flesh-colored rubber glove adds a reasonable approximation to human skin. They operate on a voluntary closing principle. The dexterity they afford is less than that of the hook, and being intricate devices they are subject to more frequent malfunction. Many amputees prefer the hook for everyday use and the mechanical hand for dress-up occasions.

Just as prosthesis design is more complex for the above-knee amputee than the below-knee amputee, so is it for the above-elbow amputee than for the below-elbow amputee. Elbow joint function must be replaced in order to place the hand at a desired position in space. This requires some kind of cable control to provide elbow flexion (forearm lift) and the elbow lock. Often the forearm lift is controlled by the same cable and shoulder harness as that which operates the terminal device. The elbow lock control unit is usually operated by a separate control cable.

The shoulder disarticulation prosthesis varies from the above-elbow prosthesis in only two ways. A friction joint is provided in the shoulder region that allows the wearer to pre-position the shoulder joint for special uses. There is no mechanical device that activates the shoulder joint, and most of the time the shoulder remains by the side. The second difference is that an excellent power source for operation of control cables

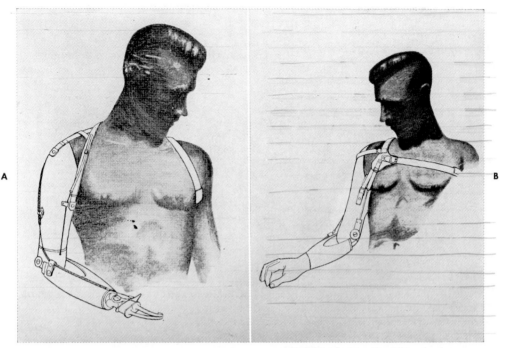

Fig. 277. **A,** Typical prosthesis for an above-elbow amputee. The voluntary opening hook is powered by a cable arrangement from the shoulder harness. Two cables are required for use of this prosthesis. **B,** The elbow-disarticulation amputee requires a slightly different elbow joint. Note the mechanical hand and the harness. (From Wilson, A. Bennett, Jr.: Limb prosthetics today, Artificial Limbs 7:1-42, 1963).

(humeral flexion) has been lost. Consequently, less convenient movements at a greater distance from the shoulder must be harnessed to operate the terminal device, the forearm lift, and the elbow lock.

The sockets for all upper extremity prostheses are usually made from plastic laminates that are individually constructed to fit each patient. Terminal devices, elbow joints, and other hardware are available in a variety of sizes. The harness is made of leather and heavy cotton-web belting. The axillary loop is coated with impervious smooth plastic because of the constant moisture and friction in the axilla. The control cables are mounted upon the harness in such a way that they derive power from the relative motion between two parts of the body.

PROSTHETIC USE TRAINING

Immediately after receiving his prosthesis, the patient should again be seen by the prescription team. The prosthesis should be checked to see that it is satisfactory in every way. The stump should be checked for edema, joint contracture, and muscle strength. If faults exist, the appropriate therapy is instituted. As soon as it is determined that the prosthesis fits properly and consists of the components prescribed, training can begin. The amputee must not be allowed to attempt to put on the limb and begin using it himself—faulty habits and pressure sores cannot easily be undone.

The therapist's first job is to teach the amputee to care for the prosthesis and how to put on and to remove the prosthesis himself. The patient should be

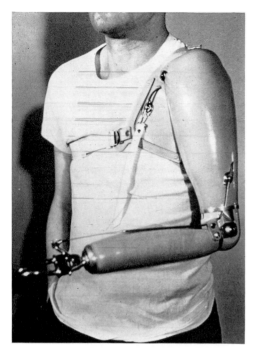

Fig. 278. The prosthesis for a shoulder disarticulation amputee has a larger, wider socket to receive the remaining shoulder. A hinge joint in the shoulder provides some passive motion. (Courtesy Prosthetic and Sensory Aids Service of the Veterans Administration, Washington, D. C.)

instructed in the mechanisms of the prosthesis; every effort should be made to give him confidence that it will not collapse. To apply the typical above-knee prosthesis, the amputee places the wool stump sock over his stump. The stump is placed in the limb socket and the wearer settles his weight into it until he feels proper weight distribution on the proper place. The pelvic belt or harness is then buckled securely.

The patient is usually given instructions by the limb maker in caring for his prosthesis or, if he is an elderly person, some member of the family may be provided with these instructions. With reasonable care the length of useful wear is greatly increased beyond that of a prosthesis carelessly worn and cared for. The patient is instructed never to allow the limb to become excessively wet because this will do irreparable damage to the appliance.

Most limb makers recommend that the prosthesis be cleaned at frequent intervals. The socket, at least, should be cleaned daily with mild soap and water. It is especially important that the socket be dried thoroughly after each use. The patient may be allowed to lubricate and to adjust the friction of certain hinges. The shoe worn on the prosthetic foot should not become excessively worn. The patient should not varnish the wooden socket himself because varnish may prove to be an irritating substance. Stockings may be held up by scotch tape or garters; the use of thumb tacks is discouraged. Hooks should not be used as a tool to pry or hammer. Anything other than the most minor repairs should be performed by the prosthetist and should be done without delay. Preventative maintenance will greatly prolong wear.

The patient will need a period of intensive practice and learning to balance himself in this new limb before he attempts to walk with it. When he has mastered balance in standing with the new limb, he will be ready to take a few steps using the parallel bars. From this he graduates to crutches or to two canes that will later be discarded, one at a time. In crutch walking, a three-point crutch gait is advised; a four-point crutch gait is rarely prescribed. The patient should not be allowed to consider crutches or canes indispensable. The artificial limb is strong enough to support the patient if he learns to use it properly.

Should a fall occur, the patient is taught how to fall as gracefully as possible and how to rise from the floor. When level walking has been mastered, ascending and descending stairs can be taught. Throughout the period of gait training, three essential points must be emphasized in teaching the patient to use the artificial limb: (1) He must learn to balance his body in good posture, (2) use steps of equal length, and (3) attain normal speed in walking.

One of the commonest errors observed in people who use artificial limbs is the rolling gait caused by abduction of the stump and prosthesis in taking a step. It is extremely difficult to overcome once it is acquired, and nurses should be alert to a tendency to walk in this fashion. The patient should not raise or hike his hip and shoulder on the amputated side as he walks.

Use training for the upper extremity amputee starts with operation of the terminal device. It may be necessary to strengthen the groups of muscles that power the terminal device. This is followed in the above-elbow amputee by learning to manage the elbow lock and forearm lift. One by one, such skills as using a knife and fork, tying shoelaces, and managing a billfold are mastered. Training emphasizes two-handed activities or those that require special techniques.

Patients sometimes become discouraged and frustrated during the period of training. The nurse should make every effort at this time to give special encouragement and commendation for his achievements. The major single cause for failure is lack of motivation.

CARE OF THE STUMP

Good care of the amputated stump is essential to continued successful use of a prosthesis. Skin problems of many sorts arise unless positive action is taken to avoid them. Enclosing the stump in an airtight container (the socket) inevitably leads to the accumulation of perspiration, skin waste products, and skin bacteria. Incubation of this mixture from normal body heat all day long pro-

duces a noxious brew. The slightest abrasion or ingrown hair quickly becomes a boil.

The stump should be washed thoroughly each night at bedtime with warm water and a mild soap containing hexachlorophene. Thorough rinsing and drying are also essential. The stump should be kept free of irritating substances such as oil, alcohol, and medicated talcum powders. Iodine and strong disinfectants are never allowed. A high quality nonmedicated talcum may be used occasionally. During initial use training especially, the stump should be inspected frequently for red spots, blisters, and boils. The patient should be specifically asked whether he has any pinched or painful areas. If the slightest skin irritation is in evidence, wearing of the prosthesis should be discontinued until the stump and the socket are checked by the doctor. Neglect of these innocent appearing friction spots can lead to serious problems that may make the fit of any future prosthesis difficult.

A stump sock, which is always worn with the lower extremity prosthesis, should be made of pure virgin wool. The patient will need two or three of these because they must be changed at least once daily. In hot weather more changes will be needed. Socks should never be used if they are torn, patched, or roughened, and they should fit snugly except at the end. Wrinkles in the sock will inevitably lead to irritation and discomfort. These socks need special washing care. They should be washed with mild soap in lukewarm water and rinsed several times. Woolite used in cold water is quite satisfactory. The wool sock should be squeezed dry, not wrung, then spread flat or placed on a sock stretcher to dry. A rubber ball of proper size will help maintain shape of the distal end. Three measurements are needed when ordering stump socks. These are the circumference of the upper rim of the socket, the circumference of the distal end of the stump, and the length of the stump (distal end of stump to the place where the upper rim of the prosthesis strikes the leg, plus a couple of inches to turn back over the socket of the prosthesis).

Some shrinkage may continue in the stump over a period of years, and it is not unusual to find patients attempting to fill the space between the stump and the socket by wearing more and more stump socks. If the nurse discovers that the patient is wearing three or four of these to raise the stump, she should advise him to contact the limb maker at once because a new socket liner or even a new socket may be necessary. The maximum number of stump socks worn at one time should not exceed two.

Phantom limb sensations are experienced by most adult amputees after removal of the limb. These are usually not distressing to the patient, and upon direct questioning he is likely to regard it as a curiosity. Over a period of years the feelings from the absent limb seem to shrink into the stump gradually until the phantom sensation is gone altogether. Distressing phantom limb pains are fortunately a rather rare occurrence —1% to 2% of all amputations. When present, the amputee often feels that the absent toes are being pinched and squeezed or being burned. The phantom limb pains may not make their appearance until years after the amputation. Invariably there is a heavy emotional overlay, and these patients can think and talk of nothing else. The cause of phantom limb pain is not clear. Many types of operative procedures have been devised, but little seems to benefit the wretched condition of patients suffering from this sensation.

On the other hand, true neuroma formation is a fairly frequent condition. Actually, this is the natural reparative reaction (attempted regrowth) of any peripheral nerve that has been cut. If the neuroma is in a location subject to pressure or trauma, it may become quite sensitive. It is characterized by electric or lightning-like pains that are triggered at one well-localized spot. Surgical removal of the offending neuroma is usually very beneficial.

In children with amputations bony overgrowth of the amputated limb is a common complication. The explanation for this phenomenon is not clear, but the bone simply outstrips the surrounding soft tissue in its growth. Again, resection of the excessive bone is usually necessary, and this may have to be repeated several times until growth of the skeleton ceases.

The public health nurse inspecting a prosthesis on a home visit should observe the apparatus for loose or worn joints, for signs of deterioration in rubber, leather, or other fabrics, and for signs of wearing or cracking in the wood or plastic. Any of these are indications that the prosthesis should be seen by the limb maker at the earliest possible moment. The nurse should also observe the number and condition of the stump socks that the patient is using. The skin of the stump should be inspected for swelling or irritation, and the nurse should inquire about the stump hygiene routine. The patient should be reminded that any abnormality or discomfort— such as swelling, redness, blisters, irritation, or induration—is a danger signal that needs immediate attention. When these things occur, he must stop weight bearing until suitable adjustment can be made in the socket of his prosthesis.

The nurse may also observe the patient's walking habits to see that he is making the best mechanical use of the prosthesis. Poor walking habits that are acquired early by the wearer of an artificial limb are extremely hard to overcome, but considerable improvement is often possible if the patient understands what is expected of him and if he is given practical suggestions for increasing his ability to use the limb more effectively.

REHABILITATION OF THE AMPUTEE

Rehabilitation ideally should start before the patient enters the hospital for his amputation. As previously stated, psychologic problems in the well-prepared patient are minimal. The average patient of today is likely to be much more cooperative and less subject to emotional shock if he is provided in advance with a reasonable expectation of what he is to experience. Often the surgeon will provide the patient with a general explanation of this, including not only a rough timetable of events during hospitalization but also the postoperative office visits up to the time when the stump is ready for limb prescription. The doctor will also tell the patient in a general way what activities he can reasonably expect to do after training with his new limb. It is not within the scope of a nurse's training or responsibility to provide this information. She should be prepared, however, to answer the patient's direct questions as honestly as possible. If any doubt exists, the questions should be referred to the doctor, but cheerful reassurance can be a source of great comfort to the patient at this time. On the other hand, unfounded optimism can be extremely cruel.

The young person who has had a single limb amputation and who has been fitted with a prosthesis and trained in its proper use should be able to carry on an active self-supporting life. His family and friends should recognize that the greatest help they can give him is to treat him, as nearly as possible, as though the amputation had never occured. The problem of the person with two amputations is manifestly more complex. It is absolutely necessary that such persons be given the benefit of specialized therapy—physical, occupation, and vocational—that will enable them to attain the maximum degree of independence.

When amputation has resulted from some systemic disease, vitality is usually lowered and habits of invalidism are easily acquired. This kind of patient

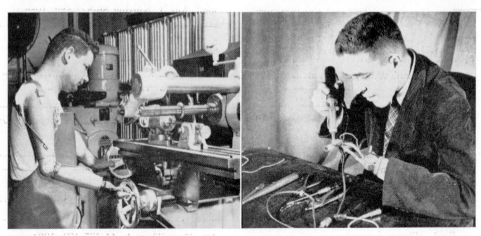

Fig. 279. Upper extremity amputees receiving specialized vocational training. (From Wilson, A. Bennett, Jr.: Limb prosthetics today, Artificial Limbs 7:34, 1963.)

may tend to prefer a wheelchair rather than to struggle with the problems associated with the use of an artificial limb. As the general health improves, however, the patient should be encouraged to resume his normal activities insofar as is possible. Sensible goals set for him to work toward, accompanied by encouragement and an attitude of hopefulness on the part of the public health nurse, will often pay dividends in the patient's increased capacity and willingness to care for his own needs.

Amputees as a group offer better results in terms of returning to social and economic independence than do patients with many other major maladies, for example, blindness and paraplegia. The chief cause for failure in rehabilitation of the amputee is motivation. In this regard the nurse can be of enormous benefit to her patient.

STUDY QUESTIONS

1. What common deformity often occurs after midthigh amputation?
2. Discuss nursing measures that will prevent flexion contractures of the hip following midthigh amputation.
3. Describe the method of applying a compression bandage to the stump.
4. What will you teach the amputee pertaining to the care of his stump and prosthesis?
5. How is the suction type prosthesis applied?
6. How will you give back care and change the bed linen for the patient in balance traction?
7. Describe the optimum position for the affected extremity after a cup arthroplasty.
8. Describe exercises prescribed for the patient with a cup arthroplasty. Why are these exercises so important for this patient?
9. Why may it be harmful to elevate the backrest of a patient newly operated on for cup arthroplasty?

REFERENCES

Aufranc, O.: Constructive surgery of the hip, St. Louis, 1962, The C. V. Mosby Co.

Baker, L.: Out on a limb, New York, 1946, McGraw-Hill Book Co.

Brooks, M. B., Beal, L., Ogg, L., and Blakeslee, B.: The child with deformed or missing limbs, his problems and prostheses, Am. J. Nursing 62:88-92, 1962.

Daniel, E. H.: Amputation prosthetic service, Baltimore, 1950, Williams & Wilkins Co.

Glattly, H. W.: A preliminary report on the amputee census, Artificial Limbs 7:5-10, 1963.

Glover, J. R.: The major amputation, Am. J. Nursing 50:544-550, 1950.

Halpern, C. D.: The child with the upper extremity amputation, Am. J. Occup. Therap. 10:50-56, 1956.

Lineberger, M. I.: Habilitation of child amputees, J. Am. Phys. Ther. A. 42:397-401, 1962.

May, B. J.: Stump bandaging of the lower-extremity amputee, J. Am. Phys. Ther. A. 44:808-814, 1964.

Moskopp, M. E., and Sloan, J.: Nursing care for the amputee, Am. J. Nursing 50:550-555, 1950.

Newman, R.: Internal derangement of the knee joint, Am. J. Nursing 56:577-582, 1956.

Psaki, R. C., Strobel, P. R., and Keys, J. J.: Postoperative management of patient with lower extremity amputations, J.A.M.A. 156:1070-1076, 1956.

Slocum, D. B.: An atlas of amputations, St. Louis, 1949, The C. V. Mosby Co.

Spittler, A. W., Woodward, G. S., and Cleland, C. K.: Cineplasty for arm amputees, Am. J. Nursing 53:802-805, 1953.

Yue, Shyh-Joug: Arthroplasty of the hip: pre- and post-operative management by physical medicine and rehabilitation, Arch. Phys. Med. 37:267-275, 1956.

Wilson, A. B., Jr.: Limb prosthetics today, Artificial Limbs 7:1-42, 1963.

Wilson, A. B., Jr.: Limp prosthetics today, J. Am. Phys. Ther. A. 44:435-469, 1964.

Chapter 12

Trauma to the bones, joints, and ligaments

Strains, sprains, fractures, and dislocations

This chapter will deal with the damage to bones, joints, and ligaments that is produced by external forces such as a blow, twist, pinch, fall or crush. The skeletal system has a certain resilience for resisting such forces until the force from the outside becomes greater than the strength of the bones, at which point the bone will yield and break. The individual bones have differences in strength, dependent mostly on their shape and size, to resist these forces. They also vary in shape, size, and strength from one person to another and from one age to another. For example, the bones of children are more flexible and less brittle than those of adults. In the elderly person the strength of the bones diminishes as it does in disease states, such as osteoporosis, so that less external force is required to break them. These external forces will be referred to as trauma. Tissues of the body exposed to external violence or insult can be damaged. The bones, joints, and ligaments of the body are vulnerable to injury, and the effects therefrom can cause serious disablement. Therefore an under-standing of the effects of trauma to the body is essential.

The occurrence of accidental injuries is increasing each year on our highways, in industry, in the home, on the farm, and in sports. Constant attention to the prevention of injury has become a national theme. Safety belts in automobiles, safety guards on machinery, nonslip materials in the home, and improved protective gear for football players are examples of the emphasis on prevention. Plans for the care of mass casualties are a part of hospital organization today and indeed are carried out on a national scale through the Federal Office of Civilian Defense.

NURSE'S ROLE IN PREVENTING INJURIES

It would be illogical to outline ways in which the nurse may assist in preventing such conditions as tuberculosis, poliomyelitis, and back strain and then to omit emphasizing her part in the prevention of fractures. Her role as health teacher demands that she recognize some of the commonest causes of accidents, particularly in the home, and methods by which they may be eliminated.

Accidents in the home are almost as important as motor accidents, both in incidence and severity. Studies have shown that the greatest number of injuries result from falls; indeed, falls are responsible for almost one half of all injuries in the home.

Because falls play a large part in the etiology of fractures, the home hazards that frequently have been the cause of falls should be recognized by nurses. Many grave accidents take place yearly in the course of going up and down stairs. Waxed stairs and waxed landings at the top or bottom of stairs are always dangerous. The waxing process of any floor surface should be carefully done, since too much wax or too little polishing tends to make floors slippery. Floor wax on stairs may be particularly treacherous.

Stairs should be provided with handrails. If none are available, the householder should be urged to stretch a cord or rope along the stairs at a suitable level, adequately supported by firm uprights. In homes in which there are young children, gates at the top of stair flights are essential to prevent falls.

Steps should never be cluttered with stray objects, as cellar stairs, for instance, are so likely to be. They should be kept clear for traffic, and all members of the family, young and old alike, should recognize that running down steps is distinctly hazardous. All stairs that lead outside should be covered with coarse salt or sand during icy weather.

Children and adults should be alert for such objects as marbles, clothespins, pencils, and toys left about on stairs, landings, and floors. Every child and adult should recognize the great danger and threat to balance that a round rolling object, like a marble or pencil, presents to the unwary walker. They should be taught to remove them from the floor or sidewalk whenever they are observed.

Small scatter rugs can be very treacherous. They must be well anchored to prevent slipping. This may be done by rug fasteners or by the use of rubber floor mats. Scatter rugs should never be placed at the top or bottom of stairs.

To assist in preventing some of the hundreds of bathroom accidents that take place each year, a rubber mat in the tub is advisable. A railing on the wall near the tub will give more confidence and provide safety for the elderly person taking a tub bath.

Another common cause of home accidents is standing on rocking chairs or on old frail kitchen chairs to reach high shelves or to put up curtains. A small firm ladder should be available for all such household jobs.

If the household includes an elderly person who must get up at night to go to the toilet, it is important that a clear, unobstructed lane be left between his bed and the bathroom. An easily available bedlight will also discourage nocturnal journeys in the dark that are fraught with so much hazard for the elderly person.

These are only a few of the more obvious pitfalls for the person in the home. The alert and observing nurse will be quick to notice others. Most of these items seem of little importance, but it is from just this background that many severe fractures originate.

In addition to the prevention of accidents in the home, it also has become very important in recent years for the nurse to aid in the prevention of injuries to hospitalized patients. The commonest causes of injury in hospitals are falling from the bed, rolling off carts, and slipping on waxed floors. Side rails on the bed are mandatory in some hospitals for all patients and should certainly be put to use for those patients who are medicated, feeble, or confused. Transport carts are commonly equipped with straps for holding the patient to the cart, and these should be utilized. Slippery floors should be kept in mind where patients are ambulating with crutches or just beginning to ambulate. Highly waxed floors should not be permitted in the hospital area.

SPRAINS AND STRAINS

Sprains and strains are terms used to describe the damage done to ligaments in the body by an injury. Every joint in the body is protected by ligaments, and each may be subject to injury.

The nurse on the orthopedic ward will seldom have occasion to care for a patient with a sprain. The nurse in the doctor's office, however, or the nurse in an outpatient area may frequently be called upon to assist in the application of support to a sprained ligament and to instruct the patient in the care of the injured area.

A sprained ankle is the most common joint injury and occurs when the foot is inverted forcibly. Normally, the lateral ligament of the ankle is a dense fibrous structure with a set length. One end is fixed to bone at the tip of the fibula and the other end is fixed to the astragalus. When the foot is inverted, this ligament

Shave ankle.

Cover lacerations with sterile dressing before tape is applied.

Paint skin with tincture of benzoin or tincture of rosin.*

Select tape size to fit contour of ankle (1 inch to 2 inches wide).

Hold foot in neutral position in regard to inversion or eversion.

Keep foot as near right angle as pain will allow.

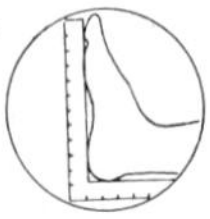

Avoid constrictive circular taping.

For subject sensitive to tape:

   use stockinet or wrap with gauze

   before taping.

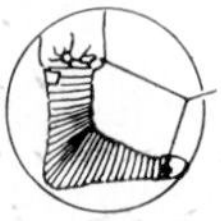

Circulation impaired

Cover skin with cotton or gauze where tape edges cross; prevents

   blisters and lacerations.

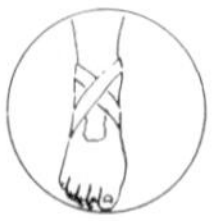

Leave no small areas of exposed

   skin between strips of tape.

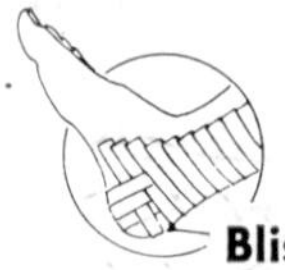

*Tincture of rosin: 1 lb. of rosin

   plus 1 gal. of alcohol (can use

   any alcohol, even rubbing alcohol)

Blister in untaped area

Fig. 280. Rules for adhesive taping used for prevention as well as treatment of sprains of the ankle. (From Paul, W. D., and Allsup, Doyle: Prevention and treatment of ankle sprains [pamphlet], State University of Iowa College of Medicine and Department of Athletics.)

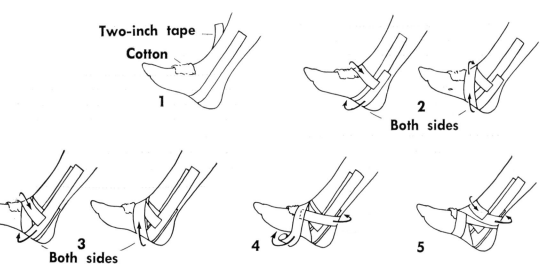

Fig. 281. Western wrap used in prevention and treatment of sprains of the ankle. This wrap is easy to apply, prevents inversion and eversion, but allows flexion and extension. It protects ankle mortise. (From Paul, W. D., and Allsup, Doyle: Prevention and treatment of ankle sprains [pamphlet], State University of Iowa College of Medicine and Department of Athletics.)

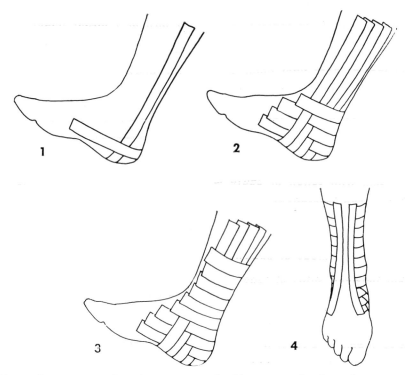

Fig. 282. Basket weave used in the treatment of ankle. It is used only in the acute stage to allow swelling but does not protect ankle mortise. (From Paul, W. D., and Allsup, Doyle: Prevention and treatment of ankle sprains [pamphlet], State University of Iowa College of Medicine and Department of Athletics.)

becomes taut and stops further inversion. If the force acting to invert the foot is greater than the resisting force or strength of the ligament, the ligament must tear. This tear is a sprain. Should the tear be incomplete or, in other words, microscopic in extent, it may be called a strain. If the ligament holds and the giving way occurs at the fixation site to bone with a small fragment of bone attached to the ligament, this would be called an avulsion fracture. Any ligament thus damaged will repair by scar tissue if the torn ends are approximated and held in place for 3 or more weeks, which is the usual healing period.

Treatment consists in providing support and protection of the ligaments until healing can take place. Support is provided by strapping the foot and ankle with adhesive tape or an Elastoplast bandage. To prevent swelling it is necessary that the extremity be elevated much of the time for the first 2 or 3 days after the injury. Also, the application of an ice bag during this time is helpful in minimizing hematoma. Although a minimal amount of weight bearing is permitted at first, this is gradually increased as the soreness diminishes. After such an injury the physician will usually request that a roentgenogram be made to rule out the possibility of a fracture.

At the end of a 2-week period, the Elastoplast support is removed, and if the tenderness has disappeared sufficiently an elastic bandage or support may be applied. This is worn to prevent swelling of the ankle and is gradually discarded as the patient's condition warrants its removal.

Occasionally, the torn ligament ends will curl just enough that the ends cannot be kept together. In such a case there is a chance that healing will be incomplete. An unstable joint or easily recurring sprain of the joint will be the outcome. Recourse to external support or surgical repair of such a ligament is occasionally necessary.

DISLOCATIONS

Traumatic dislocation of any joint occurs when the force of the injury is greater than that which would cause a sprain. A joint is protected by more than a single ligament, and if all the ligaments yield or tear under pressure of the force the entire joint can separate so that the surface of one bone making up the joint no longer meets or opposes the surface of the other bone making up the joint. This is called a dislocation and is ordinarily described in terms of which way the acting force displaced the distal portion of the joint, for example, posterior dislocation of the hip, which means that the head of the femur comes to lie outside of and behind the acetabulum. In order that any dislocated joint can function properly again the dislocated portion of that joint must be relocated to its original anatomic relation with its articulating member. Usually, an anesthetic is required to relax the muscles which in their spasm tend to hold the bones in the dislocated position. On rare occasions the dislocation cannot be reduced by simple manipulation because a portion of the torn tissues or some associated soft tissue such as tendon becomes wrapped about the dislocated part in such a fashion as to prevent relocation. In this event a surgical operation (open reduction) is necessary. Once the dislocation is reduced, whether by open or closed reduction, the damaged joint must be immobilized for 3 or more weeks to allow the torn ligamentous and capsular tissues to heal.

FRACTURES

A fracture is a break in the continuity of a bone. To understand and discuss fractures it is necessary to use terms that describe type, location, and other features pertinent to the problem.

Mode of production of fractures. Each bone in the body is highly developed to carry out a specific purpose. It is logical, therefore, that each bone has its own characteristics. In general, the long bones (femur, tibia, humerus, radius, and ulna) are tubular with variations relating to internal stress patterns of trabeculae as well as variations in cortical thickness from one end to the other. These variables are explainable on the basis of stress since nature provides the necessary strength (resistance) when it is needed to bear weight, resist muscle pulls, etc. The cortex of the tibia in a football player or weight lifter will be thicker than that in a man of similar size in a sedentary occupation. If such tibiae were tested by strain gauges and breaking points determined, it would require more force to break the tibia with the thicker cortex. Nonetheless, every bone has a point at which it can no longer resist applied force without breaking. This is the basis of all fractures. Because our bones are adapted to ordinary stresses of day-to-day living, it would take a stress greater than that to produce a fracture. Most fractures are the result of instances in which there is no control of the amount of force involved.

Since injuries are not deliberately applied, they occur when least suspected and when one is not prepared to resist them. Consequently, the forces that occur come from any direction and in variable amounts. This accounts for the fact that of the thousands of fractures that occur no two are exactly alike. Another factor that adds variability is that of muscle pulls in effect at the time of the fracture. An example of the latter accounts for the gymnast who can dive over a bar to a hard floor and absorb enough of the shock by well-timed muscular relaxation to break the impact. The type of fracture produced in this instance would be by indirect force and could be located at any point from the wrist to the shoulder. The direction of the line of fracture would most likely be long oblique.

Direct force, such as that supplied by a lead pipe falling across the forearm, allows more accuracy in the prediction of a transverse fracture line exactly at the point of impact of the lead pipe.

When a bone is fractured, it means automatically that a single unit becomes two units, and each unit is spoken of as a fragment. The fragment nearest the cephalad end of the body is referred to as the proximal and the other as the distal fragment. These two fragments ordinarily become separated at the site of the fracture in various ways. Imagine a piece of bamboo 2 feet long with a strong rubber band stretched from one end to the other and fastened. On the other side another but weaker stretched rubber band is placed. If the bamboo were cut transversely in its middle, it would bend immediately from the overpull of the stronger elastic. This is the mechanism of a transverse fracture. The angle at the fracture site will furnish the identifying description for this particular fracture, for example, a transverse fracture in the middle third with lateral angulation (if the apex of the angle points away from the midline of the body) of 30 degrees (or whatever angle the distal fragment has moved from the original bone alignment).

To construct another possibility, return to the bamboo and this time cut the bamboo on a 4-inch diagonal instead of transversely. Upon completion of the cut, the two fragments will slide by one another until the original length of the bamboo becomes shortened enough to release the tension in the elastic bands. Because one band was stronger than the

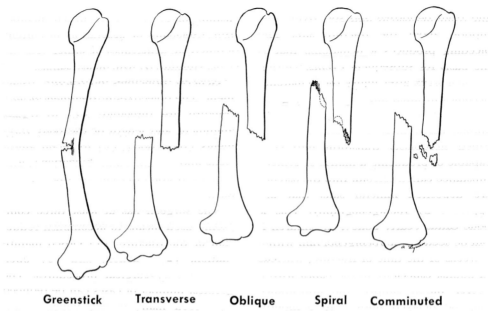

Greenstick   Transverse   Oblique   Spiral   Comminuted

Fig. 283. Fracture types.

other, the stronger side will also angulate similarly but less than it did with the transverse cut. This fracture will be described then as an oblique fracture of the middle third with a 2-inch overriding (or whatever amount the total length has been shortened) and lateral angulation of 10 degrees.

These two examples will account for the majority of fractures, but because minor variations are possible additional descriptive terms are needed. The fracture site may be splintered, in which case there may be multiple fragments. Instead of a transverse or oblique fracture, it would be called a comminuted fracture. Should the fracture line be oblique and follow a spiral course as it involves a tubular bone, it would be referred to as an oblique spiral, followed by the usual description of location, overriding, and angulation.

Occasionally, when a long bone is fractured, the fractured end of one fragment will be driven into the surrounding muscle mass. It will not only override and angulate but will also be displaced

sideways a bone's width or more from its fellow fragment. In this instance it will be described as a transverse fracture with overriding, angulation, and 1 inch (or whatever amount) lateral (medial, anterior, or posterior referring to the distal fragment) displacement. In a vertebral body in which the diameter of the bone nearly equals the length and the most force applied is compression (as one would squeeze an orange between two hands), the bone will yield by collapsing into itself. This is described as an impacted or compression fracture. In disease states in which bone is weakened, such as in osteoporosis, metastatic bone lesions, or osteogenesis imperfecta, a fracture can occur with as little force as that required during a sneeze or a twist in bed. This is termed a pathologic fracture.

Fracture healing. The sequence of events in tissue repair from the time of injury to complete healing of the fracture is quite well understood. Immediately as the bone fractures, bleeding occurs from the damaged bone ends and from periosteal and soft tissue disruption about the fracture site. The bleeding produces a hematoma that is the basis for subsequent events. During the first week after injury the hematoma becomes invaded and replaced by granulation tissue that is organized into fibrous tissue after 3 weeks. The cells called fibroblasts transform into cells capable of producing a matrix or cement substance called osteoid. Into the osteoid are deposited mineral salts that are apparent by roentgenography. This is bone callus (early bone). In children it can be seen in the roentgenogram within 3 weeks of the time of fracture, whereas in adults, especially in the bones with a poorer blood supply, the appearance may be delayed until 2 to 3 months after injury. The callus is usually fusiform in shape and forms a continuous bridge across the fracture site. After the callus has made its appearance, it then becomes remodeled into a stress pattern that resembles that of the parent bone. The callus is often more abundant than is seemingly necessary, but in the remodeling stage (which may require a year) the excess amount is absorbed, leaving only an amount sufficient to withstand the stress needs of the bone.

Certain factors are known that can disturb this healing process. It is called delayed union when the healing process is slowed to the extent that months are required to complete union. In some instances firm union is never produced (nonunion), and a false joint with fluid present as well as motion (pseudarthrosis) may actually tend to form. Repeated manipulations of the fracture after the first 7 to 10 days is one such factor, and inadequate immobilization is another. Inadequate immobilization can be a matter of degree since it is quite impossible to ensure absolute immobilization by any means. The occurrence of infection will delay and sometimes prevent

healing of fractures. Disturbed metabolism, especially of protein as in chronic debility, or deficiences of either vitamin C or vitamin D will delay callus.

General principles of fracture treatment. The objectives of treatment of any fracture are threefold: (1) to regain alignment and length of the bony fragments (reduction), (2) to retain alignment and length (immobilization), and (3) to restore function to the injured part.

The surgeon has at least three commonly used means to accomplish reduction of the fracture: (1) closed manipulation, (2) traction, and (3) open reduction by surgical procedures. The greatest number of cases can be reduced by closed manipulation, which means that the fracture ends can be brought into apposition by manual manipulation. The muscle spasm that tends to shorten the bone by overriding must be overcome. This can be acomplished by traction alone if it is maintained long enough to fatigue the muscles. However, the swelling, stretching, and rubbing of the periosteum at the site of injury is painful. In order to spare pain and also obtain muscle relaxation, an anesthetic is most often employed. It is seldom under these circumstances that reduction cannot be accomplished. If for any reason reduction cannot be performed as soon as the patient has been evaluated, the fractured part should at least be immobilized until reduction can be carried out.

Traction becomes the treatment of choice when the surgeon finds that any reduction he is able to obtain cannot be maintained by a plaster cast. This situation is common in fractures other than the transverse variety. Surmising this difficulty, the surgeon may elect to utilize the traction not only to maintain but also to accomplish the reduction, thereby obviating the need for closed reduction and anesthesia. The traction is provided by a Kirschner wire or other metal pin placed through the bone distal to the fracture and through which constant weighted pull can be maintained for weeks if necessary. This is known as skeletal traction. There are many modified methods of use, some of which are incorporated in combination with plaster casts. However it is used, the traction pin need be used only until sufficient callus is evident to maintain alignment. Plaster cast immobilization will be sufficient to complete the healing process.

To reduce a fracture by surgical methods is seldom necessary except in those fractures that are known to be impossible to reduce or maintain with either closed or traction methods. Intraarticular fractures, fracture of the medial epicondyle of the humerus in children, fractures of both bones of the forearm in adults, and fractures of the neck of the femur are examples. Except as indicated, open reductions are practically never indicated in children. Many surgeons elect open reductions at times when other methods would give satisfactory results. These are justified on the basis that hospital time will be reduced, and joints above and below the fracture can be kept mobile since immobilization is provided mechanically by rods, plates, screws, and other devices rather than by plaster casts, which must extend to immobilize the joint above and below the fracture. The advantages must outweigh the possible complications of operative infection and delayed union, which are hazards in any operative attack on the fracture site.

Restoration of function is as important as any other part of treatment. Well-planned treatment and avoidance of complications give a head start toward regaining function of a fractured extremity. Prolonged immobilization that allows for atrophy of disuse and stiffening of joints to occur is to be avoided. Although a fracture heals in good position, the function is not restored until the soft tissues are free of contractures and have regained flexibility and strength. This process, if well managed, can be accomplished in weeks. If it is neglected, a patient can be handicapped for months. Well-directed physical therapy is helpful at this stage.

Fracture complications. Fracture complications include nonunion, malunion, infection, nerve damage, circulatory disturbance, epiphyseal damage, posttraumatic arthritis, kidney stones, and emboli.

Nonunion. Nonunion may be caused by any one of several factors. Inadequate immobilization can cause delayed union or nonunion of the fracture. Inadequate reduction may be a factor. If less than one half of the bone ends are in contact with each other, nonunion usually results. If the bone ends are held too far apart by traction, it is evident that callus formation will not span the space. If the blood supply to the fracture line has been damaged, it is possible that the nutrition to one of the bone fragments may be inadequate and callus formation will not take place. When fracture occurs in certain areas (the lower one-third of the tibia, neck of the femur, and carpal scaphoid bone), healing may be slow or difficult to accomplish because of the disturbed blood supply and poor nutrition of the affected area. Also, if soft tissue becomes lodged between the bony fragments, union is not likely to take place.

To correct nonunion, the surgeon may perform a surgical procedure to freshen the bone ends and drill numerous holes near the fracture site in hopes of improving the circulation. In some instances the extremity may be braced and activity increased in order that the blood supply to the part may be improved. Bone grafting to the affected area may be necessary. Bone from the tibia or the iliac crest is placed across the fracture site. This is known as an onlay graft. Another method of bone grafting is that of inserting the graft directly into the medullary canal.

Malunion. With the complication of malunion, union of the bony fragments takes place but in a position of deformity. Numerous factors, such as inadequate reduction, an improperly applied cast, or a cast that has softened and permitted movement of bony fragments, may cause this.

Infection. Infection is always a possibility when a compound fracture occurs. Also, with open reduction of a fracture there is some risk that infection can occur and complicate the healing process.

Nerve damage. Nerve damage may be caused by the sharp edges of the bone fragments or by the injury that caused the fracture. Motor power of the muscles of the extremity and the sensitivity of the skin should be checked carefully. Damage to the peroneal nerve may result in drop foot, or injury to the radial nerve may result in wrist drop.

Circulatory disturbance. Circulation in the part distal to the fracture should also be checked carefully. This is particularly important with fractures about the elbow. Volkmann's contracture may result from a disturbance of the circulation in the elbow region. Nail beds of the fingers of the affected extremity should be observed, and the radial pulse should be taken at frequent intervals.

Damage to the epiphysis. If the fracture causes damage to the epiphysis of a child, growth may be arrested in that extremity or in a portion of the extremity. This, of course, results in deformity as the child grows.

Posttraumatic arthritis. When an intraarticular fracture causes damage to a joint surface, a painful posttraumatic arthritis may result. In some instances an arthroplasty or an arthrodesis may be performed to alleviate the pain.

Kidney stones. Kidney stones can occur when total body immobilization is carried out. They result when disuse causes excessive loss of calcium from the bones. Maintaining a high fluid intake is helpful in eliminating the calcium, but maintaining prophylactic muscular activity is better treatment.

Emboli. Occasionally, in compound fractures or in simple fractures in which clotting has taken place in a vein, a portion of the clot may break off and be carried throughout the circulation to various parts of the body. Air emboli also occur. If an embolus makes its way to a vital organ, such as the lung, heart, or brain, there may be disastrous consequences, even death.

The patient usually develops a rapid pulse and evidences of shock that come on abruptly. Death may occur within a few minutes or within a few hours after the onset of symptoms. Treatment other than preventive by adequate immobilization is of no avail. Those patients with emboli in the less vital areas may have the symptoms and signs in a milder degree and yet recover. The emboli are more frequently pulmonary than any other type and may occur as late as 6 to 8 weeks after the injury.

EVALUATION OF THE INJURED

The trauma resulting from a single force, such as a blow to the forearm, is a matter for examination of the single injured part. Such a direct blow can be expected to break the bones at the site of impact and produce an angulation the same as a bent twig. Landing on both feet in a fall from a height produces indirectly transmitted forces that can injure bones and joints at a distance from the point of impact, such as the collapse of a vertebral body in the upper lumbar spine. Crushing injuries from cave-ins increase areas of damage further because they involve both direct and indirect forces. Crushing injuries commonly involve tissues such as internal organs in addition to bones, and thus internal hemorrhage can occur and produce shock that demands immediate detection and treatment. An associated head injury may render the person unconscious, which complicates the picture of shock. The forces on the chest might have fractured enough ribs to produce paradoxical breathing that interferes with proper ventilation. With poor ventilation unconsciousness and shock present simultaneously, the evaluation and treatment of the injured bones and joints are of secondary concern. Any person with multiple injuries requires immediate evaluation by a physician well versed in all aspects of trauma, and seldom in medicine does the situation call for more astute, careful, complete, yet quick analysis to institute proper treatment in proper sequence to ensure first things first.

First aid and compound fractures. There are a few simple rules that apply to first aid in fractures.

1. Keep the patient at rest in a horizontal position as long as he is unconscious or until the extent of his injury can be determined.

2. If he must be transported while still unconscious, continue the horizontal position until consciousness is regained sufficiently for the injured person to signify points of pain and tenderness.

3. In a person with a back injury every precaution should be taken to avoid motions of the spine, particularly such as would occur if the person were brought into a sitting position, because this may lead to damage of the spinal cord by fragments of bone protruding into it or pressing upon it.

4. When there is injury to the spine or to the limbs, it is of particular importance that the surgeon know definitely whether or not any paralysis was present immediately after the injury. This cannot be determined in the unconscious patient who has a head injury, but it can be determined in other patients. The knowledge of this fact may decide the ultimate recovery or loss of function in a limb or limbs. This is also true in compound fractures. Written records of what has been found and done should accompany each patient to the hospital or surgeon's office.

5. There is considerable debate at present as to the advisability of using a tourniquet, since the prolonged use may lead to death of the tissues in the extremities beyond its point of application. In compound fractures it is preferable to use a piece of sterile or clean bandage or string to tie off the bleeding vessel if it is exposed or to apply local pressure to the vessel by means of a pad of sterile gauze and a sterile bandage. If a tourniquet must be used on a patient with violent bleeding, it should be removed every 20 to 30 minutes and the bleeding should be observed. If coagulation has occurred in the vessel, the tourniquet may be left loosened but there should be constant observation for return of bleeding.

6. Emergency immobilization and transportation depend on the anatomic location of the injury.

(a) In injuries of the spine or head the recumbent position is essential. If a rigid stretcher such as a plank, a door, a ladder, or two poles and a blanket cannot be obtained, it is advisable to roll the patient horizontally onto his face and transport him in the arms of two or three persons to a truck or the back seat of a car. He should never be brought into a position that will flex the spine.

(b) In injuries of the clavicle, ribs,

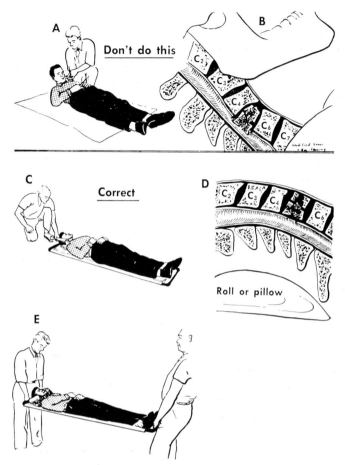

A Don't do this B

C Correct D

Roll or pillow

E

Fig. 284. Do's and don't's in the transport of patients with injuries of the cervical vertebrae. (From White, J. C.: Injuries to spinal cord and cauda equina. In Cave, E. F., editor: Fractures and other injuries, Chicago, 1958, Year Book Medical Publishers, Inc. Illustrated by Mrs. Murial McLatchie Miller.)

shoulder, and elbow, splinting can best be done by bandaging the arm to the side of the chest. This may be done with any materials obtainable, such as a torn sheet, a shirt, or other clothing. Two triangular slings work well if obtainable.

In fractures about the elbow and forearm, one or two wooden splints from the axilla to the fingertips may be tied to the arm with handkerchiefs or strips of clothing.

(c) In injuries of the hip, thigh, knee, and leg, immobilization may be obtained by narrow boards placed on either side of the leg and held together by a bandage or strips of clothing. When the hip is injured, the splinting should extend from the heel up to the side of the chest and the bandages should encircle the chest and the leg. All injuries of the bone should, if possible, be immobilized to include the joint above and below the injury. If no splinting material is available, fairly adequate immobilization can be obtained by tying the injured leg to the uninjured one with a series of bandages from the thigh to the foot.

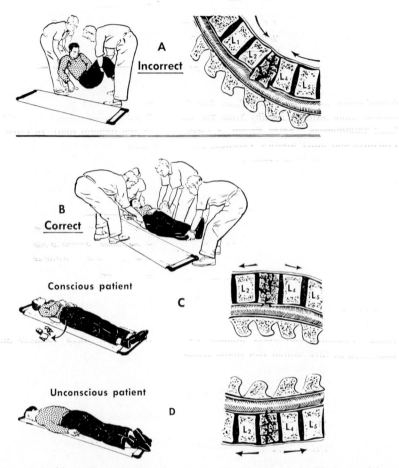

Fig. 285. Do's and don't's in the transport of patients with injuries of the lumbar and lower thoracic vertebrae. (From White, J. C.: Injuries to spinal cord and cauda equina. In Cave, E. F., editor: Fractures and other injuries, Chicago, 1958, Year Book Medical Publishers, Inc. Illustrated by Mrs. Murial McLatchie Miller.)

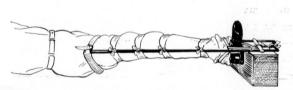

Fig. 286. Keller-Blake splint for first aid immobilization for a fractured femur. The ankle is carefully padded, and the leg is supported in the splint by encircling strips of cloth. The shoes and clothing are not removed in order to avoid unnecessary painful movement of the damaged extremity. Traction is maintained by means of a strip of cloth that is secured around the ankle, tied over the end of the splint, and twisted taut by means of a stick. The distal end of the splint is supported to give some elevation. (From Brown, T.: Fractures of the femoral shaft. In Cave, E. F., editor: Fractures and other injuries, Chicago, 1958, Year Book Medical Publishers, Inc. Illustrated by Mrs. Murial McLatchie Miller.)

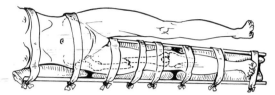

Fig. 287. Improvised splint using boards or sticks for fracture of the femoral shaft. The lateral splint extends distally from just below the axilla and is secured to the trunk, the medial splint extends distally from the groin. All splints are padded to avoid pressure over bony prominences. (From Brown, T.: Fractures of the femoral shaft. In Cave, E. F., editor: Fractures and other injuries, Chicago, 1958, Year Book Medical Publishers, Inc. Illustrated by Mrs. Murial McLatchie Miller.)

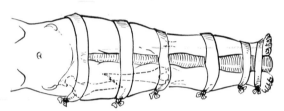

Fig. 288. Improvised immobilization for fracture of the femoral shaft when no splints are available. Legs are secured together with padding in between. Feet are also bound together in order to control rotation. (From Brown, T.: Fractures of the femoral shaft. In Cave, E. F., editor: Fractures and other injuries, Chicago, 1958, Year Book Medical Publishers, Inc. Illustrated by Mrs. Murial McLatchie Miller.)

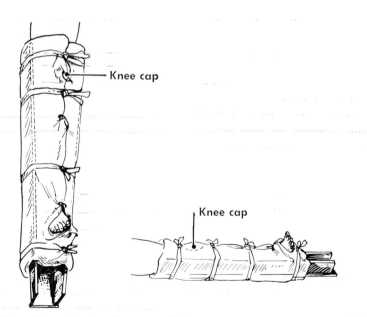

Fig. 289. The pillow-and-side splint as applied to the ankle. One strap extends above the knee and one below the foot. (From Aufranc, O.: Ankle injuries. In Cave, E. F., editor: Fractures and other injuries, Chicago, 1958, Year Book Medical Publishers, Inc. Illustrated by Mrs. Murial McLatchie Miller.)

(d) For fractures of the ankle and the lower leg the most satisfactory temporary splint is the pillow bandage. The limb is laid longitudinally on a pillow so that the heel is just above the edge. The lateral edges of the pillow are then brought together over the limb and pinned. When the ankle is reached, the lower ends of the pillow are crossed under the foot, brought upward, and pinned so that a compact splinting effect is obtained. In all splinting of fractures the bony prominences should be protected by cotton batting if obtainable or by any soft material.

(e) The Thomas splint for the leg and the Jones splint for the arm are easily applied and give good immobilization for transportation. They are carried by almost all first aid stations and ambulances, either civil or martial.

(f) Shock is the result of a disturbance in the vasomotor system that allows relaxation in the peripheral circulatory system, thereby decreasing the amount of blood returning to the heart. The heart pumps from an empty system and is unable to fulfill the requirements for blood exchange to itself and other parts of the body. Shock may be the result of hemorrhage or a complete temporary disarrangement of the nervous system as a result of the injury. Fear may be an element in its production. It may be fatal. The blood pressure is greatly lowered, and the pulse is rapid and weak. The skin becomes pale, and the injured person may become listless or even unconscious. If hemorrhage is the cause, it should be stopped as promptly as possible and fluid should be administered in replacement. Stimulants such as coffee or tea may be used. Morphine and its derivatives tend to restore the balance between the peripheral and central circulations. Complete rest must be given in a recumbent position. As soon as infusions and blood or plasma transfusions are available they should be given. Shock is usually caused by pain due to movement at the point of fracture and from hemorrhage rather than from malposition.

In first aid any contaminated compound fracture should be dressed and splinted in the exact position in which it was found so that proper precautions can be taken when the patient reaches a hospital or other point where he can receive adequate surgical attention. Some surgeons contend that because a thorough debridement is necessary in any compound fracture, the additional amount of contamination occurring when the bones are pulled into line when first seen does not materially increase the chances for infection of the compound wound. This contention is doubtful.

It is preferable that a clean dressing, handkerchief, or sheet be applied at the site of injury and that the limb be splinted in the position of the existing deformity. The use of strong irritating antiseptics such as iodine, Lysol, or carbolic acid is contraindicated. Alcohol, Mercurochrome, Mercresin, or Scott's solution may be used with little chance of local damage or coagulation of the tissues.

If the patient is in shock, all attention should be paid to this. Intravenous saline infusions, transfusions, or blood plasma may be necessary.

To prepare a compound wound for operation soap and water should be used. A brush or sponge will help the effectiveness of this. Benzine is used to dissolve greasy materials. The skin and wound are then painted with a noncoagulating antiseptic, and draping is applied. The wound is flushed clean with several quarts of saline solution under low pressure. This is done with an elevated bottle and a glass nozzle on the end of rubber tubing. All loose, bruised, or contaminated portions of tissue are then removed with knife or scissors. Bone should be preserved if possible.

The antibiotic drugs have aided greatly in lessening the fight against infection. They are placed directly into the wound after the cleansing and debridement. In addition a specific antibiotic is given orally or intramuscularly over a period of 3 to 7 days after the injury. They have served to lessen the occurrence of infection tremendously.

This should not be considered a substitute, however, but merely an adjunct to adequate debridement.

Antibiotics do not eliminate the necessity for giving both tetanus antitoxin and gas bacillus antitoxin as prophylactics for all patients with compound fractures. Immobilization after open reduction of compound fractures is an essential part in the avoidance of infection and other complications. All patients with compound fractures who arrive at the hospital for treatment within 6 hours after injury are considered clean and are treated by debridement, flushing with quantities of sterile saline solution, instillation of an antibiotic, reduction, closure, and the application of a cast.

Compound fractures occurring longer than 6 hours before the patient gains admission are considered primarily infected in spite of the most careful debridement and other precautions, including antitoxins. In these patients, drainage is instituted and, if necessary, because of pain and elevation of temperature for a 24- to 48-hour period, the cast should be bivalved or a window made and the wound inspected. Otherwise, the open wound is left undressed within the cast.

The odor of gas infection is characteristically sweet and pungent, and air bubbles may be seen exuding from the wound. The presence of air in the tissue may also be demonstrated roentgenographically. The pulse is rapid, and the temperature is variable. This complication may call for intensive radiation treatment and further administration of gas antitoxin. The removal of the cast may be necessary. The fracture is now of secondary importance. Multiple incisions into the tissues for adequate air penetration and drainage may be needed.

Fractures or dislocations of the face, jaw, and skull, the clavicle (collar bone), and the shoulder

In the statistics of World War II fractures of the skull were relatively infrequent, and when they occurred they were problems for the neurosurgeon and required special instruction from him concerning nursing care. Similarly, serious injuries to the face involving the nose and sinuses were problems for the nose and throat specialist, whose ingenuity was often taxed in evolving methods and apparatus capable of restoring and maintaining the position of misplaced fragments.

Fractures involving the jaw usually call for the special attention of a dental surgeon. However, there are certain principles in the treatment that might be mentioned. Loose teeth near the fracture line should not be removed unless it is absolutely necessary. Sometimes the alignment of the teeth and jaw may be obtained by wiring together the teeth of the upper and the lower jaw. Occasionally the fragments of the jawbone may have to be held together by wires through the bone. Sometimes metal bands may be required to supplement wiring, and sometimes plates fastened along the teeth, attached to a plaster of paris headgear by means of wires and elastic bands, may be used for adequate correction.

DISLOCATIONS OF THE JAW

Cause. Dislocation of the jaw is usually caused by violent yawning or yelling or by blows against the chin.

Anatomy. The dislocations may be unilateral or bilateral and consist usually in the forward or inward displacement of the condyles of the mandible from their articulating surface on the skull.

Symptoms and signs. Forward protrusion of the chin and inability to close the mouth are symptoms of dislocation of the jaw. If the dislocation is unilateral, the chin is displaced away from the dislocated side. There is usually rather severe pain and muscle spasm, and the lips and tongue become dry.

Treatment. Simple dislocations of the jaw can usually be reduced without anesthesia. The surgeon swathes his thumbs in gauze and bandage to prevent being bitten. Pressure is exerted against the lower molars with increasing force downward and backward until reduction takes place. Following reduction, the upper and lower jaw should be held together by bandages around the head (Barton four-tailed bandage) for a period of 2 to 3 weeks so that habitual dislocation does not develop.

FRACTURE OF THE CLAVICLE (COLLAR BONE)

Fracture of the clavicle is one of the commonest of fractures. It may occur in any part—inner, middle, or outer. Treatment may be different for each type.

Cause. A fall on the shoulder or outstretched hand, exerting the entire force on the clavicle, and occasionally a direct blow may cause a fracture of the clavicle.

Anatomy. The pectoral muscles and weight of the arm bring the shoulder downward, inward, and forward, with overriding of fragments. The clavicle is the only bony connection between the chest and shoulder girdle.

Problem. The length of the clavicle must be maintained by keeping the shoulder up and backward during healing.

Healing period. A healing period of from 4 to 8 weeks is usually required for fractures of the clavicle. Children under 10 years of age heal rapidly.

Treatment. In children the figure-of-eight dressing will usually suffice for the full treatment until union is shown to be present clinically and roentgenographically. The dressing is changed for cleanliness only. Zinc stearate powder is used to prevent chafing.

In adolescents and adults it is usually preferable to use a Velpeau dressing for 10 days to 2 weeks. This can be followed by a figure-of-eight dressing.

In obstinate cases, adolescent or adult, and especially in girls, when perfect alignment is necessary, side traction should be used for 3 to 4 weeks and followed by a figure-of-eight dressing.

Occasionally, when proper alignment cannot be obtained conservatively, an open reduction may be performed. Wiring with stainless steel or the use of Kirschner wire inserted into the medullary canal can, except for the scar, give perfect results.

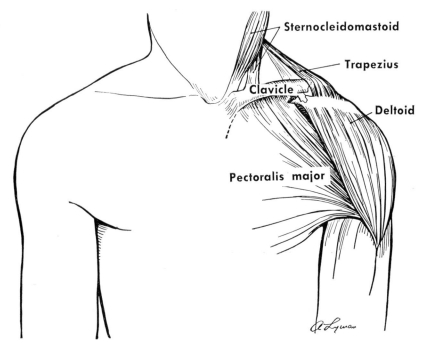

Fig. 290. Muscle mechanics of fracture of the clavicle. The sternocleidomastoid pulls upward on the proximal fragment while the weight of the shoulder pulls down and the pectorals pull inward and forward, tending to override the fragments.

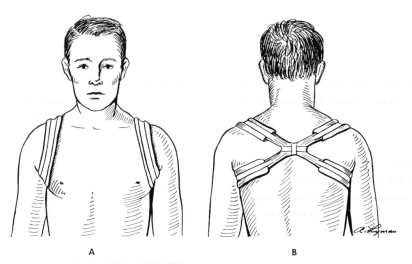

Fig. 291. A, Front view of figure-of-eight dressing. **B,** Back view. Felt, bias flannel bandage, and adhesive tape are used. Dressing should be changed every week or 10 days for cleanliness.

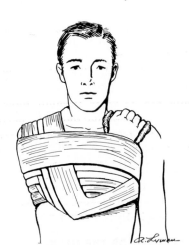

Fig. 292. The Velpeau bandage is used temporarily to immobilize clavicle, shoulder, humerus, elbow, or forearm. Wherever skin comes in contact with skin, a protective pad should be inserted.

FRACTURE-DISLOCATIONS AND DISLOCATIONS OF THE ACROMIOCLAVICULAR JOINT

Fracture-dislocations and dislocations of the acromioclavicular joint are the result of the same type of injury as that causing fracture of the clavicle. Roentgenograms frequently do not show the extent of the injury.

Problem. The shoulder must be kept upward and backward.

Treatment. A figure-of-eight bandage

with adhesive strapping from the chest to the back and a pad over the clavicle is frequently employed in treatment of these fractures. The use of compound tincture of benzoin aids greatly in preventing skin irritation from the use of adhesive tape. Adhesive tape is changed often to prevent skin irritation. Immobilization must be maintained long enough to allow complete healing (6 to 10 weeks).

Patients with severe cases may require operative repair of the acromioclavicular joint as well as the ligament between the clavicle and the coracoid process.

In chronic painful dislocations the resection of the outer inch of the end of the clavicle usually leads to relief of symptoms and restoration of function (Mumford). Recovery occurs in about 3 weeks. Metallic fixation by a nail or Kirschner wire may be used in some instances.

DISLOCATION OF THE HEAD OF THE HUMERUS

There are several types of dislocation of the head of the humerus, but the most common is a forward and downward displacement.

Cause. Dislocation of the head of the

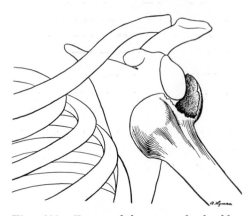

Fig. 293. Fracture-dislocation of shoulder. Greater tuberosity is torn off (subglenoid type).

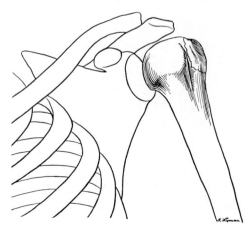

Fig. 294. Dislocation of shoulder reduced. Tuberosity has resumed normal position.

humerus is usually caused by a fall on the outstretched arm. Abduction of the shoulder joint is only possible to 90 degrees. At this point the humerus presses against the acromion process. This levers the head of the humerus downward or forward. The capsule of the joint is torn either anteriorly or at its attachment to the glenoid fossa. The head of the humerus enters the space below the glenoid fossa and rests under the coracoid process.

Symptoms and signs. The major symptom is pain. The arm cannot be brought against the side of the body, and there is a depression under the acromion process where the head of the humerus should be. The dislocation may be accompanied by fracture of the tuberosity.

Reduction. Reduction should be performed with the patient under complete anesthesia to prevent further damage to the head of the humerus and to allow free movement so that the capsule will again close over the head allowing it to fall back into its normal position.

Problem. It takes about 3 to 4 weeks for ligamentous structures to heal. Motion that does not put strain on the healing area in the torn capsule, however, does not retard healing but maintains flexibility. Therefore, the problem with simple dislocations of joints is to begin motion within a few days. In dislocation of the shoulder the problem is to keep the elbow constantly forward of the shoulder plane on the affected side. If there is a detached fragment from the head of the humerus, it usually falls back into position during the reduction.

Treatment. Frequently a Velpeau dressing is used for a few days after reduction, and then this may be replaced with a neck-wrist strap. This strap must keep the wrist close to the chin so that only forward flexion and forward rotation can be accomplished.

As more complete healing takes place this distance between the neck and wrist can be increased.

When habitual dislocations occur through placing strain on the healing capsule too early or through repeated dislocation, operative repair is needed. This may be done by passing the tendon of the long head of the biceps muscle through the head of the humerus (Nicola), or by suturing the capsule and labium to the anterior inferior lip of the glenoid fossa (Bankart).

FRACTURES OF THE NECK OF THE HUMERUS

Cause. Usually a fall directly against the shoulder with the arm against the chest or incompletely abducted is the cause of fracture of the neck of the humerus.

Anatomy. The pectoral muscles pull the distal (controllable) fragment inward and forward, and the deltoid pulls it upward. They are the strongest muscles of the shoulder girdle group. The three types of fracture of the neck of the humerus are transverse, oblique, and comminuted.

Reduction. In all patients except those

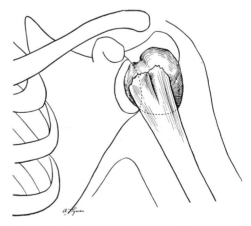

Fig. 295. Fracture of the neck of the humerus showing anterior and upward displacement of the distal fragment. The fracture line of the head is angled forward.

without displacement there should be an immediate attempt to restore perfect anatomic replacement under general anesthesia. With the transverse type this can usually be accomplished. In the other types, however, reduction may be difficult or impossible by this means.

Problem. The elbow must be kept close to the midline of the body to relieve the pull of the pectorals. Some form of traction that will relax the deltoid and thereby prevent overriding and anterior angulation, the two salient factors necessary to reduction, must be provided.

Treatment. In fractures within or in close proximity to the shoulder joint early motion is of great importance. Whenever anatomic reposition can be accomplished, motions can be started 10 days or 2 weeks after injury. In some instances, however, reductions are difficult to obtain and maintain, and it may be necessary to use a Velpeau dressing for 3 to 4 weeks or a lateral traction apparatus that maintains forward flexion and traction.

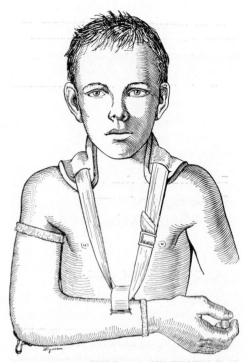

Fig. 297. The pendulum method of treatment of fractures in the region of the shoulder or shaft of humerus; this is the so-called hanging cast. Frequently, the cast is unessential, and efficiency depends on the neck-wrist strap combination. Loop at elbow for night traction.

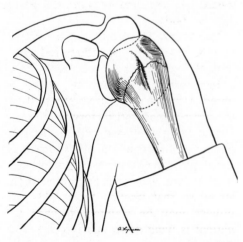

Fig. 296. Fracture manipulated under anesthesia and pendulum cast applied. For additional traction along with a neck-wrist band 3 pounds of lead were incorporated in the cast at the elbow.

As soon as gluing of the fracture is present after the most nearly perfect position has been attained, active motion is started. This may require 2 to 4 weeks, depending on the appearance of the primary and subsequent roentgenograms and the estimated mechanical difficulties.

Usually a cast extending from the axilla to the wrist with a neck-wrist strap can be applied early. The weight of the cast (which can be augmented by sheet lead at the elbow) will give the necessary traction, and the neck-wrist strap can be adjusted to give the required anterior flexion of the shoulder. In this way early motion without strain in the fractured area may be started.

Healing period. The healing period is from 6 to 10 weeks.

STIFF SHOULDER

In all fractures of the shoulder, arm, elbow, forearm, and wrist, delayed return of function is frequently caused by adhesions about the shoulder joint as a result of disuse. It is best, therefore, with the approval of the surgeon in charge, to begin shoulder motion early in all patients with fractures of the extremity. This should consist of external rotation and forward flexion of the arm two or three times daily.

Fractures of the arm, forearm, and wrist, including nursing care

FRACTURE OF THE SHAFT OF THE HUMERUS

Cause. Direct violence, such as a blow from the side, or indirect violence, such as a fall on the outstretched hand, may cause fracture of the shaft of the humerus.

Anatomy. There is usually overriding, especially when the fracture is above the attachment of the deltoid muscle. There is also a tendency toward outward bowing. If the fracture is in the middle third of the humerus, special observation is indicated at once because of the proximity of the radial nerve to the bone. If the radial nerve is injured, it may be in one of three ways, which may be recognized as follows: (1) Immediate severance of the nerve may be recognized by immediate inability to extend (raise) the hand at the wrist. Prognosis is poor for recovery without suture. (2) Contusion is made obvious by paralysis which may gradually occur with wrist drop as soon as the swelling and edema have reached a sufficient stage. Prognosis for recovery is good with rest. (3) Paralysis as a result of bony overgrowth in healing is evidenced by the gradual development of wrist drop 2 to 3 months after injury. Prognosis is good with removal of bony overgrowth freeing the nerve.

Problem. Maintaining traction and restoring the best alignment of the fragments are usually the chief problems in treating this type of fracture. There is often a tendency toward outward bowing that can be overcome either by more traction or by a pad between the elbow and the body.

Treatment. This fracture, if transverse, may be treated by immediate reduction with the patient under anesthesia, or in a few instances it may be plated or wired. Usually, a cast from the axilla to the wrist is most satisfactory to the comfort of the patient and adds to the simplicity of treatment in all fractures in the shaft of the humerus. A loop of webbing or tape may be incorporated at the elbow so that traction by weights and pulleys may be maintained when the patient is lying down (Griswold). (Fig. 297.)

Those fractures that occur a few inches above the elbow must have special consideration, since there is a

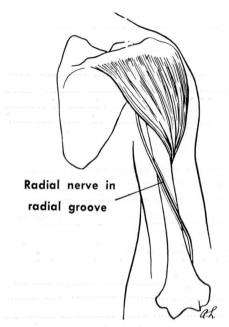

Radial nerve in radial groove

Fig. 298. Diagram showing the proximity of the nerve to the bone with accessibility to injury.

great tendency to angle outward as a result of the combined pull of the biceps and triceps muscles. This causes a loss of the carrying angle at the elbow if it is uncorrected. The tendency may be overcome to some extent by applying a cast from the axilla to the fingers with the forearm in a position of extreme and forced pronation (palm down).

Healing period. Fractures of the shaft of the humerus may be slow to heal. In about 10% of the patients either delayed union or nonunion occurs. Ordinarily, however, a fracture of the humerus will heal sufficiently for elbow motion in about 4 to 8 weeks. Complete recovery may occur in 8 to 10 weeks. In delayed union it may take as long as 3 to 6 months. In nonunion a bone graft operation is usually the most satisfactory way to obtain union.

When patients are in casts, usually little is required of the nurse except to watch for complications. She should at-

tempt, however, with the consent of the surgeon, to maintain freedom of motion in as many of the neighboring joints as possible by means of massage about the joints and assisted active motions.

FRACTURES ABOUT THE ELBOW

Fracture about the elbow is most common in two forms of injury: (1) in falls with the elbows extended (children) and (2) direct violence exerted against the elbow (adults). There may be the impact from a passing car when the elbow is out of the window or there may be a fall on the elbow. The type of fall that in an adult would likely cause a dislocation of the elbow as a result of leverage of the olecranon process in the olecranon fossa would cause a supracondylar fracture in a child.

Anatomy. The elbow cannot normally extend beyond 180 degrees. Forcing beyond this point will cause either a dislocation of the elbow joint or a fracture just above the joint. The ulnar nerve runs downward just behind the inner posterior side of the joint and the medial nerve just in front of the joint. Either is

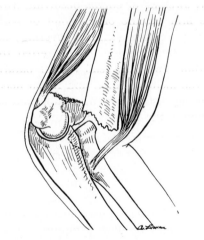

Fig. 299. Supracondylar fracture of the humerus. There is posterior displacement of the distal fragments with tension on nerves, tendons, and vessels. The fracture is within the capsule of the elbow joint.

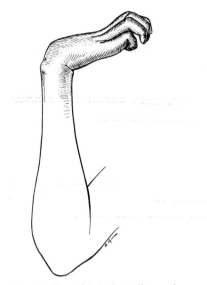

Fig. 300. Well-established Volkmann's contracture with clawhand and flexion of wrist and fingers. Note atrophy of forearm.

likely to be damaged at the time of injury or in reduction. With ulnar injury there may be an immediate or a delayed loss of sensation in the little and ring fingers. With medial injury there may be an immediate or delayed loss of sensation in the index and middle fingers. Any swelling or edema occurring within the firm capsule of the joint or within the aponeurosis (muscle covering) may cause great tension to be exerted from within. This may lead to (1) paralysis of the median, ulnar, and radial nerves, causing disturbance of motion and sensation in the forearm and hand, and (2) extravasation of blood into the fibers of muscle tissue so that they go through a stage of swelling and, later, scar formation (Volkmann's contracture). There is frequently much swelling after fractures and other injuries about the elbow joint, and therefore symptoms of constriction of vessels and injury to muscles may be apparent within 4 to 48 hours after injury. Patients with injuries about the elbow joint, therefore, should be under hourly observation for at least 48

hours whether the fracture has been reduced or not. During this time notation by the nurse of any excessive swelling or loss of sensation should be made constantly. If such should occur, there should be immediate release of tension by complete freeing of any pressure from the cast or by incision of the superficial tissues by operation. The fracture should be disregarded until a circulatory balance is reestablished.

Some of the most severe and complicated fractures the surgeon has to deal with occur in the elbow side-swipe injuries. They are usually compounded, and the humerus, the ulna, and the radius may be shattered. Nerves and tendons are frequently damaged. The repair is tedious and must consist in thorough debridement, suture of nerves and tendons, and restoration of bone and joint alignment. The latter frequently requires internal fixation with wires, screws, or plates. Some patients, however, may be treated after repair by lateral traction in recumbency.

Treatment. Supracondylar fractures and dislocations should be reduced with the patient under anesthesia. It is usually necessary to place the elbow in a position of flexion to maintain reduction. The amount of flexion must be determined by the ability of the circulation to tolerate it. In fractures in young children the flexed position may be necessary for only 2 to 3 weeks. This is true of dislocations in young and old, but older persons may need a longer period for complete bone healing. If swelling is severe in patients treated early or if reduction has not been accomplished to a satisfactory degree after 7 to 14 days, lateral traction either by adhesive traction or skeletal traction through the olecranon process should be instituted. In the majority of patients it will be successful, provided the surgeon and nurse are vigilant in the application of forces to correct the deformity.

Healing period. Motion should be begun within 3 to 6 weeks, depending on the stabiilty at the time of reduction. Complete healing of the fracture requires approximately 8 weeks, but return of complete motion may require 3 to 6 months.

FRACTURES OF THE OLECRANON PROCESS

Cause. Fractures of the olecranon process are usually caused by a direct blow.

Symptoms and signs. Pain, swelling, and inability to extend the elbow forcibly are symptoms of fracture of the olecranon process. Before swelling has occurred a groove may be felt between the fragments.

Treatment. Open reduction is the treatment of choice in all patients who manifest any perceptible separation of the fragments. Reduction may be obtained by wiring or nailing, or it may be maintained by a removable beaded screw.

FOREARM FRACTURES

Cause. Forearm fractures may be caused by either direct or indirect violence, usually the latter.

Anatomy. Pronation and supination are the essential functional motions in the forearm. To preserve these motions after fracture the bones must be replaced so that they will be parallel to each other and of equal length. There must be no obstacle or obstruction between them. The width of the interosseous space varies according to the tension or relaxation of the controlling muscles that rotate the forearm from pronation to supination. Therefore, when the fracture occurs near the elbow, in the midarm, or near the wrist, the governing factor determining the position in which the controllable distal portion of the fractures is placed in relation to the uncontrollable or fixed proximal frag-

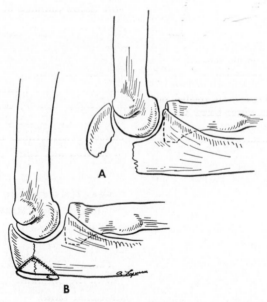

Fig. 301. Fracture of the olecranon process, which always requires open reduction if the fragments are separated. **A,** Fracture. **B,** Wire suture that should be fairly superficial for best results.

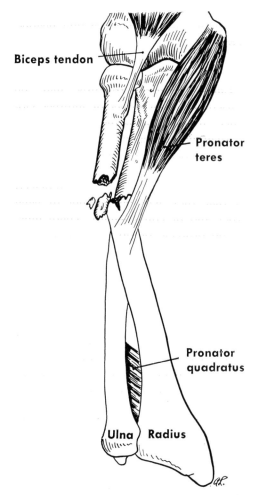

Biceps tendon

Pronator teres

Pronator quadratus

Ulna **Radius**

Fig. 302. The anatomy of the muscles of the forearm that influence pronation and supination. In fractures above the pronator teres the uncontrollable upper fragment is rotated outward (supinated). In fractures below the pronator teres the upper fragment is rotated inward (pronated). Fractures are placed in the fixed position to meet the upper fragment accordingly. The pronator quadratus always has a tendency to pull both bones together.

ments depends on the location of muscle attachments and the various tendencies of their pull.

In fractures above the pronator radii teres there is outward rotation of the upper fragment of the radius by the biceps tendon. Therefore, the forearm must be placed in outward rotation

(supination). In fractures below the pronator radii teres the forearm must be placed in a position of inward rotation (pronation) to match the muscle action above.

The radius, probably because it has a better blood supply, usually heals faster than the ulna, but nonunion in the bones of the forearm is not uncommon and may require bone graft operations to stimulate bone union. Some unreducible fractures may be treated by bone plating or by intramedullary nailing.

Problem. Rotary motion of the forearm must be restored as soon as sufficient union to tolerate the strain has been demonstrated roentgenographically. The cast must extend from the fingers to the shoulder. The nearer the fracture is to the wrist the sooner the cast can be cut to below the elbow. Daily full ranges of motion of the shoulder and, as soon as possible, of the elbow should be carried out to prevent adhesions.

Healing period. The healing period varies considerably with the amount of soft tissue damage at the time of the injury, the age of the patient, and the individual speed of healing (factors unknown). Solid union cannot be expected (except in children) in less than 8 to 12 weeks. In some patients in whom there is delayed union, immobilization must be maintained for 3 to 4 months. This causes considerable delay in the return of motion and function in the joints and muscles.

FRACTURE OF THE WRIST (COLLES' FRACTURE)

Colles' fracture is one of the most common and classic fractures.

Cause. Colles' fracture is caused by a fall or by breaking a fall with the outstretched hand.

Anatomy. The far end of the radius is broken off and displaced backward. The typical silver fork deformity results. Muscles play no particular part except to cause overriding by spasm. With the posterior displacement of the end of the radius, several other complications usually occur, such as (1) shortening of the forearm, tending to make the ulna impinge on the carpal bones, (2) fracture of the styloid process of the ulna, and (3) posterior facing of the wrist joint that interferes with action of the flexor tendons.

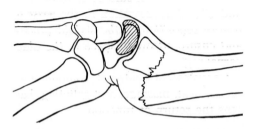

Fig. 303. Colles' fracture. Lateral view showing overriding and posterior displacement of controllable fragment.

Problem. Reduction may be maintained by the use of (1) the circular cast; (2) anterior and posterior splints that are molded and held in the correct position by bandage, preferably bias flannel or elastic; (3) commercial splints, which as a rule are not dependable except in a few patients with fractures in which fragments are not much displaced and forcible maintenance of corrective position is not necessary; or (4) skeletal traction that may be essential to good reduction in some cases of patients with comminuted fractures. A Kirschner wire may be passed through the olecranon and another through the metacarpal bones of the hand. These are incorporated in the cast after reduction. This method may also be used when both bones of the forearm are broken.

Anesthesia. One of several types of anesthesia may be used: (1) local injection of Novocain, 1% to 2%, into the

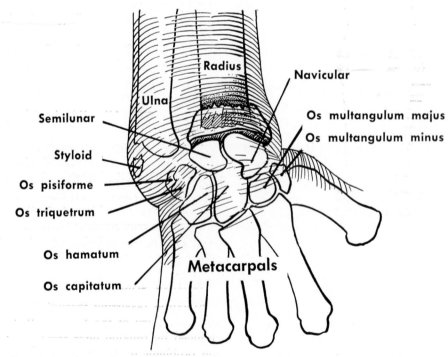

Fig. 304. Anteroposterior view of Colles' fracture showing shortening of radius, posterior facing of joint, and fracture of styloid process.

area of hemorrhage within the fracture site, (2) intravenous injection of Pentothal sodium, and (3) general anesthesia with gas, gas-ether, or ether.

In a few patients who are given treatment immediately reduction may be performed without anesthesia because of nature's temporary anesthetizing effect.

These methods may be employed in the reduction of all fractures and may be selected according to the condition of the patient. The level of blood pressure, senility, and length of anesthesia time must be taken into consideration.

Treatment. In reduction it is important that the lines of the deformity be the determining factor in the application of the traction force. The flexed elbow offers a satisfactory means of countertraction when a nurse or assistant applies a firm grip there. Traction on the fingers and hand must be exerted first

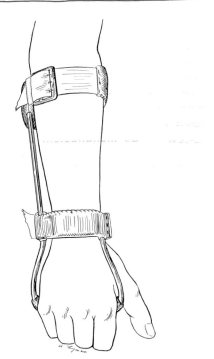

Fig. 305. Three-point splint for wrist drop; also used for protection of the wrist after fractures of the carpal bones on lower end of the radius. Allows free use of fingers and thumb.

in the line of the deformity. When sufficient traction has been obtained to overcome muscle spasm and to free the impacted serrated bone ends, correction of the deformity will be easy if the distal portion is brought into a position that meets the proximal portion of the fracture. It is essential to proper reduction that these three requirements be fulfilled: (1) restoration of the length of the radius, (2) restoration of forward facing of the joint surface of the radius, and (3) ulnar deviation of the wrist to restore reposition of the styloid process and ensure adequate space in the ulnocarpal region.

Convalescent treatment, combining exercise, heat, massage, and splinting, hastens the return of function.

ROUTINE TREATMENT FOLLOWING FRACTURES

In all patients with fractures ice bags should be employed in the region of fractures to lessen swelling and relieve pain.

As a general principle cold applications or icecaps should be used in all injuries—fractures and sprains—within the first 24 or 36 hours to prevent swelling and edema. After this, heat is more soothing.

In most patients with bone and tissue injury, aspirin or some form of salicylate is effective for relief of the aching pain. When muscle spasm is present, however, some of the morphine derivatives or Prostigmine may be used fairly freely at first. This is particularly true when the injury is associated with shock.

NURSING CARE

Fractures occurring through the neck or upper third of the humerus that are reduced by traction offer some perplexing problems to the nurse. For traction the bed must have a firm hard mattress, and some method of countertraction

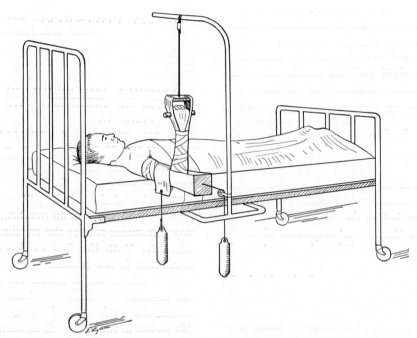

Fig. 306. Side-traction apparatus. Adaptable to fractures of the clavicle, head and neck of the humerus, shaft of the humerus, and supracondylar fractures.

must be devised. Usually, elevating the bed by shock blocks under the head and foot of the affected side will provide sufficient countertraction, although occasionally some type of restraint jacket secured to the unaffected side may be necessary also. The traction is applied in two parts with the arm flexed. Two adhesive straps that extend to a board and pulley extending from the side of the bed are used for the upper arm. Another set of adhesive straps is applied to the forearm and attached to a spreader that is a considerable distance beyond the ends of the fingers. From this spreader a rope extends to an overhead pulley and then to the weights. Some type of padded handle suspended from this spreader is useful, inasmuch as it enables the patient to flex his fingers and hand over it. Extension on the forearm is used to eliminate its dependent weight as well as to relax muscle spasm in the upper arm.

Although the rest of the patient's body is unencumbered, he is usually not permitted to turn, and for that reason considerable discomfort in the upper back and shoulders may occur. Frequent alcohol rubs for these areas will be of use in eliminating this discomfort. Changing the undersheet must be done with great dexterity to prevent movement of the patient's body and disturbance of the traction. Because pressure points tend to form rather easily around the bony prominences of the wrist, this area should be inspected frequently.

Fractures above the condyles of the humerus—the elbow fracture of common parlance—are very common in active youngsters. Such patients do not often remain long in the hospital. They are frequently brought in for reduction and dismissed in a few hours. It is essential that the parents be warned of the danger of circulatory impairment from subsequent swelling and that they be told how to detect such a complication. They must understand that the fracture itself should not occasion severe discomfort for the child and that continued crying or repeated complaints may indicate that there is an obstruction in circulation. Not long ago a small boy with such a fracture was taken to his home 5 miles out of town after reduction of a supracondylar fracture that had been performed in the hospital outpatient department. The child complained bitterly for 24 hours before the parents realized this was not the normal sequence of events after a fracture. When he was brought back to the hospital, a fully developed ischemic contracture of the kind described by and named by Volkmann had occurred, and 10 months of constant treatment were necessary to bring back even partial use of the hand.

Coldness, pallor, and cyanosis of fingers may be the first indications that there is circulatory impairment. Swelling and pain often follow rapidly, and some paresthesia may be detected on touching the digits. Since all fractures are accompanied by some degree of swelling, observation should be constant and vigilant in these cases. Too often this may be neglected because the patient seems to need relatively little nursing care and, for the most part, looks after his own wants.

A good test for circulation is the blanching sign that determines patency of blood flow. The nail of the thumb is momentarily compressed, and the return of blood to the nail is observed. If the return is immediate, circulation is thought to be adequate. Sluggishness in the return of the blood to the part is indicative of some degree of impairment and should be reported to the physician. One authority warns in huge letters in his textbook on fractures: "WATCH THE HAND FOR SWELLING AND BLUENESS OF THE NAILS. CAUTION ALL CONCERNED THAT IF THIS OCCURS THE FIXATION APPARATUS SHOULD BE REMOVED AND THE ARM BROUGHT INTO EXTENSION. THE FRACTURE CAN ALWAYS BE REDUCED THE SECOND TIME BUT A VOLKMANN'S CONTRACTURE IS A PERMANENT DISABILITY."* Surgeons make it a rule to disregard the fracture in any circulatory emergency.

Elevation of the arm by pillows or by suspending the arm in an overhead sling may sometimes reduce the swelling considerably. With the first evidence that circulation is not normal, however, the nurse needs to be on guard. No excuse can possibly be made for delay in reporting the condition to the surgeon, and this means at night as well as during the day. When no doctor is available, the nurse may have to split the cast throughout its entire length. The constriction may be caused by tight bandages or padding beneath the cast, and so these also must be cut. The skin must be visible from one end to the other. The cast, once split and spread, can be taped together temporarily, because it usually does not need to be removed to relieve the symptoms. Nurses are warned not to be satisfied with splitting the cast halfway, since this is usually inadequate to release the constriction. Unless specifically ordered by the surgeon, windows should not be cut in casts. The swelling and edema that may occur through the window will only exacerbate the existing trouble.

Releasing the constricting cast and bandages may not reduce the symptoms, particularly if they are caused by callus formation that involves the nerve. For this reason frequent inspection of the

---

*From Magnusson, Paul B.: Fractures, Philadelphia, 1949, J. B. Lippincott Co.

digits should follow the spreading of the cast.

Occasionally, the surgeon will order a small window cut out over the radial artery before the patient is brought back from the plaster room after reduction of such fractures. This allows the nurse caring for the patient to check frequently on the circulation in the extremity. It is of great importance that the pulse be carefully taken and recorded at stated intervals, perhaps as often as every 15 minutes. A faint disappearing pulse may indicate pressure on the artery and should be reported. Comparison with the pulse of the unaffected arm will be of assistance in gauging the seriousness of the constriction.

Nurses notifying physicians of circulatory impairment should chart the notation and the time at which the physician was called.

A word should be said in regard to slings that are frequently used after injury to the forearm or wrist. If the sling is applied in the common fashion with the long bias edge encircling the wrist and the ends going over alternate shoulders, do not use a knot to fasten the ends at the back of the neck. Such a knot places considerable strain on the back of the neck, and for relief the patient allows his shoulders to droop forward. Small safety pins used to pin the ends distribute the weight of the sling more evenly. Some surgeons object to a sling being passed around the neck at all. They prefer that it be passed over the

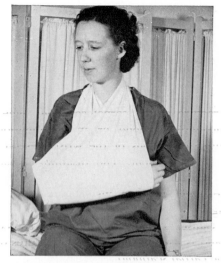

Fig. 307. Correct application of arm sling. Note support of wrist. The sling ends are crossed on the posterior aspect of the neck and pinned in two places. The double pinning helps distribute the weight, and there is no pressure from a knot.

opposite shoulder and under the arm, because if the sling is placed around the neck it is possible for the patient to lower his arm by simply lowering his head. A sagging sling that does not support the wrist and allows the forearm to droop beyond a right angle is a very sloppy, inefficient apparatus. The patient who is wearing a sling to support the arm must be given instructions regarding movement of the shoulder joint. This joint should be taken through a normal range of motion several times daily to prevent tightness or limitation in shoulder motion.

Fractures in the hand

FRACTURES OF THE CARPAL SCAPHOID

Fracture of the carpal scaphoid, when encountered alone or in combination with dislocations of the wrist, deserves special comment. The disabling possibilities are often underestimated, and treatment is often insufficient or lacking.

Cause. Falling on the outstretched hand is usually the cause of fractures of the carpal scaphoid.

Anatomy. The bones of the wrist are peculiar in that the greater part of their surface is covered with articular cartilage. This means that the supply of circulation is correspondingly limited.

An interruption of the circulation by fracture or loss of continuity means starvation to one or another portion of the injured bone with resulting disintegration or death of bone (aseptic necrosis).

Diagnosis. Diagnosis is based on roentgenographic findings. Four views should be taken. Sometimes, the fracture line does not show up for 2 or 3 weeks. There are pain and tenderness in the "snuffbox."

Treatment. Complete reduction by adequate manipulation is the first requirement. Adequate and prolonged immobilization in a cast or splint is next. If nonunion should occur, drilling holes through the fracture line or a bone graft may lead to healing; or the removal of one or both of the fragments may improve function and relieve pain.

Healing period. A fracture of the carpal scaphoid requires immobilization in a cast or splints for 8 to 10 weeks for union to take place.

FRACTURES OF THE METACARPALS

Cause. Fractures of the metacarpals are caused by (1) direct violence or crushing injuries, and (2) indirect violence, such as striking a blow with the closed fist.

Anatomy. Most of the muscle power in the hand is on the palmar surface (interossei and lumbricales). These act to bow the metacarpal bones backward in the event of fracture.

Problem. The metacarpals must be immobilized adequately in a position that will overcome the tendency toward posterior bowing.

Reduction. Manipulation under anesthesia is often necessary to restore normal position. To maintain this, several methods are used.

A plaster cast may be employed to apply pressure posteriorly along the shaft and anteriorly on the palmar surface under the head, or the metacarpophalangeal joint.

Skeletal traction is another method used to maintain reduction of the fracture. By passing a small pin through the phalanx or by using the miniature icetong apparatus, sufficient traction may be applied through elastic bands and the banjo splint to maintain proper position of the fragments. This is particularly adaptable to the overriding oblique or spiral fracture.

At the critical time of about 3 weeks, roentgenographic examination must be carried out to see that proper reduction has been maintained.

Healing period. The healing period is 4 to 5 weeks.

FRACTURES OF THE PHALANGES

Fractures of the phalanges comprise two types: the transverse and oblique fractures of the phalanges and the chip fractures of the posterior surface of the distal fragment of the distal phalanx.

Transverse and oblique fractures of the phalanges

Anatomy. The lumbrical muscles tend to cause palmar angulation of the fragments.

Treatment. The problem of reduction as well as treatment is to keep the fingers in flexion until the critical time has passed. This may be done by binding the fingers over a rolled bandage. When removed, motion should be reestablished.

Chip fractures of the posterior surface of the distal fragment of the distal phalanx

Anatomy. To the posterior surface of the distal fragment of the distal phalanx is attached the tendon of the long extensor. Injury causes an inability to extend the distal phalanx and grave loss of an important function. A stiff joint or an amputation is less disabling than this deformity (baseball finger).

Treatment. Complete exaggerated, and prolonged (4 to 6 weeks) hyperextension of the distal joint of the finger is the treatment of choice. This gives, as a rule, sufficient time for complete reattachment of the tendon and a return of function. Suture by operation is occasionally necessary.

Fractures and dislocations of the spine and pelvis, including nursing care

Fractures or dislocations of the spine are divided into the following groups in the order of severity: (1) fractures or dislocations with extensive displacement and immediate paralysis of the nerves below the point of fracture, (2) fractures or dislocations with displacement and delayed paralysis below the point of fracture, (3) fractures with compression of the vertebrae but with no neurologic disturbance, and (4) fractures of the accessory processes (such as spinous or lateral processes) without any evidence of nerve pressure.

Cause. Causes of fractures of the spine are as follows: (1) a fall in the sitting or stooped position, (2) a jackknife type of injury such as occurs when force is exerted against the shoulders and pelvis

at the same time, (3) a direct blow against the back or flank, and (4) certain diseases that cause softening or disintegration of the bones of the spine, such as hyperparathyroidism and malignant metastases. In this last the break may occur spontaneously or with minimal strain.

First aid. There is a great lesson to be learned in the treatment of acute injuries that is particularly exemplified by fractures of the spine. Usually, such injuries occur in auto accidents, in athletics, or as the result of falls in construction work or under similar circumstances.

The treatment should be started at the scene of the injury. Obviously, the victim of such an accident may have spicules of bone that could result in further

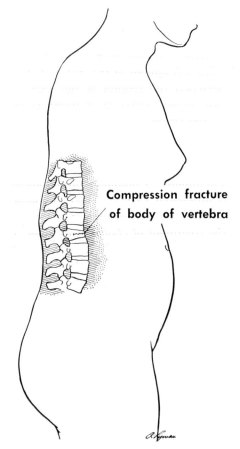

Compression fracture
of body of vertebra

Fig. 308. Compression fracture of the spine. Angulation or gibbus may occur over the spinous process of fractured vertebra or the one above.

damage to the tissues of the spinal cord.

Anatomy. The spinal cord is encased in a tube or channel of bone. The abnormal position of the vertebra may cause complete shearing severance of the cord at the time of injury, or it may be subjected to damage from spicules of bone or the pressure from surrounding hemorrhage and congestion. If severance occurs, paralysis is immediate below the fractured vertebra. If the damage results from pressure alone, the paralysis is delayed in its development.

Problem. If paralysis occurs but is not immediate or complete, laminectomy

(decompression of the spinal cord) and the removal of bone fragments are sometimes indicated.

In complete immediate paralysis laminectomy has no value.

In uncomplicated compression fractures the problem is to restore the normal contour of the spine by producing hyperextension.

Following injuries to the spine there is almost invariably a shock to the sympathetic nervous system. With this shock comes disturbance of intestinal and bladder activity, and the most serious immediate problem of the patient with spine fracture often directly results from these factors.

The presence of pain often requires morphine sedation, which exaggerates internal stasis and sluggishness of bladder muscles to such an extent that enemas and catheterization are frequently necessary for several days. Strong cathartics should not be used because they may cause increased discomfort. The use of hot fomentations, rectal tube, and gastric lavage is advocated. An indwelling catheter is occasionally necessary for 5 or 7 days.

Treatment. Hyperextension and traction may be accomplished in several ways.

A frame or Gatch bed may be used in the treatment of these patients. Its angle is gradually increased within 4 to 14 days. Maintenance of reduction is checked roentgenographically. After reduction a body cast is applied.

Early reduction under anesthesia is accomplished with the patient suspended by his feet and shoulders, face down. Pressure is exerted on the spinous processes at the point of fracture until correction has been obtained. Roentgenographic examination may be used to confirm the reduction before the cast is applied. The cast should extend from the hips to the neck to maintain correction. The higher the fracture in the spine, the more difficult it is to maintain the correction. In fractures above the fifth dorsal vertebra, it is necessary to carry the cast on up to the head and chin.

Some spine fractures that have healed with persistent pain need internal fixation by some form of bone fusion or graft or other apparatus to stabilize the spinous processes and laminae in the correct position.

Fractures or dislocations of the cervical spine are best treated by the use of the Crutchfield tongs. These allow weights of 30 to 40 pounds to be used for reduction.

Treatment in the hyperextension cast is usually carried out for 3 to 6 months, according to the severity of the fractures. This is followed by a hyperexten-

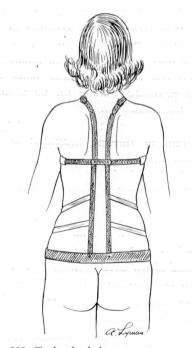

Fig. 309. Taylor back brace used for support of the spine in many conditions, such as convalescent fractures and tuberculosis, epiphysitis, arthritis, malignancy, and round-shoulder deformity.

sion brace such as the Taylor back brace for an additional 4 to 6 months.

Healing period. The healing period of vertebrae is from 6 to 12 months.

FRACTURES OF THE SACRUM AND COCCYX

Cause. Fractures of the sacrum and coccyx are usually caused by direct violence and are very painful. Falling on the ice in a sitting position is a common cause.

Symptoms. Pain that is aggravated by sitting down or arising and tenderness over the sacrum or sacrococcygeal joint are symptoms of fracture of the sacrum and coccyx.

Treatment. After the patient has spent a period of rest in bed with the affected area supported on a rubber ring and much time lying prone, low adhesive strapping or a low girdle may be used to relieve muscle pull. Sitting on hard surfaces should be avoided. Repeated massage of the piriformis muscles (rectally) often gives relief. Occasionally, the coccyx may be removed as a last resort.

NURSING CARE OF THE PATIENT WITH FRACTURE OF THE SPINE WITH CORD INJURY

World War II brought about a great change in the attitude of medical people regarding the treatment of patients with spinal cord injuries. Before the war spinal injuries were often fatal, and treatment of patients who did survive was usually limited to the complications and infections that seemed to be inseparable from the condition. Very little was done in the matter of total rehabilitation. One or two such patients in a community might constitute all that were seen during a single season. But during the war the injury was a fairly common one. It became evident early that an intensive reconditioning program would be necessary if these unfortunate victims were to be salvaged for anything resembling a useful life. The accomplishments that came out of this program have been little short of heroic.

This program of physical, social, and vocational rehabilitation was built on the conviction that the task, however difficult, could be done. From the outset the attitude of the workers was one of determined hope. The pessimism that had always undermined the treatment of this type of patient was vigorously combated in all phases of the work. As General Kirk pointed out early in the war, nothing less than an active, self-supporting wheelchair life could be considered for these patients; walking with the aid of splints and crutches was the goal in all possible cases. The time taken to accomplish these things was not to be considered a factor. At the outset, everyone involved in the process had to be brought to recognize that fact—and this meant the entire medical team, the patient himself, and the family. As great a degree of independence as possible was the goal to be worked for with all patients.

Most of the patients with this type of injury whom nurses will care for in civilian hospitals will be boys or young men who have been injured in a swimming mishap, automobile crash, football, or trampoline accident. They have been active and energetic all their lives, and the sudden forced helplessness and inactivity may produce profound personality changes. Moroseness, depression, sullenness, and unwillingness to cooperate in treatment frequently occur. Threats of suicide are not uncommon when the period of recumbency goes on month after month without apparent progress. It takes considerable emotional maturity to understand such attitudes and yet maintain an unwavering determination to guide the patient toward more con-

structive thinking so that he is willing to do his utmost toward attaining independence. Probably the most important single feature in preventing despair and depression is early mobilization. The fact that he is not to be confined to bed and complete helplessness for a prolonged period will aid the patient immeasurably by giving him something to live for. It will also play a most important part in preventing loss of muscle tone, stiff joints, and contractures such as occur in the plantar fascia, causing pes cavus, or in the gastrocnemius and Achilles tendon, causing drop foot.

Nurses in small hospitals and small communities will feel particularly helpless in attempting to plan a program of activities to fit the paraplegic patient's needs. Nevertheless, there are often resources within the community that can be called upon for assistance if the nurse recognizes their existence and their potentialities. It is particularly important that this assistance be solicited at the earliest possible period after danger to life is past. A long period of idleness in which the patient becomes more and more pessimistic about his lot is often the forerunner to severe personality changes that could be prevented by a program of therapy instituted at the earliest possible moment.

But where is the nurse to obtain help in planning such a program if there is no physical or occupational therapist or physical education consultant on her agency or hospital staff?

The physician is, of course, the chief adviser in all such matters and should direct the patient's activities in the projected recovery program. However, he cannot be expected to work out the details of such a program or to be on hand to direct every feature of it. He will expect the nurse to explore community resources and to make sensible use of them under his direction.

All nurses should know the location of their state services for crippled children in order to call upon them for assistance when the need arises. The orthopedic nursing consultant employed on these services will be able to give valuable suggestions as to how to obtain assistance in planning such a program. In some instances she may be able to share in this work directly. The facilities of the state rehabilitation services should be explored and the patient given the opportunity to learn what this organization can offer him. The local or state chapter of the National Society for Crippled Children and Adults may be able to give suggestions. The principal of the local high school can often give suggestions as to personnel on the school faculty who would be of assistance in developing skill in certain arts or crafts for which the patient displays interest or ability. The teacher of physical education might be willing to assist with a program of physical reconditioning to fit the patient's needs. Since community interest in this type of patient is always high, the alert nurse should be able to interest civic groups in aiding her to solve some of the problems in rehabilitation that she is not capable of working out alone.

Nursing problems. A patient with a fractured spine with spinal cord involvement presents what may be truly called a major nursing problem. Fractures of the spine may, of course, exist without cord injury, but these patients do not constitute the great nursing problem that fracture with cord injuries do. Attention will therefore be fixed primarily on the more severe type of injury where some degree of cord involvement is present.

Injury to the spinal cord is almost invariably accompanied by disturbances of the bowel and bladder. In fractures of the lower dorsal and lumbar vertebrae, these disturbances are especially acute because the spinal segments that control these reflexes are so near the site of injury. Cervical and upper thoracic injuries are a more serious immediate threat to life, but if the patient survives, the resulting bladder complications may not be so severe.

Nurses caring for patients who have paraplegia from spinal cord injury must constantly consider the following: (1) Urinary sepsis is the primary cause of death after paraplegia. (2) Trophic ulcers and bedsores are the second most common cause of death in the condition. Armed with this knowledge, nurses are better able to play an intelligent part in the effort to salvage these patients.

Management of the bladder. Opinions as to the management of the bladder in patients with paraplegia vary somewhat. Some physicians feel that every patient with spinal cord injury should be catheterized and an indwelling catheter should be secured in place at the earliest possible moment. It is felt that retention of urine, combined with overdistention, may produce considerable permanent damage to the muscle fibers of the bladder. In addition, residual urine adds to the danger of urinary tract infection. It is of the utmost importance to use the most careful aseptic technique in catheterization procedures. Even the compelling necessity for haste and the conviction that the patient will not survive are no reasons for using careless methods in catheterizing a patient after cord injury.

Other physicians object to urethral catheterization for these patients. They feel that the problem of retention is not as urgent as was formerly thought. They believe that overflow incontinence will cause no permanent ill effects and point out that the catheter has long been considered the "grand executioner" for patients with paraplegia. They have observed that the bladder goes through three periods following cord injury: (1) complete retention of urine, (2) retention with overflow, and (3) periodic reflex (automatic) voiding. When this sequence is not complete, these physicians tend to prefer suprapubic aspiration or cystotomy rather than urethral catheterization.

The establishment of the automatic bladder is frequently part of the management of patients recovering from spinal cord injury. When it seems evident that voluntary control of the bladder is not going to be attained, manual expression of urine is attempted. At stated intervals, pressure is exerted upon the abdominal wall over the bladder, and this pressure is continued until the bladder contracts by reflex action powerful enough to cause the sphincter to relax and the bladder to empty itself. This is done at intervals of 4 to 6 hours. It has been found that less pressure is necessary after the bladder becomes accustomed to this system, and the patient may carry out the manual pressure by himself.

In the army it was customary to perform cystotomies on all paraplegic patients within 5 days after the injury. A suprapubic catheter was placed in the bladder. Tidal drainage may be instituted.

Tidal drainage resembles the natural physiologic functioning of the bladder. It consists in filling the bladder with liquid at a rate of 40 to 60 drops a minute. It is arranged to provide gravity and siphonage, with automatic emptying of the bladder every 2 or 3 hours. It has not, however, been found wholly effective in the paraplegic patient with complete cord transection.

As has been stated, the problem of bladder management is always a major one in this condition. To eliminate the possibility of infection careful preparation of materials, the nurse's hands, and the area must be made before implementation. The patient's liquid intake should be high—at least 2500 ml. and preferably nearer 5000 ml. daily. And last but not least, the patient's position should be changed at frequent intervals to eliminate stasis of the urinary tract that might contribute toward the formation of renal stones.

Gastrointestinal complications. The patient with compression fracture of the spine may frequently have a troublesome stasis of the gastrointestinal tract. The abdomen may be ballooned to drumlike tenseness by distension of the bowel, and respiratory embarrassment may be present because of the crowding of the chest. Hot fomentations to the abdomen for relief of distension are sometimes ordered. The danger of too excessive heat must be borne in mind, for if the patient has sensory loss he will not complain that the packs are too hot, and blistering of the skin may follow. Rectal tubes may sometimes afford considerable relief. Enemas must be given with extreme care because the intestine of the paraplegic patient distends very easily if too much liquid is given or if it is given too rapidly. It is always wise to measure the amount of fluid given by enema and to record the amount of fluid that the patient expels. All patients with spinal cord injury must be watched constantly for fecal impaction.

Prevention of bedsores and trophic ulcers. The problem of bedsores in the paraplegic patient is undoubtedly the most serious consideration from the nursing standpoint. Pressure areas develop with a speed that will seem unbelievable to nurses who have not worked with such patients before. Some physicians prefer that patients with spinal cord injuries be placed on air mattresses immediately so that the pressure of the bed will not be concentrated on certain vulnerable parts of the body, such as the sacrum or the heels. There is no general agreement on this subject, however, for other physicians are strongly opposed to this type of mattress. The use of rubber rings and doughnuts is considered unwise because window edema so often develops from their use. Window edema will, of course, cut off circulation to the threatened part and thereby add to the damage.

Frequent changes of position are imperative. Orders will often be written to turn the patient as frequently as every 1 to 2 hours, day and night. Even if this is done, intelligent understanding of the dangers of side-lying and prone-lying is necessary, for congested areas often develop on dependent parts and bony prominences even though the patient lies on these areas only for an hour. The ingenuity of the nurse will be taxed to the utmost to find positions that will not cause undue pressure on any body area for too long a period.

Pads of thick porous sponge rubber may be placed under the sacrum and heels when the patient lies on his back or under the ilium, trochanter, and malleolus when he lies on his side. These pads should be large enough to extend under a wide area. Large squares of unclipped sheepskin will also be helpful. This material can be washed daily in warm water with a mild soap. It should be rinsed thoroughly and dried in the sun if possible.

The linen used for the paraplegic patient should be carefully inspected; no new or stiff, harsh sheets should be used. Drawsheets should be placed on the bed to facilitate changing of linen, for a wet bed is a great menace to the paraplegic patient's skin. He should never be allowed to lie in a wet bed for even a short period. Wrinkles in bed linen will also contribute toward the development of pressure sores.

Patients with paraplegia are unable to feel cold in the paralyzed extremities, and circulation in these parts may be very poor. Hot-water bags, even of fairly mild temperatures, may produce blisters that are almost impossible to heal. Death from infected bedsores can come about in a very few days. They are not merely a troublesome complication in paraplegia; they may very easily be fatal. It is best to depend on sufficient wool covering for warmth rather than to risk using external heating equipment on such patients.

In recent years many patients with paraplegia have been cared for on special types of apparatus, such as the Foster bed, the Stryker frame, or the alternating pressure pad. This apparatus has been designed primarily to prevent pressure areas and to facilitate nursing care.

Alternating pressure pad or pneumatic mattress. The alternating pressure pad is made of air cells 1¼ inches in diameter, running transversely or longitudinally of the bed. Every other cell is connected to an air tube that comprises the edge of the mattress. This arrangement provides for two systems of air cells. These air cells are alternately inflated and deflated by an electrically driven air pump. The air is shifted first into one system and then into the other. This means that the patient's body is alternately resting on the odd-numbered cells and then on the even-numbered cells. The cells are inflated and deflated at intervals of 2 to 3 minutes. This interchange of air in the cells is so smooth that it is barely perceptible to the hand. It produces a massaging effect to the cutaneous tissues and provides for a continuous change of pressure points. With improved circulation to the skin and the changing pressure points, the danger of decubitus ulcers is somewhat lessened. This pad not only facilitates

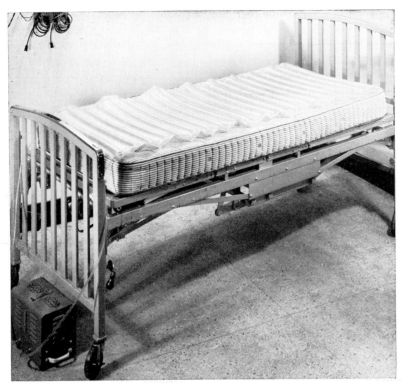

Fig. 310. Alternating pressure pad. The pad is placed on top of the regular mattress. A Pliofilm apron that is attached to the head end of the pad tucks beneath the mattress and maintains the pad in position. (Courtesy Grant-Messenger and Associates, Cleveland, Ohio.)

the care of the patient in the hospital but it also may be used in the home to help prevent pressure areas.

Alternating pressure pads for use in wheelchairs are now available. These can be most helpful to the paraplegic patient by enabling him to remain in a sitting position for longer periods without developing pressure areas.

Nursing care of the patient on a Foster bed. During recent years many patients whose care has necessitated the use of a frame have been placed on a Foster or Stryker frame. This apparatus is similar to the Bradford frame, except that both the anterior and posterior frames have been fitted on a standard that has a pivoting device. This pivoting device makes it possible in many instances for one nurse to turn an adult

patient. Not only is it easier to turn the patient but better immobilization is secured; consequently the patient experiences less pain in turning. These frames are used primarily in the treatment and nursing care of patients with various back conditions. The patient with spinal cord damage may be placed on this type of bed. Good position can be maintained, and it is possible to turn the patient frequently, thus changing the pressure points.

Canvas covers are used with these frames, the same as with the Bradford frame. They may be fastened with buckles or with lacings but must be firm and taut continuously. Divided covers are frequently used. This can vary, however, depending on the diagnosis and the purpose for which the frame is being used.

The divided cover for the upper half of the posterior frame should extend from the top of the frame to the level of the patient's buttocks (gluteal cleft). A space of approximately 4 inches is left for the perineal opening. The lower half

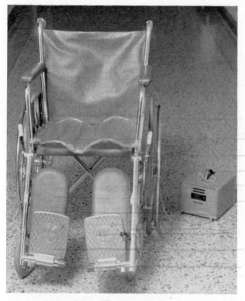

Fig. 311. An alternating pressure pad for use in a wheelchair. The paraplegic finds this helpful in preventing the development of pressure sores over the ischial tuberosities.

of the posterior cover extends to the end of the frame. The upper portion of the divided cover for the anterior frame will extend from the patient's shoulders to the symphysis pubis. Again a space of 4 inches is maintained for the perineal opening, and the lower portion of the anterior cover extends to the level of the patient's malleolus. This arrangement permits the patient's feet to extend over the frame cover when he is lying in the prone position. Some type of support must be arranged for the patient's forehead or face. This usually consists of a narrow canvas strip buckled at the top of the anterior frame. When caring for a patient with incontinence on the frame, it will be necessary to protect the canvas covering around the perineal opening with a waterproof material such as Pliofilm. A narrow canvas strip is buckled across the perineal opening when the bedpan is not in place. This prevents the patient's buttocks from sagging and helps to maintain a good back-lying position.

The frame may be padded with cotton blankets folded to fit the frame, or strips of sponge rubber cut in the desired size

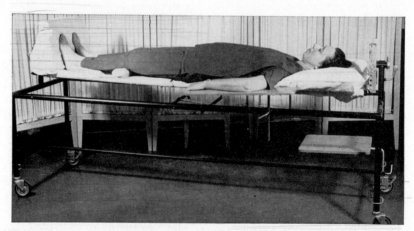

Fig. 312. Supine position on the Foster bed. Note the footboard maintaining neutral position of the feet, the small pad to prevent pressure on the heel, and the roll placed beneath the head of the tibia to prevent hyperextension of the knee joint. The rack to hold the bedpan is hooked over the frame edges beneath the divided frame cover.

can be used. The outer linen covering is made to fit the frame and is held in place by tying it on the underside. When the patient is being turned from the supine to the prone position, a pillow should be placed crosswise above the dorsum of the feet. The top frame is fastened in place so that the patient is held snugly between the two frames.

Two or three canvas turning straps are buckled around both frames and the patient. This gives the patient added security and will prevent the limbs from slipping during the turning process. The arm boards are removed, and the screw or spring lock that keeps the frame from turning is released. The patient is instructed as to which way he will be

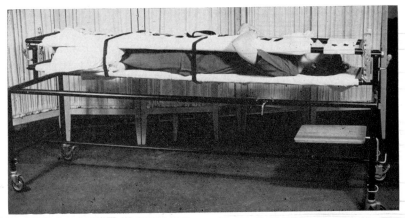

Fig. 313. The anterior frame has been fastened so that the patient is held snugly between the two frames. Turning straps have been applied to give added security. The adjustable arm boards have been removed in readiness for turning. Note the pulley at each end of the frame. These may be used in the application of cervical or leg traction. Also, note pegs in the legs of the frame that permit elevation of either end of the bed.

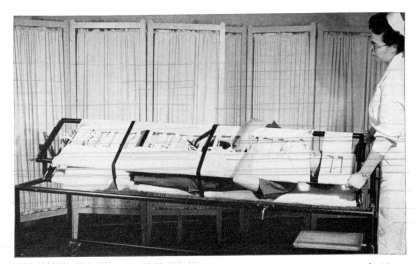

Fig. 314. The screw lock has been loosened and the turning process started. Note ties of muslin sheet covering the canvas frame cover. Also, note the narrow strip of canvas used to support the patient's forehead when in the prone position.

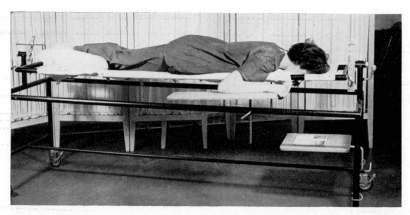

Fig. 315. Prone position on the Foster bed. The posterior frame has been removed and will have needed linen changes while the patient is on the anterior frame. In this position the patient can use the lower shelf for holding reading material or the diet tray may be placed here.

turned. If he is being turned by one nurse, it is best that she move to the side of the frame. The turning should be done quickly and smoothly. After turning the patient the screw or spring lock must be in place before the nurse's grasp on the frame is released. This screw or lock holds the frame firmly and prevents turning. The straps and upper frame are removed, and back care can be given. The covers and linen are changed when that half of the bed is not in use.

These frames may be used even when it is necessary for the patient to have traction applied. The frames are constructed so that traction can be applied to the patient's lower extremities or to the cervical region.

The general nursing care of the patient is the same as for other bed patients. Skin care, change of position, prevention of deformity, and maintenance of normal joint motion are essential for his rehabilitation.

Treatment of bedsores and trophic ulcers. Treatment of pressure sores and trophic ulcers in the patient with paraplegia should be directed by the physician, for the problem is too serious to be left entirely to the nurse's judgment. Pressure sores in other conditions may safely be considered more or less a nursing problem, but in paraplegia the patient's life may depend upon the kind of treatment he receives for this condition.

Except for the universal acknowledgment of the need for frequent turning of the patient, there is no unanimity of opinion regarding the treatment of established pressure sores. There are numerous types of ointments, pastes, and lacquers that may be used. Irrigation with antiseptic solutions is frequently ordered for the deep decubitus ulcers. Bactericidal lamps and sunlight have sometimes brought about surprising improvement. Sulfonamides and penicillin, either in ointment or solution, may be helpful in combating infection. Cleaning the wound with soap or pHiso-Hex followed by alcohol and a thin layer of boric acid ointment is used in many places. Immersion of the patient in a Hubbard tank is recommended by some workers. After this last treatment the affected area is dried with a hair dryer and local ultraviolet irradiation is given.

Large bedsores that heal slowly are sometimes treated by surgical closure. To ensure the success of this treatment, the patient should be given a high protein, high vitamin, high caloric diet before surgery is undertaken. Intravenous amino acid therapy is also sometimes used to prepare the patient for skin grafting. Following surgery the patient may be placed on a Stryker frame for easier handling.

It has been found that fully developed, deep decubitus ulcers are a source of great loss of body protein. It is therefore important that any patient who is receiving treatment for bedsores and trophic ulcers should have a diet high in protein. A diet containing 150 to 200 mg. of protein daily is considered essential. The salt intake should be increased, and large amounts of all vitamins, with particular attention to vitamin C, are usually considered important.

Prevention of deformities and joint contractures. When caring for the patient with paraplegia it is imperative that the nurse understand and apply the principles of body alignment. She must also have an understanding of normal joint motion. These patients must have the joints of the affected extremities taken through a range of motion daily. This activity is usually ordered and supervised by the attending physician. In some of the larger hospitals the physical therapist is assigned this responsibility, but in smaller hospitals the nurse is the person who must assume the task of preventing joint contractures. Fibrosis of ligaments and ankylosis of joints will occur within a short time if joints are not exercised. Body alignment and normal joint motion have been described in an earlier chapter.

Cord transection. The patient with cord transection presents a more difficult problem. Traction, frames, splinting, and even positioning in bed are of doubtful value, for they seem only to stimulate the mass reflex that brings about contractions of muscles around joints. Furthermore, apparatus applied forcibly to maintain a desired position almost always causes pressure sores to develop. As the patient improves generally the tendency toward flexion and adduction deformities becomes a most perplexing problem. Even turning the patient in bed may set up abnormal motor impulses that are almost impossible to control.

Because this mass reflex is so difficult to combat and is so distressing to the patient, surgery is sometimes performed to eliminate it. Surgery may consist in cutting the anterior spinal roots from the twelfth dorsal to the first sacral segment intraspinally on both sides. This produces a flaccid paralysis that eliminates the constant tendency toward flexion and adduction that the mass reflex brings about. Since the bladder is no longer constantly stimulated by contraction of the abdominal muscles, tidal drainage may be instituted. It is then possible to care for pressure sores more adequately because the bed can be kept dry and the patient can be turned frequently. Physiologic bed positions are also possible, the patient can be made comfortable, and deformity can be prevented with the usual supports for feet, knees, and back.

Patient with cervical cord injuries. A patient with a cervical fracture with some cord injury will have quadriplegia of varying degrees of severity. Frequently, these persons who survive present a picture of spastic rather than flaccid paralysis with involvement of all four extremities. They are entirely dependent upon others for assistance during the early stages of their illness, and the outlook may seem particularly black and hopeless to both nurse and patient. Nevertheless, many of these patients regain partial independence and have

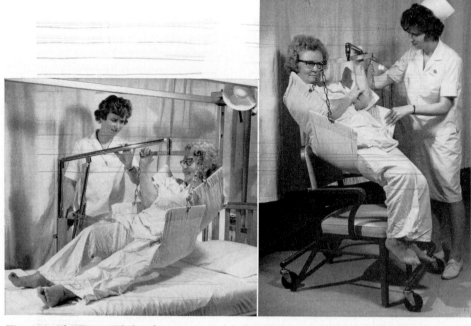

Fig. 316. The Porta-Lift has become a useful device in the hospital as well as in the home for lifting and moving helpless patients. This device makes it possible for one person to move a patient from the bed to a wheelchair and vice versa.

been able to live a fairly normal life.

Quadriplegic patients will not be able to perform the sitting-up, pushing-up, or rolling exercises as efficiently or as quickly as the paraplegic patient whose arms are not involved. The whole program of reconditioning must be built on the patient's potential ability and modified from day to day to meet his needs. Unless the condition is complicated by debilitating diseases, such as hypostatic pneumonia to which these patients are particularly vulnerable, attempts should be made to get the quadriplegic patient in a chair or on his feet as soon as possible. When involvement is not too severe, he may learn to master the four-point gait.

NURSING CARE OF THE PATIENT WITH FRACTURE OF THE SPINE WITHOUT CORD INJURY

Bed positions in fractures of the lumbar and thoracic regions of the spine. In fracture of the spine that is not accompanied by permanent cord injury or spinal fluid block the patient is sometimes placed on a sponge rubber mattress that is superimposed on an ordinary firm felt mattress and bed boards. The feet are kept in the normal physiologic position, the knees are relaxed with a knee roll, and the limbs are cradled so that the weight of the bedclothes is eliminated. Sometimes spinal hyperextension is ordered. This may be obtained by placing a blanket roll beneath the felt mattress at the desired position, or the patient may be placed in a Gatch bed with his head at the foot of the bed and the knee rest elevated. This will provide hyperextension of the spine and has the advantage of being easily alterable. The elevation of the knee rest is usually around 3 inches at the beginning of the treatment. It may be increased 2 inches daily until a maximum elevation of approximately 10 inches has been reached. Occasionally, reverse peristaltic action accompanied by vomiting may

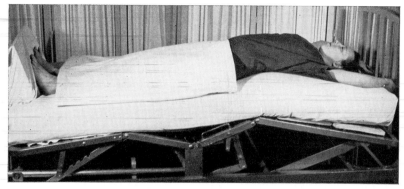

Fig. 317. Maintaining a hyperextended position of the spine by use of the three-crank Deckert bed. The amount of hyperextension can be increased or decreased according to need. The same position can be secured with the ordinary Gatch bed by placing the patient's head at the foot and then elevating the knee rest.

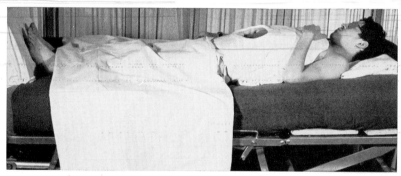

Fig. 318. A body cast that has been applied to maintain the spine in a hyperextended position.

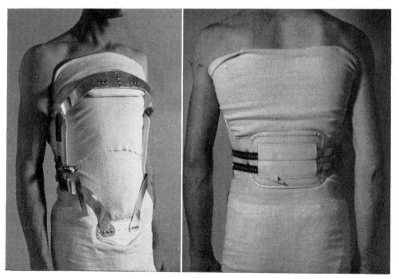

Fig. 319. A hyperextension brace commonly used in the aftercare of fractures of the spine. Anterior and posterior views.

occur during this process. If this happens, further elevation of the Gatch bed should not be attempted.

The patient may be kept in a position of hyperextension for approximately 2 months. At this time if roentgenograms show satisfactory results, he may be allowed out of bed in some type of back brace prescribed by the physician. The Taylor back brace is frequently used. If bowel and bladder disturbances were present at the outset, the patient will usually have regained control by this time.

Patients in hyperextension casts may be given a regime of exercises designed to strengthen the body musculature, particularly the back extensors, which will be of great importance when the cast is finally removed.

Fracture or dislocation of the cervical spine. Skeletal traction, applied by tongs inserted in the parietal eminences of the skull, is frequently used for reduction of

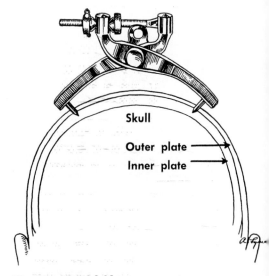

Fig. 321. Crutchfield tongs apparatus.

fractures and dislocations of the cervical vertebrae. In some instances it may be necessary to use rather large amounts of weight to reduce the fracture. Progress of reduction is checked roentgenographically, and when complete reduction has been obtained the amount of weight is usually decreased.

The nursing care of the patient with traction in the skull is not as difficult as it is when some type of chin or occipital halter is used. When the latter is used, the skin tends to break down easily because of the large amount of weight that must be used to obtain reduction of the fracture. Furthermore, turning the patient is not permissible since traction efficiency must be sacrificed during the process. With the Crutchfield skull traction, however, careful turning of the patient for back care is permitted. (Permission and instruction pertaining to turning should be obtained from the attending surgeon.) The patient must be watched for signs of cyanosis during the process or for dyspnea that might indicate further damage to the cord.

Body alignment should be carefully maintained during the turning process,

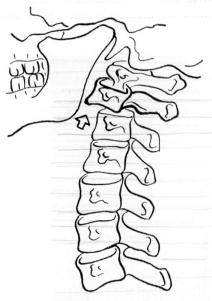

Fig. 320. Dislocation of the cervical spine. (From Kenney, William C., and Larson, Carroll B.: Orthopedics for the general practitioner, St. Louis, 1957, The C. V. Mosby Co.)

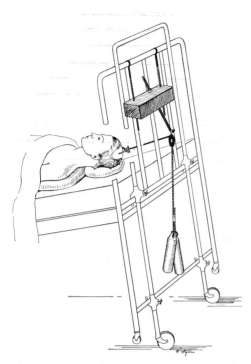

Fig. 322. Crutchfield tongs. Head should be low and shoulders high. The upper end of the bed should be elevated. Traction weights of 25 to 35 pounds may be applied safely and comfortably.

and the patient should be turned as though he were a log and would not bend. Head, shoulders, and pelvis must be turned simultaneously. Flexion of the cervical spine is not permitted. A pillow should be placed in front of the patient's chest to support the shoulder and arm, and another should be placed between the thighs and legs to prevent sagging of the hip. Either of these conditions, sagging of the hip or shoulder in the side-lying position, will inevitably alter the position of the spine and should be avoided.

It is sometimes necessary to provide spinal hyperextension in conjunction with the skeletal tongs. For this two mattresses may be placed on the bed; one in the usual position and another— the upper one, which may be a rubber or air mattress—so placed that it reaches only to the patient's shoulders. Hyperextension of the cervical spine is obtained by allowing the head to fall back over the upper mattress and rest on the lower one. The same effect can be obtained by placing a firm pillow under

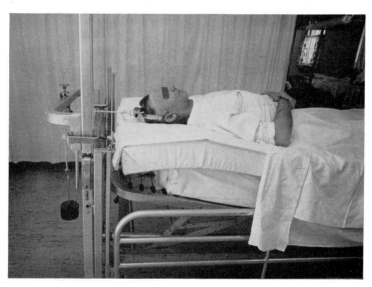

Fig. 323. Vinke tongs applied to patient with cervical fracture. Note arrangement of mattresses to provide for hyperextension of the cervical region.

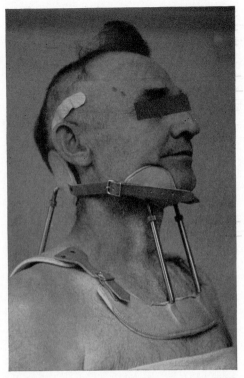

Fig. 324. After removal of the Crutchfield tongs the patient is fitted with a brace designed to provide support and immobilization of the cervical vertebrae.

the patient's back from the sacrum to the shoulders. A thin pillow or pad may be used for comfort under the head.

The stab wounds through which the tongs are introduced into the skull are usually dressed with small circular sponges saturated with collodion to make a waterproof dressing. Very little danger of infection exists, although occasionally this does occur. Inspection of the wound dressings should be made each day, but the dressings are not disturbed without order of the surgeon. Tightening of the tongs is usually done by the surgeon or his assistants.

Although such emergencies are not common, skeletal traction in the skull has sometimes become loose and actual slipping out of the tongs may result. For this reason a set of alternate equip-

ment should be kept on hand that the nurse may apply until she can reach the physician. A chin halter, a spreader, some rope, and a few sandbags will suffice to maintain hyperextension until the tongs can be replaced in the skull.

Changing the bed linen is easier if two drawsheets are used instead of one full-length sheet. Pillowcases or towels may be placed at either side of the head. When these are soiled, they can be changed without disturbing the head position. The patient in cervical traction will need help with his diet, and he needs food that can be chewed easily. Because of the large amount of weight applied, the jaws may become sore and ache. Swallowing in this position is difficult, and care should be taken to avoid choking. If choking occurs, the head cannot be raised or turned. Therefore, it is advisable to have a suction machine available. Because the amount of movement permitted the patient in head traction is markedly limited, deep breathing and coughing need to be encouraged and supervised at frequent intervals throughout the day. This will help considerably in preventing lung congestion.

During this period of bed rest active or passive exercise of the arms and legs (as prescribed by the surgeon) is necessary to ensure maintenance of normal joint motion. Time passes slowly for this patient. Prism glasses may help him to read and to watch television or other activities in the area.

When roentgenograms indicate that sufficient healing has taken place to permit ambulation, the patient is fitted with a neck brace. When the traction is removed and the brace is applied, it must be worn continuously until permission for its removal is given by the surgeon. Ambulation for this patient must be a slow and gradual process. Assistance

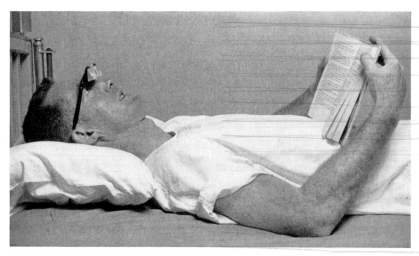

Fig. 325. The use of prism glasses makes reading and watching television possible for the patient who cannot have the backrest elevated.

with walking is necessary until all danger of falling is past.

FRACTURES OF THE PELVIS

Cause. Fractures of the pelvis usually result from crushing between two forces with considerable violence.

Anatomy. The pelvis is a ring composed of the sacrum posteriorly, the ilia on either side, and the symphysis pubis in front. The weakest spots in this ring are the rami of the pubis. Most of the pelvic fractures occur in the rami, but they may occur in the ilia with displacement of the pelvis.

Complications. At the time of injury there may be damage to the pelvic organs as a result of the direct force or spicules of bone. The urethra is most frequently damaged; the bladder is next. There may be damage to the rectum. If the bladder is full at the time of injury, damage is more likely.

Problem. There are two main reasons for restoration of the symmetric ring of the pelvis: (1) to avoid future abnormal strain on the sacroiliac joints and (2) to restore the normal birth canal in women.

Treatment. Overriding of the frag-

ments may be overcome by the use of Buck's extension or skeletal traction on the leg of the fractured side. Traction automatically causes abduction and pull at the same time, although side traction may also be necessary.

When sufficient correction has been obtained through traction, a hip spica of plaster of paris is applied with the hip in abduction. It is usually necessary to apply it only down to the knee.

Healing period. Healing usually takes place in 6 to 8 weeks. Weight bearing

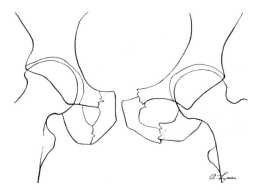

Fig. 326. Fracture of both rami of both sides of the pubis. Note the asymmetry of the pelvis. Abduction of both thighs is necessary for correction.

on the affected side should be avoided during that time. Crutches may be used. Patients with this injury are likely to have persistent trouble in the sacroiliac joint. It is wise to use some form of pelvic girdle for protection during the early months of weight bearing to prevent permanent damage to the sacroiliac joint.

Nursing care. Under the classification of pelvic fractures are fractures of the ilium, pubic bone, sacroiliac, and acetabulum. They are of varying degrees of severity, but in all the nurse should be aware of the danger of internal injuries, particularly to the bladder, urethra, or rectum. A urine specimen is usually ordered immediately by catheterization. A soft rubber catheter should be used—never one made of metal. A rectal examination is also carried out by the physician to rule out injury to the lower bowel.

The most common fracture of the pelvis is that occurring in the pubic bone, and it is often caused by a compression between two solid objects or a fall in which the patient lands on the hip.

After reduction of a fracture of this nature the patient may be placed in a canvas sling attached to an overhead frame. Buck's extension is usually applied to the leg of the injured side. Compression of the pelvis is obtained by fastening the ends of the canvas sling together over the front of the patient. If compression is not desired, the canvas sling may have wooden spreaders at either side and be supported by separate ropes and pulleys on the overhead frame. The hammock should be about 5 feet long and 2 feet wide. It should extend from the upper border of the lumbar vertebrae to midthigh. Just enough weight to keep the pelvis off the mattress is used, and for nursing care the hammock may be pushed or folded back over the buttocks. This type of hammock-sling accomplishes lateral compression on the sides of the pelvis, forcing the separated pubis together at the symphysis. It is usually continued for about 6 weeks.

When there is no separation of the fragments, the patient may be placed on a hard bed or Bradford frame with

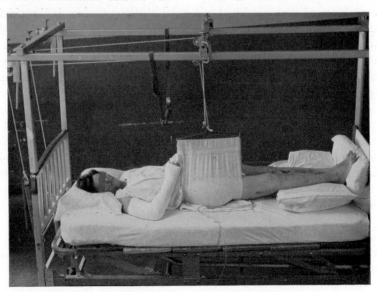

Fig. 327. Pelvic sling used in the treatment of fractures of the pelvis.

Buck's extension applied to the legs. Unless orders are specifically given to turn the patient, back care is given by elevating the patient either with the aid of an overhead trapeze or with the assistance of another nurse.

Scultetus or abdominal binders are sometimes used instead of hammocks, particularly if there has been no involvement of the acetabulum. The binder should extend from the iliac crest to 2 or 3 inches below the pubis. If the binder is made of canvas, it is wise to insert a lining of silence cloth or other soft material between the skin and the binder. Instructions given for application of the binder in different types of pelvic fractures are usually as follows: (1) For fracture of the iliac bone, the binder is applied without snugness. (2) For fracture of the ischium or pubic bones, it is applied snugly. (3) If there is separation of the symphysis pubis, the binder is applied as tightly as possible.

Fractures and dislocations of the hip, including nursing care

FRACTURES ABOUT THE HIP

Cause. Fractures in the upper end of the femur may be near the head. These are called intracapsular. If they occur further out in the neck of the femur, they are called extracapsular, and if they occur still further out in the region of the trochanters, they are called trochanteric or intertrochanteric. To the laity, all of these are broken hips, but to the orthopedic surgeon, they are very different in regard to treatment and prognosis.

Anatomy. The hip is a ball-and-socket joint. To allow free ranges of motion the capsule that surrounds the joint is quite flexible and extends a considerable distance out along the neck. This means that the blood vessels that supply nutrition must enter outside the point of attachment of the capsule. Unfortunately, the ligament between the head and the acetabulum (cotyloid ligament) carries little or no circulation to the head. Most of the circulation enters the neck of the femur through nutrient foramina and reaches the head inside the bone. Fractures of the neck cause a tearing of these vessels, and the head within the capsule may be left with little or no circulation. This anatomic fact is the chief cause of the percentage of nonunions that occur in spite of perfect reduction (20% to 25%). This is also the cause of the necrosis and disintegration that may occur in the head of the femur. When the fragments have been separated by the injury, the strong gluteus medius muscle pulls the distal portion upward. The iliopsoas tends to rotate outward, as does the gluteus maximus. Immediately after the accident, therefore, the leg is usually found in the position of helpless eversion. There is shortening of the extremity and considerable pain and muscle spasm on any attempt to move the patient.

Reduction. Reduction is accomplished by applying traction, preferably the Rus-

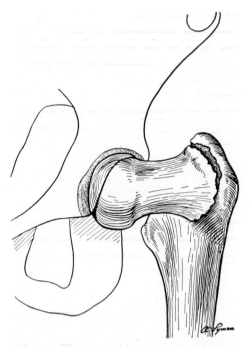

Fig. 328. Fracture at base of neck of femur (intertrochanteric type). Note decrease in angle of neck and eversion. The lesser trochanter shows up prominently denoting outward rotation.

sell traction (Fig. 86), maintaining the alignment of the knee in a neutral plane and the hip in flexion. About 10 pounds of weight are used (20 pounds' pull). Reduction usually takes place automatically in 3 to 5 days. During this time the patient is likely to have a great deal of abdominal distress and possibly some difficulty in voiding, as do patients with spinal injuries. Sedatives that tend to make elimination more sluggish should be avoided if possible. By the injury, the patient has in most cases been forced abruptly from an active to a completely inactive existence, adding to the digestive difficulties. Foods that tend to form gas should be avoided.

Treatment. After reduction by traction or by the manipulative method of Leadbetter, the type of treatment must be determined by the proximity of the fracture to the head, the estimated amount of damage to the circulation to the head, and the general condition of the patient.

When there is a fair amount of neck connected with the head fragment, nailing the femur with a three-flanged Smith-Petersen nail offers many advantages. Complete union may be possible in 5 to 8 months.

After the nailing the patient may be allowed in a wheelchair for well-tolerated intervals on the first or second day. In a few weeks he may be allowed on crutches without weight bearing. Weight bearing should not be allowed for 3 to 5 months and then only if roentgenographic examination shows sufficient union.

When the fracture is very near the head or when circulatory damage ap-

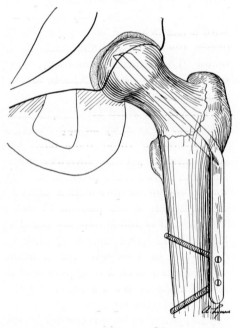

Fig. 329. Open reduction of intertrochanteric fracture with Neufeld nail inserted into neck and head and down shaft of femur with divergent screws. The nail is a one-piece stainless steel nail with v-shaped flanges into the neck and head.

pears to be severe, it is advisable, if the patient's condition is satisfactory, to treat the fracture by bone graft. The graft may be taken from the upper part of the same femur, from either tibia, or from the bone bank. It is passed through a drill hole of appropriate size, through the trochanter and the neck, and well into the head. In addition to acting as a circulatory stimulus, it also acts as a means of fixation. Beaded wires or a Smith-Petersen nail may be used for better stabilization, and when these are used the cast may be avoided. Otherwise, after the operation a plaster of paris spica is applied from the axilla to the toes. Union usually occurs, sufficient for bivalving the cast and exercise, in 10 to 12 weeks. Union sufficient for weight bearing does not usually occur sooner than 4 to 6 months.

Intertrochanteric fractures almost invariably heal. With the strong pull of the muscles, however, they tend to heal with a loss of the normal angulation between the shaft and the neck of the femur. This leads to deformity. There is shortening, external rotation, and adduction.

Problem. To avoid deformity the fracture must be held by an apparatus that will overcome these tendencies until solid union is present. Intertrochanteric fractures have been a problem from the standpoint of hospitalization and also of the health of the patient, because a safe amount of union may not occur before 10 to 12 weeks, and complete union requires 4 to 8 months. The treatment of choice has been a long period of immobilization in the Russell traction or in an adduction hip spica cast.

Several types of apparatus for internal fixation have been devised. Most notable of these are the Neufeld angled nail, the apparatus of Austin Moore, and the multiple pin technique of Roger Anderson and others. When the Neufeld nail

or the Smith-Petersen nail with the McLaughlin attachment is inserted into the neck of the femur after reduction, the handle is fastened to the shaft of the femur by means of thread-cutting screws. The patients may be allowed to be in a wheelchair in 2 to 3 days and to go through the same routine of convalescence as those patients with nailing of fractures of the neck of the femur.

Early ambulation. The early ambulation of postoperative patients as described by Leithauser cannot be entirely adapted to orthopedic patients because his problem is concerned with abdominal operations whereas ours is concerned chiefly with conditions involving the extremities (see Fractures about the hip). Fracture treatment requires a complete immobilization of the part. The general condition of the patient must, of course, be taken into consideration. The mobilization of patients as related to their general health must be considered first. The things most feared are (1) atelectasis, (2) embolism, and (3) thrombosis. Most of these can be avoided by early ambulation. This does not necessarily mean getting the patient out of bed immediately after operation, but it does mean putting the patient in the most erect position possible after recovery from anesthesia and frequent turning after operation.

The patient does not feel the development of lung complications, and the doctor may be unable to detect rales until there is a cough. The cough may be painful and the patient may resist it, but the accumulation of mucus in the bronchi may still be present in the form of increasingly solid masses. The longer the process goes on the more difficult it is to get rid of the plugs by coughing. Often, coughing causes pain at the operative site, and the patient resists the coughing mechanism. The erect position of the body stimulates the elimination of these bronchial plugs. Hence, it is especially important in postoperative patients to avoid this serious complication by early institution of the erect position of the body. If standing is possible it is preferred, but this is not always tolerable to the orthopedic patient, especially if he is in a hip spica or body cast. In such patients frequent change of position from back to abdomen and, if therapeutically possible, to the side is necessary.

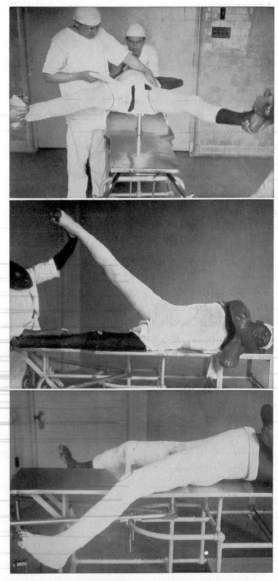

Fig. 330. Casts used in fracture of the femur, showing abduction, internal rotation, and slight extension of the limb; sometimes called the Whitman cast, or the method of external fixation in fracture of the femur. (From Conwell, H. E., and Reynolds, F. C.: Key and Conwell's management of fractures, dislocations, and sprains, ed. 7, St. Louis, 1961, The C. V. Mosby Co.)

Internal fixation in fractures of the neck of the femur and intertrochanteric fractures of the hip has made it possible to mobilize patients at a very early period. The patient who is classified as a poor surgical risk may be up in a chair as early as the following day, occasionally the same day. Postoperative deaths have been cut by more than half, and the danger of operation upon the aged person has been minimized.

Nursing care. Since fracture of the upper end or neck of the femur, the hip fracture as it is commonly called, presents more nursing problems than any other type of femoral fracture, emphasis will be placed on the nursing care required for this condition. Fracture of the femur at other levels will not vary greatly from this.

The methods of reduction and of maintaining reduction are still complex and various. The patient may be placed in a hip spica or well-leg cast, he may be placed in one of a half-dozen types of suspension traction, or he may be treated surgically by internal fixation. If he is obviously moribund, treatment may be palliative, with simple traction of 10 to 15 pounds applied merely to relieve the pain and muscle spasm and to enable him to be moved in bed without too much discomfort.

Probably the most common method of treatment in the past was the method of Whitman. It is sometimes spoken of as the method of external fixation, in contrast to later methods of internal fixation. In this treatment a double hip spica cast was used, extending from the nipple line to the toes on the affected side and usually to the knee on the unaffected side. Since the care of patients in casts is discussed in detail in another chapter, it will not be repeated here, except to emphasize the necessity for sealing cast edges so that plaster crumbs are not allowed to get inside the cast.

Raw cast edges are extremely hazardous for the skin of elderly patients.

The Whitman cast made frequent turning of the patient possible and the ever-present danger of congestion of the lungs was obviated somewhat by conscientious care. It was possible in some cases to get the patient on his feet with crutches soon after reduction.

Nursing care in internal fixation. Internal fixation apparatus (the Smith-Petersen flanged nail, the Neufeld nail, the Jewett nail, or the Austin Moore pins, to mention only a few) has become the accepted method of treating hip fractures. Nursing problems after such procedures are greatly simplified. The operation itself is not considered a serious threat unless the patient is in very poor physical condition. The complications of old age, however, such as kidney dysfunction, cardiac impairment,

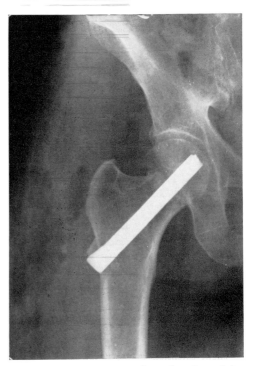

Fig. 331. Smith-Petersen flanged nail used for internal fixation of fractures of the neck of the femur.

and hypostatic pneumonia, make any operation somewhat hazardous and should not be lost sight of in any method of treatment.

Aftertreatment when internal fixation is used may vary considerably. Buck's extension or some type of suspension traction in combination with a Thomas ring splint may be applied for a brief period. The patient is usually given much latitude in regard to movement in bed. As early as the first postoperative evening, the patient may be turned for back care. If turning is done toward the extremity operated upon, the bed supplies a type of splint, and the patient will be fairly comfortable. There is no danger to bone fragments involved in moving about in bed, for fixation is complete. Such traction as is employed is usually a temporary measure for overcoming muscle spasm and making the patient more comfortable.

In turning a patient after a recent fixation, when he is somewhat apprehensive about being moved, it is usually preferable to stand on the side of the fractured hip and place the hands on the opposite hip and shoulder by reaching across the patient. He may then be gently turned onto the fractured extremity and toward the nurse. Segmental bending should be avoided. When the patient is turned on the unaffected leg, the fractured limb should be kept at the same level as the trunk. This can be accomplished by the use of pillows placed between the legs before the turning process is begun. Carelessness in supporting the uppermost limb will be a source of considerable discomfort to the patient. If the patient desires further support as he turns, he may steady himself by placing his upper hand on the nurse's shoulder. If the fractured leg is suspended in a sling or splint after internal fixation, the patient is usually turned on the normal leg and firm pillows are used to support the leg in the suspension after the patient is turned.

Postoperatively, if there are no contraindications and the patient has not been placed in traction, the surgeon usually requests that elderly patients be up in a chair the morning after surgery. There is no weight bearing on the affected extremity; the patient is lifted or assisted to the chair. This procedure alone does much to prevent postoperative pneumonia.

Many physicians instruct the patient to begin knee movement the day after fixation of the hip. The patient is turned to the side of the fractured extremity so that the knee may be flexed while the hip is kept in the extended position. There may be muscle spasm in the muscles of the thigh, particularly in the quadriceps, when this is first attempted. Nurses should seek complete instruc-

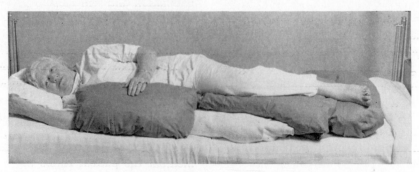

Fig. 332. Good side-lying position for the patient who has had an internal fixation of a femoral neck fracture. The pillows between the thighs prevent adduction of the involved limb.

tions from the surgeon regarding this treatment and the rate of progress expected.

If secondary deformities are to be prevented, maintenance of good body alignment and frequent changes of position are mandatory. Flexion and adduction contractures of the hips, flexion contractures of the knees, and drop-foot deformity may develop in a relatively short time if the elderly patient is permitted to remain in one position for long periods. Full extension of the hip and knee joints should be encouraged and maintained part of the time. In the side-lying position pillows should be used to support the uppermost limb. This will help to prevent adduction contractures. Many of these patients seem to be more comfortable with the extremity supported by a pillow, with the hip and knee flexed and the leg in external rotation. This pillow must be removed at frequent intervals and the patient encouraged to extend the hip and knee. Some provision should be made to prevent drop foot and external rotation of the limb during the patient's days in bed. A bedroom slipper with a thin strip of wood, 1 inch by 8 inches, nailed to the heel will effectively prevent outward rotation of the leg. A footboard or pillow may be used to prevent the development of an equinus deformity.

Care and prevention of complications

Pneumonia. A high percentage of the patients with fractured hips are elderly. The problems involved in this type of nursing are geriatric as well as surgical in nature. Many complications of advanced age may be present, including cardiovascular disease, renal dysfunction, diabetes, and obesity. Hypostatic pneumonia is always a threat if these patients are put to bed even for short periods. We are told that one half of the deaths that occur after fracture of the femur in elderly patients are brought about by pneumonia. For this reason, prophylactic antibiotic therapy is sometimes instituted after fractures and continued for a week or longer. Frequent turning, elevation of the head of the bed, protection from drafts, and solicitude in keeping the patient well covered during bathing and turning are essential nursing measures. This patient should be encouraged to breathe deeply and to cough up mucus. Frequent observation must be made to detect evidences of beginning cyanosis and dyspnea. Another common cause of death after fracture of the femur in elderly patients is thrombophlebitis with embolus. As a prophylactic measure against this, Dicumarol may be given 10 to 14 days after the fracture if the patient is being kept at bed rest.

Prevention of decubitus ulcers. Skin care for the older patient is of the utmost importance. A daily bath and the use of strong soaps may increase the dryness of his skin and tend to cause discomfort. A complete bath every other day or twice a week is usually sufficient. Frequent cleansing of the hands, however, and of the perineum and buttock's region is essential in the care of the elderly person. The use of baby oil or lotions will aid in preventing dryness and irritation of the skin. Frequent massage of the buttock's region improves circulation and will help to prevent the development of decubitus ulcers.

Maintaining a clean dry bed is essential if pressure areas are to be prevented. If the patient is very old, if evidences of chronic malnutrition are present, or if there is circulatory impairment as a result of arteriosclerosis, the fight to prevent pressure areas must be particularly vigilant. It must be begun the moment the patient enters the hospital. Patients of this type are not usually placed in an apparatus that would make turning them too difficult, and the responsibility for seeing that decubitus ulcers do not develop is completely in the hands of the nurse. Where circulatory impairment is present, it is an extremely difficult problem. Nothing, of course, will be as beneficial as frequent changes of position. This means that the patient must be turned every 2 hours or even more often. Rubber rings must be used with caution because a too highly inflated ring sometimes serves to cut off circulation in the buttock's area. An air mattress may be useful in preventing excessive pressure at any one point of the body. Airfoam sponge rubber under threatened areas has proved very helpful in preventing pressure sores on the sacrum and heels, and unclipped sheepskin is also excellent for this purpose. The sheepskin should be washed frequently with a mild soap and water, rinsed carefully, and dried in the sun to keep it soft and pliable.

Gastrointestinal disturbances. Obstinate constipation is almost invariably present in these patients. The management of this feature can be extremely troublesome if strong cathartics have been used too frequently during the early course of immobilization. Distension is not infrequent, and rectal tubes and hot fomentations or stupes may sometimes be necessary to overcome this. Careful attention to the patient's diet for roughage, vitamins, and elimination of foods that cause distress will help to overcome constipation. Enemas may be necessary occasionally, and a laxative may be ordered as needed. Attention to regularity is, of course, essential.

Nutritional problems. A large number of these patients will have eating problems. They have no teeth and are unable to see or hear well. They have definite food likes and dislikes, and it is difficult for them to understand hospital routines and methods. The thoughtful nurse can help to make mealtime a pleasant occasion for these older patients.

Because the rate of repair in fractures has been shown to be greatly influenced by deficiency diseases and malnutrition that are so often present in elderly patients, considerable thought must be given to the diet to include the necessary food elements. Sufficient vitamin and protein intake is particularly important. To build tissue resistance and hasten repair protein supplements may be given. Protein hydrolysates and amino acid mixtures are procurable for this purpose when the patient is unable to eat sufficient foods containing these substances. Vitamins B and C are also considered important in fracture healing. If these patients are unable to take sufficient diet orally, supplementary feedings containing the essential proteins and vitamins may be given in a formula through a polyethylene tube. The polyethylene tube is a small plastic tube that is inserted through the nostril into the stomach. This tube is taped to the nose and is left in place.

It must be remembered, also, that anything that affects the patient's general condition will be likely to affect the healing of his fracture. Age, of course, plays a large part in the rate at which a fracture will heal. A fracture of the femur in a very young baby will heal firmly in 4 weeks, whereas in a person 50 years of age or older the time required may be 3 or 4 months or longer. As has been stated, deficiency diseases, cachexia, and senile osteoporosis will definitely retard the rate of bone union. Blood chemistry determinations are ordered by the physician when the progress of healing is slow. Serum calcium of 10 to 12 mg. per 100 ml. of blood and phosphorus concentration of 3.5 to 4 mg. are considered normal. Milk and a calcium medication or a parathyroid solution and synthetic vitamin D are sometimes ordered. Vitamin D is usually considered not to be effective unless a sufficient intake of phosphorus-containing foods is given.

Urologic complications. Elderly patients are particularly prone to develop urologic complications during a period of immobilization. This is sometimes caused by an unwillingness to take sufficient fluids and to an already existing renal impairment. Scantiness of output, discomfort on voiding, concentrated urine, suppression, incontinence, or edema should be reported to the physician at once. Intake and output should be estimated daily in elderly patients with fracture of the femur until it has been ascertained that kidney function is normal.

All patients, whether young or old, are in danger of developing renal stones if they are extensively immobilized for a considerable period of time. This is true whether the immobilizing apparatus is a cast or traction or merely continuous bed rest. Intelligent nursing care can play an important part in diminishing this danger. A large fluid output is essential to overcome renal stasis and to ensure a steady flow of urine. The nurse will need to encourage the patient to take an adequate diet and increased amounts of fluids. This is not always an easy task since the appetite is often very sluggish. Furthermore, the patient must be moved frequently and with sufficient variation in bed or chair posture that no part of the urinary tract is left undrained for too long a time.

In addition to these measures some type of chemotherapy may be ordered to combat the development of stones. The regime described is usually continued for as long as 3 months after the patient is ambulatory, and roentgenograms every 3 to 4 months thereafter may be ordered. Any symptoms of pain or distress referable to the urinary tract should be reported at once. Renal stones may occur as early as a month after recumbency.

Mental aspects in the nursing care of the patient with a fractured hip. Frequently the older patient with a fractured hip becomes disoriented. The pain and shock suffered coupled with a strange environment are sufficient to cause mental confusion. This confusion may not be apparent in the daytime, but at night the patient will attempt to get out of bed and his speech will be incoherent. The nurse must realize that this may be expected and that she should provide side rails or other protection for her patient.

Elderly patients with fracture of the hip rarely escape serious mental depression. The prospect of inactivity is in itself a heavy burden to bear, and when it is accompanied by financial worry, as it almost always is, it is extremely difficult to prevent attitudes of depression and melancholy. Furthermore, these patients frequently have a pessimistic outlook regarding their own recovery. The nurse caring for them needs to develop considerable understanding and sympathy for their problems. She will be confronted by sessions of tears and hopelessness, not once but periodically during the time the patient is inactive. Good mental hygiene demands that the patient be given something to do, and constructive occupational therapy is almost indispensable in caring for these patients. Although the trained occupational therapist is highly desirable for assisting with the daily program of the fracture patient, the bedside nurse can help by urging him to do as much as he can for himself, even though he is confined to a chair. It is not always easy to secure cooperation, because considerable apathy and indifference may exist. If the nurse makes it clear to the patient that her desire to have him do things for himself stems from her interest in his progress, he will be much more likely to cooperate with her and less likely to feel neglected when he is urged to care for his own wants as far as it is possible for him to do so. Many physicians order a series of gentle bed exercises to be carried out under the nurse's direction several times during the day to prevent loss of muscle tone and to prepare the patient for successful ambulation at as early a date as possible.

Preparation for weight bearing. The amount of time the patient will be kept without weight bearing varies according to the progress of union. It may be from 12 to 16 weeks or longer. As has been stated, bed exercises are frequently prescribed. These may be muscle-setting exercises for the abdominal, gluteal, and quadriceps muscles, dorsiflexion and inversion exercises for the feet, and rhythmic breathing exercises. Exercises to strengthen the arms and shoulder muscles are usually added before the patient is ready to walk to prepare these muscles for crutch walking. But since the period of inactivity is long, considerable encouragement may be necessary to motivate the patient to continue the exercises over the period when he is nonambulatory. Explanation of the importance of these exercises may need to be repeated at frequent intervals.

Even though exercises are faithfully carried out, there is still a tremendous hill for the patient to climb. Unexpected weaknesses and stiffness of many parts of the body that were not involved in the fracture may be present. These will alarm and depress the patient if he is not forewarned of them. For instance, it is not uncommon to have the patient complain that his knee feels worse than the hip that was fractured. This may be a source of great concern to him, and nurses should take the opportunity to teach the patient something about the mechanics of the quadriceps muscle and its action on the knee and hip in walking.

If the nurse can help the patient understand that his weaknesses and the stiffness in his joints are the natural outcome of his fracture and inactivity and are not a permanent sequela to it, she will aid greatly in bolstering his failing courage. She must be very careful not to do anything that will make him more apprehensive. Sudden jarring of the bed, for instance, will be enough to undermine his confidence considerably. Any rough or hurried movement while carrying out the prescribed exercise for increasing motion in hip or knee or any enthusiastic increase in the range of motion beyond which the patient has previously gone will also be conducive to much loss of courage. Furthermore, acute muscle spasm around the hip will make it impossible to do anything further in the way of mobilization at that time. Support should be placed under the lumbar spine, the knee, and at the foot, and the limb should not be allowed to lie in outward rotation.

Helping the patient to be ambulatory. Physical therapy treatments given by a trained therapist can at this time make the ordeal easier for the patient. Heat, special types of massage, and exercise will aid in promoting normal circulation in the injured limb and will hasten absorption of traumatic exudate. In addition, pain and discomfort are lessened through release of the protective muscle spasm around the joint, and joint function necessary for walking is reestablished. If such treatments must be given by the nurse, they should first be demonstrated by the physician, and every detail of the treatment should be clearly pointed out.

When the order has been given for the patient to sit on the side of the bed

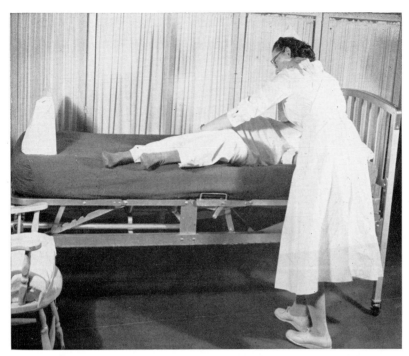

Fig. 333. Assisting the bed patient to a sitting position. The patient is turned to her side with hips and knees flexed. The nurse places one arm beneath the patient's shoulders and the other one under the knees. She stands close to the bed with one foot forward, knees and hips flexed slightly, and trunk in good alignment. Note that in this picture to show the position of the patient the nurse has stepped to one side.

preparatory to being up, he should first roll onto the side of the sound leg. When this has been accomplished, the knee and hip of the normal leg should be flexed to a right angle, approximating the position of the body in sitting. If the patient is able to partially flex the hip and knee of the affected side, this should be done, but it must be remembered that this leg will require the most gentle handling at all times and that the joints should never be forced beyond the point of pain. Some physicians prescribe the application of an elastic bandage to the injured extremity before the patient is allowed to sit. This support prevents the troublesome edema and mottling that occur when the extremity becomes dependent.

To bring the patient to the sitting position, the nurse places one arm under the patient's shoulder and the other arm under the knees, gently swiveling the patient to the sitting position. If the fractured leg is extremely sensitive, another nurse may need to be on hand to support it.

The nurse should check her own body mechanics carefully for this procedure, being sure to assume the foot-forward position with knees and hips flexed and back straight. Considerable strain and torsion may be placed on her back if she encounters resistance from the patient, and she should be prepared for this before beginning the procedure.

The patient is pivoted, or swiveled, to the sitting position, slowly at first in order to prevent faintness. When the sitting position has been obtained, the nurse should continue to support the patient's back until he is steady. The ini-

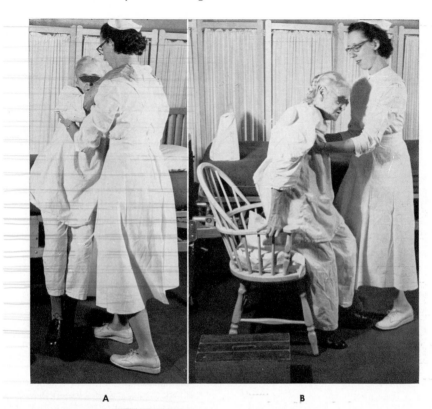

A   **B**

Fig. 334. A, When assisting an elderly patient from the bed to a chair, it is important for the nurse to know whether there is to be any weight bearing on the affected extremity. If no weight bearing is permitted, it is best not to use a footstool but to have the patient slide off the bed in the manner illustrated, taking weight on the normal extremity. A bed that can be raised and lowered is very helpful in getting orthopedic patients in and out of bed. B, The chair is placed parallel with the bed. After the patient has gained her balance in the standing position, she pivots on the normal extremity and is in position to sit in the chair. Note that the nurse has a firm grip on the patient and is in a position to support a great deal of the patient's weight without strain to her own back.

tial period of dangling is usually very short, and the patient is then returned to the side-lying position that he assumed before coming to the upright position. This dangling procedure may be ordered frequently during the day, with gradual increase of the time spent in the sitting position. The patient may be instructed to lift the chest, to practice breathing exercises, and to contract the gluteal and abdominal muscles after he has become accustomed to sitting. The almost universal tendency of the elderly patient is to sit on the side of the bed with shoulders sagging, chin on chest,

and head and shoulders drooped. Unless efforts are made to overcome this at the outset, this type of posture may become permanent.

To assist the patient to the standing position and then into a chair, the nurse should place her hands under the axillae and allow the patient to place his hands firmly on her shoulders. In this way he is assured of adequate support for his first standing experience. The chair should be parallel to the bed, and the patient is gently guided toward it by the nurse, who turns him in such a fashion that his back is toward the chair seat. If he is very weak, the nurse should flex her knees and hips sufficiently to allow the patient to retain his hold on her shoulders until he is safely seated in the chair.

Later the patient can be taught to come to a standing position from the chair without too much difficulty, and his confidence in his ability will be greatly increased once he has accomplished this. The chair must be steady, propped against the bed or wall. The patient is instructed to bend forward from the hips, to place the unaffected leg backward until an acute angle of the knee is formed, and to have the knee on the affected side flexed as much as possible with the foot flat on the floor. The patient places his hands on the armrests of the chair with the elbows slightly flexed to assist in elevating himself. Weight is taken entirely by the normal foot as the patient comes to the erect position. If the crutches are near at hand, the patient can steady himself with one hand on the back of the chair as he reaches for the crutches with the other. Care is to be taken that no weight is borne on the injured leg.

Instruction in crutch walking for the elderly patient is usually delayed until partial weight bearing can be permitted. Then the three-point gait is taught. This delay in crutch walking is necessary because the danger of falling and of bearing weight on the affected extremity is too great.

When ambulation and weight bearing are permitted, the use of a walker may be preferred to crutches. The elderly patient feels more secure with the walker and is less likely to fall.

Home care after fracture of the hip. After a fracture of the hip there is one question that always seems to arise and that causes the patient much worry: "Where does he go when he leaves the hospital?" With the increasing number

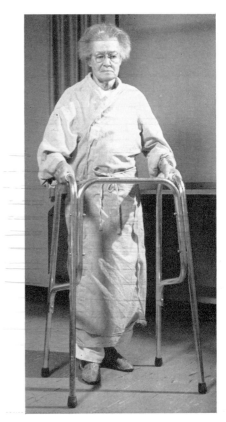

Fig. 335. A lightweight adjustable aluminum walker may be used by the elderly patient when ambulation is permitted.

of elderly persons in our population, the need for adequate convalescent care has become a major problem. The patient with a fractured hip can no longer take care of his needs and be independent. His elderly mate is physically unable to assume this added responsibility. It will be 10 or 12 weeks before he is able to begin weight bearing, barring any complications. We know that good care is essential during this convalescent period if the elderly person is to maintain his strength and the desire to walk again. Will some member of his family be able to care for him, or will plans for care in a nursing home be arranged? Whatever plans are made for his convalescent care, the assistance that the public health nurse gives the family and patient at this time may mean the difference between failure and success—a patient who later is able to walk, care for his own needs, and live a somewhat independent life.

Nonunion and aseptic necrosis. It is necessary that provision be made for adequate follow-up care of the patient with a fractured hip. Early detection of loss of position, nonunion, or aseptic necrosis makes it possible to institute corrective measures. When nonunion persists after adequate reduction, the surgeon may wish to insert a tibial bone graft in the freshened nail tract; or, when aseptic necrosis has taken place, he may wish to replace the head of the femur with a Vitallium prosthesis. The ball part of the prosthesis fits into the acetabulum. Some studies of this last surgical procedure have been encouraging. Others report that in some instances there is bone absorption resulting in loosening of the prosthesis and loss of functional results. After the insertion of a prosthesis, the patient is placed in balanced suspension traction or a hip spica cast for a period of 7 to 10 days.

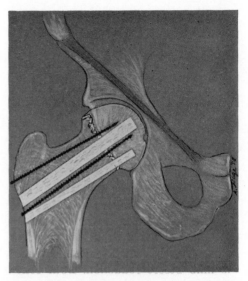

Fig. 337. Bone graft with threaded Steinmann pin fixation may be used in the absence of union after nailing procedure. (From Ziffren, Sidney E.: Management of the aged surgical patient, Chicago, 1960, Year Book Medical Publishers, Inc.)

During this time good nursing care is of the utmost importance if complications so common to the elderly patient are to be prevented. After removal of the traction or cast, crutch walking (three-point gait) with partial weight bearing is instituted, and the patient is encouraged to resume normal activity as nearly as possible.

TRAUMATIC DISLOCATIONS OF THE HIP

There are several types of hip dislocations, but the most common ones are posterior dislocation with or without fracture of the acetabulum and anterior or obturator dislocation.

Cause. Posterior dislocation with or without fracture of the acetabulum is caused by force against the knee with the hip flexed and adducted (dashboard dislocations). There may be damage to the sciatic nerve.

Anterior or obturator dislocations are caused by forced abduction of the thigh

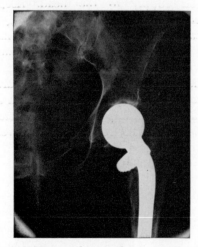

Fig. 336. Hip prosthesis. When aseptic necrosis of the head of the femur occurs after a fracture of the neck of the femur, the prosthesis may be inserted, thus making weight bearing possible.

with the hip in flexion. The head of the femur is displaced forward and enters the depression of the obturator foramen. There may be damage to the obturator nerve with weakness or paralysis of the adductor muscles.

Symptoms and signs. It is characteristic of the posterior upward dislocation that the patient cannot abduct, extend, or externally rotate the limb. This is in contrast to fractures about the hip joint. There is a mass (the head of the femur) palpable on the ilium.

With the obturator dislocation the mass is felt in the groin, and the patient is unable to abduct or internally rotate the limb before reduction. Both conditions are very painful during the period of dislocation because of muscle spasm.

Reduction and problem. In posterior dislocation, general anesthesia is necessary. Reduction can be accomplished by placing the patient on his back and exerting manual traction with the hip in full flexion (surgeon's shoulder under patient's knee). Relaxation is essential. If this method fails the method of Lorenz for congenital dislocations may be successful, that is, extreme flexion and abduction to bring the head into the cotyloid notch, then further abduction combined with a decrease in flexion to force the head upward into the acetabulum.

In obturator dislocation exertion of forceful traction in the line of deformity and then adduction as the head engages in the acetabulum accomplish reduction. All reductions of dislocations of the hip are usually accompanied by relaxation of the muscles, freedom of movement, and great relief of pain. A thud can usually be heard and felt as the head enters the acetabulum. The clinical signs should not be relied upon to indicate adequate reduction. Evidence should be established by roentgenograms taken in two directions.

Treatment. Hip dislocations are comparatively easily treated after reduction. It is comforting to the patient because of ligamentous injuries to have Buck's extension (with about 5 to 10 pounds of weight) for 2 or 3 weeks—long enough for ligamentous healing. During this time daily exercises of all joints should be carried out as soon as the patient is able to tolerate them.

In fractures of the acetabulum the same treatment is used, but traction should be prolonged for 2 to 3 additional weeks. A wheelchair, crutches, and gradual weight bearing with crutches (then cane) follow over a period of 6 to 10 weeks.

Attention has been drawn to the possibility of permanent damage to the head of the femur as the result of ligamentous tearing and disturbance in the blood supply to the head. Aseptic necrosis may occur if the damage is great. Such necrosis may manifest itself after several years by degenerative change in the joint. There may be degeneration of the cartilage and partial or complete ankylosis. Patients with dislocations uncomplicated by fracture, however, usually recover in 6 to 8 weeks without further trouble.

Fractures of the femur, including nursing care

FRACTURE OF THE FEMUR BELOW THE TROCHANTERS

Anatomy. Fracture of the femur below the trochanters is one of the most difficult fractures to treat successfully. The fracture occurs above the stabilizing attachment of the adductor muscles so that the upper fragment is controlled entirely by the intrinsic muscles of the hip. The proximal fragment is brought into acute flexion by the action of the iliopsoas. It is brought into abduction by the gluteus medius and into external rotation by both the iliopsoas and the gluteus maximus. Consequently, it tends to project forward at a right angle to the body and to abduct and rotate outward.

Problem. The problem is to bring the controllable distal fragment into a position which will meet the position of the uncontrollable proximal fragment in flexion at about 80 degrees and abduction and external rotation.

Reduction. Reduction can often be accomplished by the Russell traction method, but it is necessary to add extra traction under the knee by an independent pulley to increase the usual flexion, and 10 to 15 pounds may be required. Lateral traction of 5 to 10 pounds may be necessary to bring the distal fragment outward to engage the proximal fragment. Alignment may be obtained and demonstrated in anteroposterior and lateral views roentgenographically. If not, additional changes in the apparatus may be made.

If alignment does not take place this way, however, some means of internal fixation may be used, such as properly arranged and fixed stainless steel pins,

Vitallium or stainless steel plates, or possibly intramedullary pins.

Healing period. Healing is slow. Solid union does not usually occur in less than 10 to 12 weeks. We are, again, frequently confronted with a hospitalization problem. Internal fixation does not always obviate the necessity of immobilization but may make the treatment of the fracture a more flexible one in regard to hospitalization and the necessity for bed treatment.

FRACTURE OF THE SHAFT OF THE FEMUR (MIDDLE THIRD)

Cause. Direct or indirect violence is the cause of fracture of the middle third of the shaft of the femur.

Anatomy. The action of the gluteus medius has some tendency to pull the upper fragment outward, and the strong pull of the adductor muscle group tends to cause outward bowing at the point of fracture. In this fracture there is a general tendency to develop inward rotation of the lower fragment and outward bowing. This, if allowed to develop, constitutes an awkward deformity and is quite disabling.

Treatment. Some form of traction is required that will maintain pull. Russell traction usually fulfills the requirements. Abduction and external rotation of the distal fragment must be maintained. Roentgenograms should be taken frequently to check the position. If there is anterior or posterior angulation or if there is inward or outward bowing, the apparatus must be adjusted with proper slings and weights to counteract and cor-

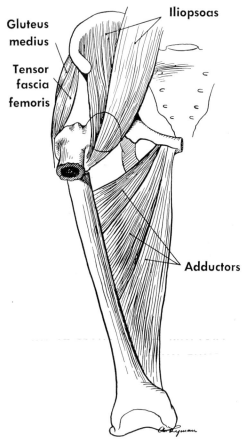

Gluteus medius

Tensor fascia femoris

Iliopsoas

Adductors

Fig. 338. Muscle action in subtrochanteric fractures of the femur.

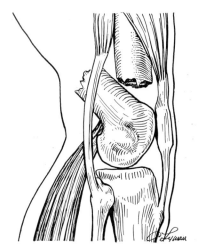

Fig. 339. Supracondylar fracture of the femur (transverse). Note the pull exerted by the gastrocnemius.

rect the tendency toward deformity. Here again the critical period is important before the callus has developed so firmly that it cannot be molded into correct alignment. Necessary correction must be made before this state occurs. Skin traction obtained by moleskin adhesive or skeletal traction obtained by use of a Kirschner wire or Steinmann pin may be used to secure the desired position of the fragments and to provide for immobilization.

Other satisfactory methods of treatment are those requiring operation. Those most commonly employed are (1) reduction and insertion of an intramedullary nail (Fig. 340), (2) reduction with internotching of the fragments so that they cannot slip off, (3) plating with slotted stainless steel or Vitallium plates and screws, and (4) distraction.

In reduction with the internotching of the fragments, stainless steel wire may be used to prevent slipping. Open reduction is followed by the application of a hip spica cast extending from the chest to the toes of the affected side with the leg in abduction and external rotation.

In plating with slotted stainless steel or Vitallium plates and screws, it must be remembered that muscular and mechanical stresses are great and that it may be necessary to have plates on two sides of the bone, preferably at right angles to each other. The screws should penetrate both cortical surfaces of the bone.

Distraction is accomplished by inserting pins above and below the fracture in such a manner that reduction is accomplished by a rachet and maintained by incorporating the pins in plaster of paris or steel bars (Haynes or Stader) so that overriding or angulation may not take place during healing. Some pressure contact must always be present to prevent nonunion.

Healing period. In children femoral shaft fractures heal quickly. There is frequently solid union in 3 to 4 weeks. In adults solid healing sufficient to avoid deformities from constant muscle pull may not take place in less than 10 to 16 weeks. The likelihood of deformity must be judged clinically according to the age of the patient, the type of the fracture, and the speed with which the individual produces callus, not only visible in the roentgenogram but also recognized clinically by its tendency to shrink and solidify.

It should be remembered that whatever the method used the speed of healing is not changed, and whatever apparatus is picked by circumstance for the individual case must be kept functioning until complete healing has occurred.

FRACTURE OF THE LOWER END OF THE FEMUR (SUPRACONDYLAR)

Cause. Direct or indirect violence causes fracture of the lower end of the femur.

Anatomy. Fracture of the lower end of the femur is a distinctive fracture because there is always a tendency toward deformity. It may be serious and permanent if the mechanical principles are not recognized. The gastrocnemius group of muscles is attached above the knee joint and between the condyles of the femur in the popliteal space. The only other muscles that influence the position of the lower fragment in this fracture are the thigh muscles, which cause overriding. Therefore, flexion occurs. This varies according to the distance of the fracture above the joint. Flexion may approach 90 degrees.

Problem. Traction on the leg must be applied with flexion of the knee joint (to release gastrocnemius pull).

Reduction. Usually reduction is accomplished by means of adhesive or skeletal traction with the knee in a flexed position.

If the fracture is of the transverse type, reduction may be accomplished immediately with the patient under anesthesia and maintained by a plaster cast with the knee in flexion. This is true also in young persons in whom there is an epiphyseal separation of the lower femoral epiphysis rather than a fracture.

Healing period. These fractures heal rather rapidly. Complete immobilization is usually necessary for only 4 to 6 weeks. Physical therapy is often valuable in restoring free motion in the joint. Full development of union and function usually takes place in 6 to 10 weeks.

FRACTURES INTO THE KNEE JOINT (FEMORAL CONDYLES)

Cause. Direct force either against the inner or the outer side of the knee joint usually causes fractures into the knee joint.

Anatomy. Such fractures may involve either condyle of the femur or may be of the plateau type involving either of the articular surfaces of the tibia. They are characterized by a tendency to produce a knock-knee (genu valgum) or bowleg (genu varum) deformity of the leg. Muscle pull plays very little part in the treatment, but the lateral and internal ligaments of the joint play a considerable part.

Problem. The contour of the joint must be restored as nearly perfect as possible, and the tendency toward deformity must be slightly overcorrected. Wherever there is damage within a joint as a result of fracture, the prognosis should be guarded, because the healing process in itself may be the source of irregularities that can lead to future irritation and disturbance of joint function.

Reduction. In some instances reduction may be accomplished spontaneously by manipulation with or without anesthesia and the position maintained by a plaster of paris cast. If the fracture is badly comminuted, the cast may need to be extended from the waist to the toes. Usually, however, it need not extend above the thigh.

Knee joint fractures heal better in traction with adhesive tape from the knee down. Often lateral traction is used to correct any tendency toward lateral deformity in the knee. This treatment has the advantage of allowing active motion of the joint during healing of the fracture, but of course it adds to the number of hospital days.

Open reduction is used in patients with severe fractures. This usually consists in the removal of small fragments that prevent apposition of the main fragments. Fixation by the use of nails or threaded wires may be necessary to hold the fragments together during healing.

Healing period. These fractures usually heal rapidly, but strength and stability are lacking for 3 or 4 months. Early motion is important in the knee joint, but protection from the development of knock-knee or bowleg deformity using a long leg brace may be necessary during the healing period of 3 to 4 months.

GENERAL TREATMENT

Use of traction in fracture of the femur. Skeletal traction and suspension applied by means of the Thomas, Hodgen, or Keller-Blake splint are frequently used for treatment of fracture of the femur. Skeletal traction is preferred to skin traction because a considerable amount of weight must be applied to overcome spasm of the thigh muscles. When reduction of the fracture has been secured, the amount of weight is reduced to prevent separation of the bone fragments. Traction must be continued until sufficient healing has taken place to permit crutch walking or until sufficient callus

has formed to permit the application of a hip spica cast. Care of the patient in traction has been discussed previously, but it should be emphasized that when traction of any kind is employed for the reduction of fracture in the aged person the likelihood of pressure areas is even greater than in the Whitman cast method. The use of the backrest to prevent pulmonary congestion means that much of the body weight is borne on the buttocks and sacrum, necessitating frequent massage of those areas. An overhead trapeze will make it possible for the patient to lift himself for back care and to be placed on the bedpan with less difficulty.

It has sometimes been considered a perplexing problem to provide for a backrest when boards are used between mattress and springs as they are on orthopedic wards. Hinged full-length boards, so constructed that the hinge coincides with the backrest elevation of the bed, are now available in many hospitals. If desired, narrow bed boards placed in stitched pockets of heavy canvas may be purchased. This type of bed board makes it possible to raise and lower the backrest as necessary. The heavy canvas also protects the hands of the hospital personnel from splinters.

Because there is evidence that a high incidence of kidney stones occurs after long periods in traction, nurses should do everything in their power to eliminate this danger. Patients in traction should have a high fluid intake and as much postural variation as is possible without disturbing the apparatus. Frequent urinalyses for patients in traction are usually considered advisable.

The child under 6 years of age with fracture of the femur is usually placed in Bryant traction for approximately 6 weeks. After this a hip spica cast is applied and is worn until roentgenograms show that there is solid union at the fracture site. Care of the patient in Bryant traction has been described previously.

Treatment by means of the well-leg splint. The Roger Anderson well-leg splint is very frequently used in treatment of subtrochanteric fractures of the femur, particularly in the elderly patient. One section of this splint is applied to the unaffected leg by means of a plaster cast that extends above the knee. A Kirschner wire or Steinmann pin is placed at the distal end of the tibia on the affected leg, and a plaster cast is applied extending to the knee. The remaining section of the splint is then attached to the Kirschner wire (or Steinmann pin). The apparatus is so constructed that screw adjustments make it possible to push the well leg upward while traction downward is made on the affected leg. This pressure and pull are exerted on the pelvis causing the well leg to be adducted and the injured leg abducted.

Textbooks on fractures claim that this method of treatment makes nursing care very simple, but as a rule nurses consider this statement a questionable assumption. The undeniable advantage, however, is that this type of treatment enables the patient to sit up in bed or in a chair very soon after the injury, thereby minimizing the danger of lung congestion. The patient may also be turned from side to side, permitting adequate drainage of the urinary system. The long immobilization of the knee joints tends to cause stiffness in the knees, but muscle tone can be maintained partly by quadriceps-setting exercises. Pressure on the medial aspect of the leg may sometimes cause thrombosis of the vessels in that area, and nurses should be alert for

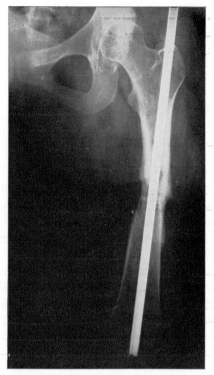

Fig. 340. Treatment of fracture of the femur by means of the intramedullary nail. Following reduction of the fracture, the nail is driven down through the shaft of the femur across the fracture site. This type of internal fixation permits increased activity and earlier ambulation.

symptoms indicating this complication.

Treatment by insertion of intramedullary nail. Fracture of the shaft of the femur may be treated by the insertion of an intramedullary nail. After open reduction the metal pin is inserted distally through the greater trochanter and across the fracture site. It extends the length of the medullary canal. With this type of fixation early mobilization and the use of adjacent joints are possible. Thus, the tendency to develop secondary deformities and contractures is not so great.

Fractures about the knee, ankle, and foot, including nursing care

FRACTURE OF THE PATELLA

Causes. Direct violence is usually the cause of fracture of the patella. Muscular action is another cause.

Types. The three types of patellar fracture are (1) transverse, (2) comminuted (stellate), and (3) linear.

Anatomy. The action of the quadriceps may separate the fragments as much as several inches when the injury occurs. It is important to recognize the significance of this in considering the damage to the capsular ligaments of the knee joint. The repair of lateral tears should be an important part of the treatment.

Treatment. Only linear fractures or stellate fractures without separation of the fragments should be treated conservatively. Conservative treatment can be accomplished by immobilization in a cast in extension for 3 to 6 weeks.

When there is separation of the fragments with tearing of the capsule, open reduction is always indicated. It is preferable in open reduction about joints to delay the operation 3 to 6 days to allow the traumatic reaction to subside and to permit tissue resistance to develop. This lessens the chance for infection. Compound fractures may need to be treated immediately.

As a rule it is best to remove small fragments of the patella and leave only one main fragment to which the patella or quadriceps tendon is sutured. There is no longer a fracture to heal, but only the ligamentous attachments. Therefore immobilization time is greatly reduced. When severe comminution with separation occurs, the entire patella is removed, with restoration of good function.

ACUTE AND HABITUAL DISLOCATIONS OF THE PATELLA

Causes. Acute dislocation of the patella is usually caused by direct force against its inner side when the knee is flexed.

Habitual dislocation may start from the same mechanism, but there may be other factors, such as (1) too shallow a groove in the femoral condyles, (2) ball-like shape of the patella, and (3) knock-knee. Here the pull transmitted from the quadriceps tendon to the attachment of the patella tendon on the tibia is not in a straight line, and therefore it places abnormal tension on the ligamentous structure of the inner side of the knee.

Symptoms and signs. The patella can be seen displaced to the outer side of the knee. There is severe pain and muscle spasm, and the knee cannot be actively extended.

Treatment. Reduction occurs automatically when the knee is extended, but sometimes an anesthetic is necessary to accomplish reduction.

When reduced, primary dislocations are immobilized in a well-molded plaster cast from the ankle to the groin. This cast should be worn about 4 weeks. After this an elastic support with stays should be worn for 2 or 3 weeks longer.

In the habitual type some form of operative fixation is necessary. The commonest methods are (1) transference of the patella tendon and its bony attach-

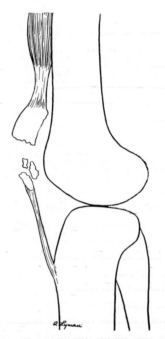

Fig. 341. Fracture of the patella with comminution of the lower fragment. This was removed.

ment inward on the tibia to create a direct-line pull, (2) osteotomy and wedging to deepen the femoral groove if it is shallow, and (3) tendon or fascia lata fixation of the patella to the inner condyle of the tibia.

FRACTURE AND DISLOCATION OF THE TIBIA BELOW THE KNEE (BUMPER FRACTURE)

Cause. Usually direct violence is the cause of fracture and dislocation of the tibia below the knee. They are frequently caused by a person stepping between two cars that are in motion toward each other and are commonly known as bumper fractures. Sometimes they are compound. The section immediately below the knee is usually involved.

Anatomy. The tibia is composed of two plates or surfaces that articulate with the two condyles of the femur. The

knee joint has four important ligaments and two semilunar cartilages. The lateral ligaments protect the knee joint from any instability when it is completely straight. When it is extended, both lateral ligaments are tight and prevent any lateral motion of the knee joint.

The internal cruciate ligaments are those in the center of the knee joint and are designed to prevent the leg from displacing itself either forward or backward on the femur. To become acquainted with the direction of these ligaments, remember the direction of the anterior crucial ligament by placing your right hand, with fingers spread, directly over the right patella when the knee is in flexion. The index finger will give the direction of the anterior crucial ligament that goes from behind forward and is attached to the anterior tibial spine. The posterior ligament goes in the opposite direction; that is, from the inner condyle of the femur backward to the

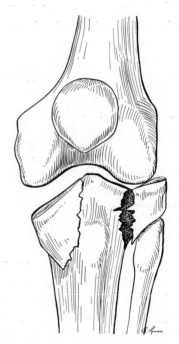

Fig. 342. Fracture of the condyles of the tibia into the knee joint. Open reduction done.

posterior spine of the tibia. These four ligaments are responsible for the stability of the knee joint in all directions.

The test for injury or tearing of the anterior crucial ligament is to force the knee completely straight into extension. The anterior ligament becomes tight and hyperextension is not possible when the ligament is intact. If the ligament is torn, however, the joint may be carried to a position beyond 180 degrees.

If the posterior ligament is damaged or torn or if there is a detachment of the ligament with a small amount of bone from the posterior spine of the tibia, the knee joint, when it is placed in a position of 90-degree flexion, may be displaced forward on the femoral condyles to the extent of ½ to ¾ inch. Rotary motions are also increased.

The tendency for deformity is toward the collapsed or fractured side of the tibial condyles. Should it be the outer condyles, there is a tendency toward the development of a knock-knee deformity. Should it be the inner condyle, there is a tendency toward the development of a bowleg deformity. Both of these are preventable.

Problem. The deformed leg must be maintained in proper alignment to the normal leg, and normal joint motion must be reestablished at the earliest possible time. Restoration of the most perfect contour of the joint surface is another important problem to be dealt with.

Treatment. In most instances when there are fractures of the upper end of the tibia involving the knee joint, conservative treatment is best.

Conservative treatment consists first in the use of moleskin adhesive traction from the knee down, with 5 to 8 pounds of weight. If there is a tendency toward knock-knee deformity, a sling may be arranged so that lateral traction may be applied at the inner side of the joint,

using 5 to 8 pounds of weight over the outer side of the bed. The side traction is flexible, as is the traction in the vertical line. Therefore, during the process of healing and repair, the patient is able to carry on motions that will greatly facilitate the speed of recovery of joint motion. As was said before, in all fractures involving any joint, the patient or his relatives should be advised of the possible difficulties in reestablishing joint motion.

In spite of the fact that the knee joint is the heaviest weight-bearing joint in the body, the results of fractures into the knee joint are often more favorable than might be expected from the severity of the fracture affecting it.

It is sometimes necessary, because of the interposition of small fragments between the main fragments of the condylar fractures of the tibia, to perform an operation in which the area is approached, the fragments are removed, and the condyles are brought together in the best possible alignment of the joint surface. Occasionally, it may be necessary to employ a threaded bolt that penetrates both condyles and buckles them together by means of nuts properly arranged and properly designed to exert their pressure. The semilunar cartilages that are frequently mentioned in the literature as a source of trouble in these fractures seem rarely to be the cause of any serious trouble. The scar developed during healing usually anchors them sufficiently to assure future stability.

In some types hospitalization time may be shortened by the application of a cast in an overcorrected position. For example, if the inner condyle is fractured and there is a tendency toward development of bowleg deformity, the cast can be applied in a position of knock-knee.

If the opposite is the case, then the cast must also be applied from high in the groin to the toes in a slightly exaggerated position of bowleg. In either case the cast should be bivalved at an early period with daily motion of the knee joint. Throughout the course of treatment positive active motion and a slight range of assisted passive motion should be practiced.

Healing period. In cancellous bone, such as is found in and near the joint, there is a stage of rapid primary healing, but the stability of the callus so formed is insufficient to withstand much strain in less than 3 or 4 months. This allows the early establishment of motion in the joint, but there is not strength enough for early stress, strain, or weight bearing without danger of the development of deformity.

Condylar fractures of the tibia may heal within 3 or 4 weeks sufficiently for guarded motion with a split cast. Weight bearing on crutches should not be undertaken until the roentgenogram shows a fair amount of union.

It is desirable at times, particularly when early weight bearing is necessary, to use a brace that extends from the ischium to the heel of the shoe with a strap on the inner or outer side of the knee joint (dependent on the tendency toward deformity) to prevent abnormal strain.

From the industrial standpoint, it usually takes from 4 to 6 months for patients with this type of fracture to recover sufficiently to return to their normal occupations. The amount of permanent disability is variable. Many patients with severe fractures may return to their normal occupations without any permanent disability. In some, however, whether mildly or severely affected, there may be partial permanent disability and the development of traumatic arthritis.

If the ligaments of the knee joint are sufficiently damaged to create permanent instability of the joint and interfere with the normal function, it may be necessary to operate, using ligamentous structures, such as tendons or tensor fascia lata (from the outer side of the thigh), to stabilize the joint. The procedure requires hospitalization of a patient for 3 to 6 weeks.

FRACTURE OF THE SHAFT OF THE TIBIA

Cause. The cause of fracture of the shaft of the tibia may be either direct or indirect violence. When there is direct violence, the fracture may be compound. A twisting injury may cause a spiral fracture. Fracture of the tibia is one of the most common in automobile accidents, and the percentage of compound fractures is greater than in almost any other region of the body. Fractures that occur in automobiles, industry, and war are most often caused by direct violence. The tibia may be broken by the direct impact of the penetrating force or may be broken in such a way that the points of the fracture penetrate the skin.

Anatomy. The tibia is the main weight-bearing bone of the leg. It is well cov-

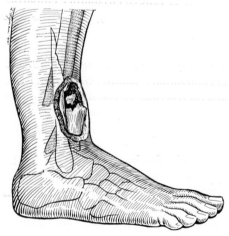

Fig. 343. Compound fracture of the tibia and fibula at junction of middle and lower thirds.

ered with muscle tissue in the upper and middle parts, except over the shin, but sparsely covered with subcutaneous tissue and skin in the lower third. For this reason circulation is poor and healing is slow. Nonunion is relatively frequent in the middle and lower portions. The relation of the planes of the knee joint and those of the ankle are important in reduction. The injured leg should be compared with the uninjured leg before reduction is attempted so that the proper position in regard to rotation may be obtained.

Problem. The problem depends largely on the nature of the fracture—whether transverse, oblique, or comminuted. The problem is to reduce the fracture and maintain reduction by the simplest possible means. Any deviation in alignment must be avoided.

Treatment. With the patient under anesthesia, simple transverse and many oblique fractures may be manipulated into position and treated in a long leg cast. Roentgenograms should be taken at frequent intervals during the first few weeks to see that slipping does not occur. If severe swelling should occur shortly after reduction, the cast should be split its full length and spread sufficiently to relieve circulatory embarrassment. It can be brought together again after swelling subsides.

If fractures of the tibia are difficult to hold in position, they may be treated by intramedullary nailing, by plating, or by skeletal traction. In the oblique type two or more screws may maintain reduction by transfixing the fracture site. In either case a cast is used for immobilization during the healing period. The fixation apparatus is incorporated.

When nonunion occurs, bone grafting will usually stimulate union. The onlay full-thickness graft held in place by metal screws seems to be the most popular method.

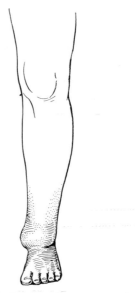

Fig. 344. Pott's fracture showing posterior and outward displacement of ankle joint. Ordinary joint contours disappear.

POTT'S FRACTURE

Cause. A blow against the outer side of the ankle when the foot is in contact with the ground or twisting the ankle when slipping or falling may cause Pott's fracture.

Anatomy. The ankle joint forms a mortice with the internal and external malleoli acting as stabilizing forces to prevent lateral motion. The astragalus acts as a gliding hinge against the lower articular surface of the tibia, allowing only plantar movement and dorsiflexion. All lateral movements occur in joints below the ankle joint. The classical Pott's fracture, frequently called trimalleolar, consists of a fracture of the internal malleolus and of the lower end of the fibula combined with a backward and outward displacement of the astragalus. Frequently, the posterior lip of the tibia (posterior malleolus) is also broken.

Problem. Proper alignment and contact of the various fragments must be restored by manipulation with the patient under anesthesia. The ease or difficulty with which this reduction may be performed depends on two main factors. (1) If the inner malleolus is fractured near the tip rather than at the base of the malleolus, the proximal portion can serve as a barrier against overcorrecting the fracture inwardly. (2) If the fracture of the posterior malleolus involves as much as one third or one half of the posterior surface of the tibial part of the joint, the difficulty in maintaining the forward reduction of the dislocation is very great and some form of open fixation is usually necessary.

Reduction. In addition to an accurate interpretation of the roentgenograms of Pott's fracture, a comparison between the fractured and unfractured sides should be made. In some persons the ankle joint and the knee joint work in the same plane, whereas in others the ankle joint may be outwardly or inwardly rotated. If reduction is attempted without taking this into consideration, the internal and external malleoli may not come in close contact at the points of fracture.

Treatment. Under fluoroscopic control the fragments are manipulated into a position that gives the closest contact. This usually consists in forced inversion, dorsiflexion, and lateral pressure through the ankle to restore accurate contact of the internal malleolus with the astragalus and of the external malleolus with the tibia. A circular plaster of paris cast is applied to maintain this position and must extend from the toes well up on the thigh with the knee moderately flexed in order to maintain the corrective amount of rotation. When the fracture line of the internal malleolus is at the same level of the joint surface or above it, fixation of the internal malleolus by nailing may be necessary.

Healing period. Healing usually requires from 8 to 12 weeks. As a rule, the portion of the cast above the knee may be removed at the end of 8 weeks, and frequently the lower portion may be bivalved for daily motion at the same time.

When the fracture is the favorable type, weight bearing with the use of a walking iron or similar device incorporated into the cast may be begun as early as 4 to 6 weeks. There may be some permanent disability as a result of traumatic arthritis in the ankle joint.

NURSING CARE IN FRACTURES OF THE BONES OF THE LOWER LEG

Nursing care of a simple fracture of either or both bones of the lower leg after reduction has been obtained and a cast applied presents no very troublesome features to the nurse. If there is considerable swelling, the patient may be admitted to the hospital for a short period before reduction is attempted. Ice bags are frequently used to reduce

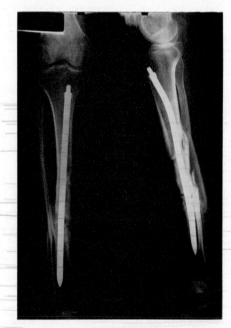

Fig. 345. Roentgenograms showing internal fixation of fracture of the tibia by insertion of an intramedullary nail (Lottes' nail). Fracture of the distal third of the tibia is frequently complicated by delayed union or nonunion.

edema. These bags should not be too heavily filled with ice, and air should be eliminated before the bags are closed. The pressure of several very tightly filled ice bags on a swollen and painful ankle has been known to cause great discomfort to the patient as well as considerable interference with circulation. Attention to the underlying skin to eliminate the danger of ice burns is important. Ice bags should not be applied without some material between the patient's skin and the rubber, even in an emergency. Heat is usually substituted for the ice after 24 to 36 hours.

Walking casts are sometimes applied to patients with simple fractures of the leg in order to allow the patient to continue his normal occupation. The manner of applying these casts varies somewhat in different clinics. Reenforcements on the sole either with additional layers of plaster or with some type of flexible wood may be used. Stirrups or walking irons of metal may be incorporated into the plaster on the plantar surface of the cast. The patient should wear some type

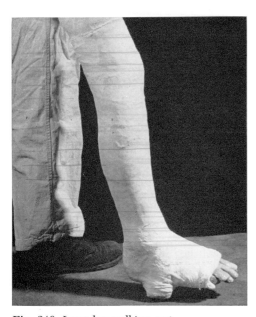

Fig. 346. Long leg walking cast.

of protective sock to keep the cast and foot clean, and a coat or two of shellac when the cast is thoroughly dried is advisable.

Complications of compound fractures. Tetanus and gas bacillus infection are two complications of compound fractures with whose symptoms every nurse should be familiar. Gas gangrene will first be noted at the site of infection as local edema, discoloration, and puffiness. Increase of the pulse rate is a constant systemic manifestation. The complete clinical picture is one of severe localized pain, increase in the size of the limb, rise in temperature, continued acceleration of the pulse rate, and a general picture of severe illness. The coppery color of the skin, which caused Velpeau to name the disease bronze erysipelas, is a characteristic of a very advanced state. Crepitation, which is caused by gas bubbles beneath the skin, is usually present. After some trauma has broken the patient's skin any of these symptoms is extremely grave and demands immediate surgical attention.

General symptoms of tetanus may be absent. The earliest symptoms observed may be muscular twitchings and spasms that are tonic in nature. Frequently, there is difficulty in opening the mouth. This symptom may occur early in the course before any other symptoms have been noted.

Both diseases are caused by anaerobic bacteria, and surgical debridement of the wound is usually performed immediately. When gas bacillus infection is suspected, the wound is opened wide and all muscle planes in the affected part are exposed. Formerly, deep radiation was employed, followed by irrigation through rubber tubes placed so that they came in contact with every section of the muscles involved. Hydrogen peroxide, Dakin's solution, and other antiseptics were used for continuous irrigation. Amputation was frequently required. Antigas gangrene (polyvalent) serum was administered intramuscularly as often as every 6 to 10 hours in doses of 10,000 units. Local use of penicillin and the sulfonamides has largely replaced the radiation treatments and irrigations formerly employed. Serum is still used in large doses, although faith in it as being of specific value to treatment is somewhat disputed.

Wounds infected by tetanus are also opened wide, and very large doses of tetanus antitoxin may be given intramuscularly, intravenously, or into the spinal canal. In both diseases supportive treatment is extremely important and intake is kept up by fluids given parenterally. In tetanus the convulsive states are managed with sedative drugs.

FRACTURE OF THE ASTRAGALUS

Cause. Usually indirect violence, such as landing on the foot in a fall, is the cause of fracture of the astragalus.

Anatomy. The astragalus articulates with several bones, and a large portion of its surface is covered by articular cartilage. The area in which the blood supply may reach it is therefore small. In many instances fractures will damage the blood supply to such an extent that healing is delayed. Disintegration of the bone through aseptic necrosis is not infrequent, or there may be nonunion.

Treatment. Perfect reduction of the fracture is essential. To maintain reduction, nailing or bone graft may be required. Occasionally, removal of the astragalus is indicated.

Immobilization in a plaster of paris cast is advocated. The ankle should be placed in a right-angle position so that, if ankylosis should occur, the best function will ensue.

Healing period. Healing is slow, and weight bearing cannot be allowed until union is demonstrated roentgenograph-

ically. However, the cast may be bivalved in 6 to 8 weeks, and some motion, heat, and massage may be started for the restoration of joint function. When the cast is discarded, the arch should be supported for weight bearing. Total healing may not occur sooner than 10 to 14 weeks.

FRACTURE OF THE OS CALCIS (CALCANEUS)

Cause. Direct violence, usually from falls in which the victim lands on his heels, is the cause of fracture of the os calcis. Frequently, these injuries are bilateral and may be associated with compression fractures of the spine. They are common in explosions on shipboard.

Anatomy. The os calcis (or calcaneus) is composed almost entirely of spongy bone. When the outer surface is broken, the inherent strength of the bone is lost.

Displacements that occur from the injury are usually in three directions. Lateral squashing shoves the fragments out under the external malleolus and tends to cause a flatfoot deformity. Upward displacement of the posterior portion tends to exaggerate the flatfoot tendency. This is increased by the pull of the Achilles tendon. Outward rotation also occurs.

In the usual anteroposterior and lateral roentgenograms of the foot and ankle, the true degree of displacement is not shown. This has led to disastrous undertreatment of these fractures. Because of their disabling effect they are usually much more formidable than they appear. Therefore, roentgenograms should be taken from behind the leg at a 45-degree angle so that a true picture of the lateral displacement and outward rotation of the fragments will be shown. The foot for this view is in complete contact with the x-ray plate.

Treatment. There are several methods of treatment, but the essential factor of all is that the bone be restored to as near its normal shape as possible. This requires lateral impaction of the fragments and downward displacement of the heel. The latter can be accomplished through lengthening of the Achilles tendon and downward replacement through leverage in skeletal traction. The arch must be restored and all corrections must be maintained by the proper application of a plaster of paris cast.

Healing period. Weight bearing cannot be allowed in less than 6 to 8 weeks and then only with the arch well supported to prevent weight being exerted on the os calcis. The degree of permanent disability is usually determined (1) by the extent of involvement of the subastragaloid joint, (2) by the amount of residual lateral displacement under the external malleolus and against the peroneal tendons, and (3) by the residual flattening of the longitudinal arch.

The rule in many clinics is that, if the pain persists beyond the 6 months' period, the accumulation of bone under the external malleolus should be removed and the subastragaloid joint, and possibly others, should be ankylosed by operation.

FRACTURES OF THE METATARSAL BONES AND TOES

Cause. Usually, fractures of the metatarsal bones and toes are caused by direct violence.

Anatomy. The metatarsal heads comprise the anterior arch and one of the main weight-bearing surfaces of the foot. The muscles and tissues here are sparse. Restoration of length and alignment, therefore, particularly in the anteroposterior plane, are the main problems of reduction and treatment because a prominence of bone on either the plantar or dorsal surface of the foot could lead to irritation from weight bearing or shoes. The treatment following the necessary

amount of reduction is usually the application of a plaster of paris cast from the calf to the end of the toes. Skeletal traction may be necessary occasionally.

Healing period. These bones usually heal in about 4 weeks. After the removal of the cast protection must be maintained for several weeks by the use of an arch support within the shoe and a metatarsal bar on the outside.

PHYSICAL THERAPY IN THE TREATMENT OF FRACTURES

Physical therapy after any type of fracture is recognized to be of great importance regardless of what type of reduction has been used. Although nurses will not be required to carry out these treatments as a rule, it is important that they have a good concept of the treatment and its purpose.

The main purposes of physical therapy after fractures are (1) to encourage absorption of traumatic hemorrhage and exudate, (2) to relax muscle spasm and thereby eliminate discomfort and possible deformity, (3) to promote normal circulation in the part and thus to hasten the healing process, and (4) to restore muscle tone and flexibility so that normal functioning is possible.

Heat in some form is almost always part of the treatment. It may be given by means of an electric light bulb suspended from a cradle, by hot packs, by a therapeutic lamp, or by means of a whirlpool bath. It is exceedingly important that nurses recognize the fact that heat has a greater value if administered at low intensity over a long period than if it is given at high intensity for a shorter period of time.

When massage is given, it is usually of the light stroking variety, with slow steady strokes given in the same direction, that is, in the long axis of the muscle and in the direction of venous flow.

Muscle stimulation to encourage muscle contraction is usually part of the physical therapy program. This may be done through electric stimulation or through the patient's own voluntary effort. (Voluntary effort is usually considered preferable.) Although this voluntary effort is possible even though the patient is encased in a plaster cast, many orthopedists provide some type of fixation that allows guarded use of contiguous joints while controlling the fracture site. Traction, hinged splints, or bivalved casts are particularly useful for this purpose.

Active or active-assistive exercises with gentle stretching are frequently prescribed for the patient in traction or splints. It is exceedingly important during the first few weeks after fracture. Development of muscle power is recognized as essential if normal function is to be regained. The method of De Lorme, known as the heavy resistance, low repetition method, has worked well in the hands of experienced physical therapists. This method differs from older methods that concentrated largely on low resistance exercises repeated a great number of times. Although this method served to develop endurance, it did not always develop muscle power sufficient for the demands of normal function.

Some type of apparatus to assist the patient in active exercise of the hip may be attached to the bed. This may consist of an overhead frame, skin or ankle traction, and a series of ropes or pulleys that permit the patient to exercise his leg in adduction, abduction, flexion, and extension. The patient is taught to do this by himself, although supervision of his activities is repeated at frequent intervals.

STUDY QUESTIONS

1. Discuss some of the home hazards that may lead to fractures.
2. List two common complications that follow fracture of the femur in the aged person. What can good nursing care do to eliminate these?
3. Discuss prevention of pressure areas in aged patients who are confined to bed with fractured limbs.
4. How would you prepare an elderly patient, recently removed from a hip spica cast, to begin functional activities such as getting up in a chair and using crutches?
5. What is the aim of all treatment for the patient with paraplegia?
6. What are the two most common causes of death in the patient with paraplegia? What can good nursing care do to eliminate these?

REFERENCES

Adams, J.: Outline of fractures, ed. 4, Baltimore, 1964, Williams & Wilkins Co.

Bardsley, C., Fowler, H., Moody, E., Teigen, E., and Sommer, J.: Pressure sores—a regimen for preventing and treating them, Am. J. Nursing 64:82-84, 1964.

Barton, B.: And now to live again, New York, 1944, Appleton-Century Co.

Beck, E. D.: General principles of fracture management in the aged, Surg. Gynec. & Obst. 106:343-346, 1958.

Blount, W. P.: Fractures in children, Baltimore, 1954, Williams & Wilkins Co.

Buchwald, E., McCormack, M., and Raby, E.: A bladder and bowel training program for patients with spinal cord disease, Rehabilitation Monograph III, The Institute of Physical Medicine and Rehabilitation, New York University-Bellevue Medical Center, 1952.

Buckley, B. R.: Feeding the aged person, Am. J. Nursing 59:1591-1593, 1959.

Cannell, J.: Decubitus ulcers—plastic spray, Am. J. Nursing 58:1009-1010, 1958.

Caldwell, J. A., and Seymour, P.: Supracondylar fracture of the humerus in children, Am. J. Nursing 57:1177-1180, 1957.

Cave, E. F., editor: Fractures and other injuries, Chicago, 1958, Year Book Medical Publishers, Inc.

Clark, J.: Modern trends in orthopaedics—fracture treatment, Washington, 1962, Butterworth Inc.

Conwell, H. E., and Reynolds, F. C.: Key and Conwell's management of fractures, dislocations and sprains, ed. 7, St. Louis, 1961, The C. V. Mosby Co.

Davenport, R.: Tube feeding for long-term patients, Am. J. Nursing **64**:121-123, 1964.

Donaldson, J. S., and Williams, M. E.: Replacement arthroplasties of the hip, Am. J. Nursing **55**:566-568, 1955.

Garrett, A., Perry, J., and Nickel, V.: Traumatic quadriplegia, J.A.M.A. **187**:7-11, 1964.

Goldstein, M. S., Beye, C. L., Bonfiglio, M., and Ziffren, S. E.: Treatment of fractures of the neck of the femur in the aged, J. Am. Geriat. Soc. **4**:75-81, 1956.

Hacker, G. I.: The medullary nail, Am. J. Nursing **50**:104-106, 1950.

Heckel, N. J.: Kidney stones, their etiology and treatment, Am. J. Nursing **55**:194-196, 1955.

Henley, B. M.: Helping the elderly find community services, Am. J. Nursing **63**:89-92, 1963.

Hicks, D., Scalisi, S., Woody, F., and Skinner, B.: Increasing upper extremity function, Am. J. Nursing **64**:69-73, 1964.

Hicks, M. L.: Decubitus ulcers—alternating pressure pad, Am. J. Nursing **58**:1008-1009, 1958.

Holdsworth, F. W., and Hardy, A.: Early treatment of paraplegia from fractures of the thoraco-lumbar spine, J. Bone & Joint Surg. **35B**:540-550, 1953.

Horwitz, I. G., and Lenobel, M. I.: Artificial hip prosthesis in acute and nonunion fractures of the femoral neck, J.A.M.A. **155**:564-567, 1954.

Hulicka, I.: Fostering self-respect in aged patients, Am. J. Nursing **64**:84-89, 1964.

Larson, C. B., and Gould, M. L.: Fractures of the hip and nursing care of the patient with a fractured hip, Am. J. Nursing **58**:1558-1563, 1958.

Lindsey, D.: Effective emergency splinting, Am. J. Nursing **56**:1120-1124, 1956.

Lonergan, R. C.: As we grow older, Am. J. Nursing **56**:736-737, 1956.

Ludlum, W. D., Jr., and McCann, W. J.: The treatment of trochanteric fractures of the femur by internal fixation, Am. J. Surg. **87**:347-350, 1954.

Martin, M. A.: Nursing care in cervical cord injury, Am. J. Nursing **63**:60-61, 1963.

Martin, J., and Craig, I.: The early care of patient with injury of the spinal cord, Am. J. Nursing **55**:936-939, 1955.

Mayo, R. A., and Hughes, J. M.: Intramedullary nailing of long bone fractures; nursing care after intramedullary nailing, Am. J. Nursing **59**:236-240, 1959.

Mendelson, J.: Sprains and strains, Am. J. Nursing **61**:45-50, 1961.

Moore, M.: Ambulation following fractures of the lower extremity, Am. J. Nursing **53**:174-175, 1953.

Moore, J. C.: Reading aids for a quadriplegic patient, Am. J. Occup. Therapy **10**:119-120, 1956.

Morrissey, A. B.: The procedures of urinary and bowel rehabilitation, Am. J. Nursing **51**:194-197, 1951.

Newton, K.: Geriatric nursing, St. Louis, 1960, The C. V. Mosby Co.

Patton, F., Behlore, D., and Pechth, P.: Treatment of hip fractures in the geriatic patient, J. Am. Phys. Ther. A. **42**:314-318, 1962.

Robinson, M., and Van Volkenburgh, S.: Intermaxillary fixation: immediate postoperative care, Am. J. Nursing **63**:71-72, 1963.

Robertson, C. A.: Manual expression of urine, Am. J. Nursing **59**:840-841, 1959.

Rusk, H.: Early management of the paraplegic patient, Armed Forces M. J. **6**:157-161, 1955.

Rusk, H.: Geriatrics and rehabilitation, Geriatrics **6**:143-150, 1951.

Sandick, H.: Priorities must be established in emergency care of the injured, Am. J. Nursing **62**:93-96, 1962.

Saxon, J.: Techniques for bowel and bladder training, Am. J. Nursing **62**:69-71, 1962.

Sister Maria Francis: Nursing the patient with internal hip fixation, Am. J. Nursing **64**:111-112, 1964.

Soller, G. R.: The aging patient, Am. J. Nursing **62**:114-116, 1962.

Stafford, N.: Bowel hygiene of aged patients, Am. J. Nursing **63**:102-103, 1963.

Stilwell, E.: Pressure sores—one method of cure, Am. J. Nursing **61**:109-110, 1961.

Talbot, H. S., Cooper, I. S., and Covalt, D. A.: Panel discussion on rehabilitation of patients with paraplegia, J.A.M.A. **162**:1203-1209, 1956.

Talbot, H. S.: Care of the bladder in neurological disorders, J.A.M.A. **161**:944-947, 1956.

Thompson, F. R.: Two and a half years' experience with a Vitallium intramedullary hip prosthesis, J. Bone & Joint Surg. **36A**:489-500, 1954.

Thompson, P. W.: Let's take a good look at the aging, Am. J. Nursing **61**:76-79, 1961.

Watson-Jones, R.: Fractures and joint injuries, ed. 3, Baltimore, 1952, Williams & Wilkins Co.

White House Conference: Problems of the aging, Am. J. Nursing **61**:55-57, 1961.

Wiles, P.: Fractures, dislocations and sprains, Boston, 1960, Little, Brown & Co.

Winter, C. C., Reehm, M., and Watson, H.: Urinary calculi—nursing care, Am. J. Nursing **63**:72-76, 1963.

Ziffren, S. E.: Management of the aged surgical patient, Chicago, 1960, Year Book Medical Publishers, Inc.

Chapter 13

Types of bone tumors, including nursing care in malignant tumors

Three types of tumors occur in bone: benign (nonmalignant), malignant, and metastatic from other tissues or organs. The benign type grows slowly and does not tend to destroy surrounding tissues or spread to other parts of the body through the bloodstream or lymphatic system. They are osteocartilaginous exostosis, enchondroma, chondroblastoma, hemangioma, osteoid osteoma, and giant cell tumor.

A malignant tumor (sarcoma) is usually rapid in growth and may be of considerable size before it is recognized by the patient. It often spreads to other parts of the body through the bloodstream before it is brought to the attention of a surgeon.

Tumors metastatic from cancer of other tissues, such as the breast, prostate, lung, kidney, thyroid, etc., are quite common because bone marrow has a rich blood supply and cancer cells are easily spread through the bloodstream.

BENIGN TUMORS

Generally, the cause is not known for all types of benign tumors. Some of the benign tumors are thought to be an aberration of the growth and development of tissues. The osteocartilaginous exostosis is considered to be caused by displacement of cartilage cells at the epiphyseal plate. As bone growth takes place these displaced cells cause an enlargement near the ends of long bones that may be bumped easily because of their prominence. Some patients may have exostoses of many bones. At times malignant change takes place in one of these tumors. All of the other benign tumors have little or no visible external manifestations because they are confined within bone.

The symptoms in these patients are generally mild pain in the affected bone or prominence, as in the patient with an exostosis. The diagnosis is made with the aid of roentgenograms and surgical biopsy.

Treatment is simple removal, excision, or curettage. Therefore, the nursing care involves routine postoperative management of a patient in a plaster dressing or soft bandages.

MALIGNANT BONE TUMORS

Most bone sarcomas are classified according to the type of tissue formed by the malignant cells; for example, osteosarcoma, fibrosarcoma, chondrosarcoma, hemangiosarcoma, and round cell sarcomas (Ewing's sarcoma, reticulum cell sarcoma, and multiple myeloma). As is true for benign tumors, the cause is

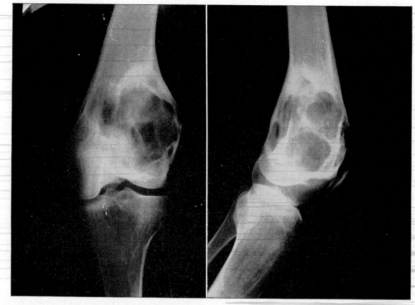

Fig. 347. Giant cell tumor (osteoclastoma). It is usually benign but difficult to differentiate from certain malignant osteogenic sarcomas even after biopsy. Characteristically, these tumors expand the shaft, show little bone reaction, involve the epiphyses of the long bones, and seldom break into a joint cavity. (From Kenney, William C., and Larson, Carroll B.: Orthopedics for the general practitioner, St. Louis, 1957, The C. V. Mosby Co.)

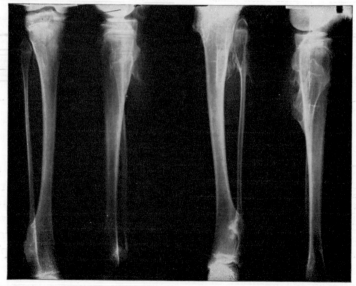

Fig. 348. Multiple cartilaginous exostoses. These exostoses are capped by cartilage that tends to mature when the normal epiphyses close. These tumors are familial and benign but can produce symptoms if mechanically injured. Rarely after incomplete surgical removal or with repeated trauma do they become malignant. (From Kenney, William C., and Larson, Carroll B.: Orthopedics for the general practitioner, St. Louis, 1957, The C. V. Mosby Co.)

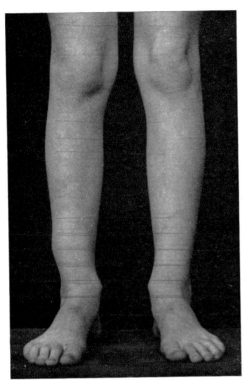

Fig. 349. Osteocartilaginous exostosis of the fibula. Note enlargement of lower end of the right leg. This tumor is painless unless bumped.

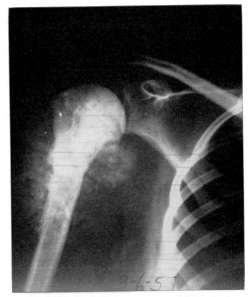

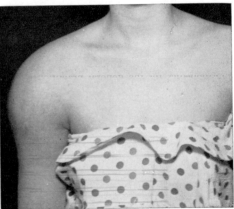

Fig. 350. Osteogenic sarcoma of the humerus.

generally not known. Certain preexisting conditions, such as Paget's disease of bone, may cause bone sarcoma to develop. At times irradiation therapy given for nonmalignant lesions may induce malignant tumors after a latent period of several years or more.

Diagnosis and treatment. A history of intermittent pain that is particularly troublesome at night, tiredness, a limp, and swelling of a part of an extremity without previous trauma or obvious infection may lead one to suspect a tumor. Such a combination of symptoms requires immediate medical attention. Sometimes the parent will belittle the symptoms as being the result of some recent fall or trauma. Needless to say, the nurse who advises the patient to seek medical attention does not voice her suspicion aloud. The patient fre-

quently looks deceptively well when admitted to the hospital for the first time. The night pain may increase in severity. Roentgenograms are a helpful adjunct to proper diagnosis. In certain of the bone sarcomas, laboratory work is of value. For instance, osteosarcomas tend to produce a high alkaline phosphatase in the blood serum. Because the treatment and prognosis of bone sarcoma vary with the type of tumor, a surgical biopsy is the surest way to establish an accurate diagnosis. A roentgenogram of the chest will help to determine whether

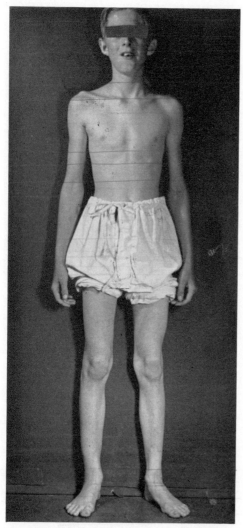

Fig. 351. Ewing's sarcoma of the lower end of the right fibula. Patient had intermittent pain and limp of a year's duration.

quently possible to perform a local resection without amputation or disarticulation. In the lower extremity when tumors are present near the knee joint, function is usually better after amputation and the use of an artificial limb. At the midshaft of the femur and the upper end of the femur, resection and replacement either with a metallic prosthesis or an intramedullary rod with supplementary bone transplants may provide function without sacrificing the extremity. When metastasis can be demonstrated, as in the chest, surgical removal of the original tumor obviously will not cure the patient, but it may be necessary to control pain and to prevent the local tumor from becoming an ulcerated fungating foul-smelling mass.

X-ray irradiation or radioactive cobalt irradiation will be used in patients in whom the tumor is radiosensitive. Some tumors, such as Ewing's sarcoma, can be controlled for many months by this treatment. Reticulum cell sarcoma may be cured by this method. Radiation is often helpful to relieve pain in tumors even though it may not be curative. In the far-advanced stages of malignant bone disease and in tumors from other parts of the body that have metastasized to bone drugs have been and are being tried in an effort to find one that might control the growth of the tumor cells.

Tumor metastatic to bone from cancer of other tissues is the most common tumor found in bone. It usually occurs in patients over 40 years of age when cancers of the breast, prostate, intestinal organs, lungs, and other tissues are most common. The cancer deposit is most frequently found in those bones rich in red marrow such as the spine, pelvis, and ribs. As a rule this site of deposit is the cause of pain, but occasionally the first indication of bone involvement comes when a fracture occurs as a result

or not obvious metastases are present in the lungs. Metastases, however, may not be visible at the time of the initial examination but may be manifested after treatment has been instituted.

The treatment of malignant bone tumors is surgical removal either by wide local resection (when it is both technically feasible and consistent with conservation of function) or by amputation. In the upper extremity it is more fre-

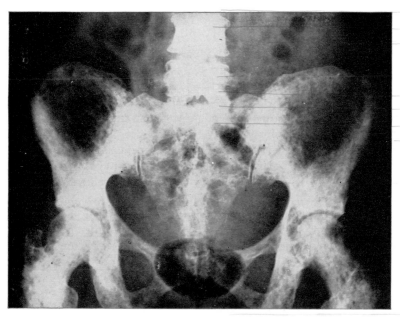

Fig. 352. Carcinoma of the breast, metastatic to bone. Solitary metastases usually to the vertebrae or femur. The more common type of lesion is osteolytic, but occasional cases show bone formation and resemble metastatic carcinoma of the prostate. (From Kenney, William C., and Larson, Carroll B.: Orthopedics for the general practitioner, St. Louis, 1957, The C. V. Mosby Co.)

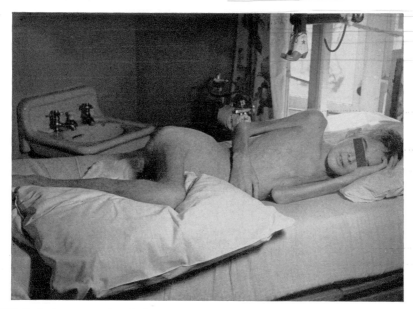

Fig. 353. Ewing's sarcoma, terminal stage.

of some trivial accident. Compression fractures of the spine are very common when cancer cells have weakened the structure of the bones of the vertebrae, or there may be pathologic fractures of the hip, shoulder or pelvis. Proper diagnosis of the type of cancer is essential to proper treatment. Therefore, one needs information afforded by the roentgenogram and, if it is possible to obtain tissue from the metastasis, the histologic diagnosis. In certain locations needle biopsy may be necessary rather than an open surgical biopsy. Metastases from breast or prostate may be controlled for variable periods of time by the use of hormones, but in most instances x-ray irradiation and analgesic drugs are necessary for control of pain.

Nursing care. Nursing care of patients with malignant bone tumors does not differ greatly from the care given to a patient with malignancy of any part of the body. Very few of the features will be unfamiliar to the orthopedic nurse experienced in the care of bone infections. The postoperative care of patients who have had amputations or disarticulations will correspond to that of patients with amputations for any cause. If a local resection has been performed, the patient undoubtedly will be in a plaster dressing and the care is the same as that for one in a plaster cast. The real problem develops in patients who have had local recurrence or metastases from the original bone tumor.

The prognosis for these patients is poor. One watches week by week the local and general progress of malignant disease. The patient's own outlook at first is hopeful. Whether or not amputation takes place, he usually displays early desire and determination to get well. Since he presumably knows nothing of the moribund nature of the disease, one wonders sometimes at the gradual change that comes about in the morale. Consciously or unconsciously, these pa-

tients seem to know the outcome. It has been said that the attitude of parents, visiting friends, and even nurses toward the patient tells him the whole story quite clearly. This is probably not entirely true. But there is enough truth in it that the nurse needs to help the relatives understand the necessity for self-control in the presence of these patients. This is a stern lesson but an important one, and it is just as important for the nurse to learn it as for the parents and relatives.

Splinting of the extremity is done to prevent pain or injury to the affected part. The chance of pathologic fracture occurring at or near the site of the tumor is to be kept in mind, for very little trauma or manipulation is necessary to bring about such fractures. This should be remembered during the bed making process or when the patient is being turned, and especially if he is allowed out of bed. In the latter case he should be carefully protected against bumps or falls.

When radiation treatment is prescribed, instructions should be sought from the surgeon regarding the patient's routine treatment. It is usually considered unwise to continue heliotherapy while the patient is receiving a course of radiation treatments because the patient's skin at this time is particularly sensitive to light. The diet is usually fortified by additional vitamins and protein and by blood-building foods to counteract the advancing anemia.

Symptoms that the nurse should recognize as particularly indicative of progress of the disease are signs of chest involvement, the most common site of metastasis. Coughing, pain in the chest, and expectoration of blood are serious and should be reported immediately. Fracture may occur from relatively trivial mishaps and, since the fracture is almost painless, may go unnoticed unless the nurse is vigilant in observation.

STUDY QUESTIONS

1. Give the main points of difference between a malignant and a benign tumor.

2. What are two complications an observant nurse might recognize in bed care of the patient with a malignant bone tumor?

REFERENCES

Clark, R. L., and Maisel, C. J.: Malignant bone tumors, Am. J. Nursing **55:**688-690, 1955.

Gilmer, W., Higley, G., and Kilgore, W.: Atlas of bone tumors, St. Louis, 1963, The C. V. Mosby Co.

Jaffe, H. L.: Tumors and tumorous conditions of the bones and joints, Philadelphia, 1963, Lea & Febiger.

Lichtenstein, L.: Bone tumors, St. Louis, 1952, The C. V. Mosby Co.

McCarroll, H. R.: Practical considerations in the management of malignant bone tumors, J.A.M.A. **152:**297-300, 1953.

McKinnie C.: Multiple myeloma, Am. J. Nursing **63:**99-102, 1963.

Mercer, Sir Walter, and Duthie, R. B.: Orthopedic surgery, Baltimore, 1964, Williams & Wilkins Co.

Pack, G., and Ariel, I.: Treatment of cancer and allied diseases, New York, 1964, Hoeber Medical Division, Harper and Row Publishers.

Shands, A., Raney, R., and Brashear, R.: Handbook of orthopaedic surgery, ed. 6, St. Louis, 1963, The C. V. Mosby Co.

Chapter 14

Neuromuscular affections

Progressive muscular dystrophy

Types. A number of neuromuscular disorders are included under the term progressive muscular dystrophy. The most common type is that of pseudohypertrophic muscular dystrophy. With this type symptoms may be noted by the time the child is 2 or 3 years of age. The mother becomes aware that the child stumbles and falls more easily than do other children. He may not be able to run, and he tends to walk on his toes with a slight waddling gait. The calf muscles become enlarged, and as the disease advances, intermittently, the waddling gait increases and an exaggerated hollow back develops. The muscles about the thighs, hips, and shoulders atrophy. The fibers of the enlarged calf muscles become displaced by fat and fibrous tissue. It is characteristic that when these children are placed in a sitting position on the floor they first arise to their knees and hands, awkwardly bring each leg up separately to a flexed weight-bearing position, and then with their hands against the knees and thighs gradually force themselves up into an erect position (Gowers' sign). Even then they have great instability, and a small blow against their knees or other parts of their bodies may throw them off balance and cause them to collapse to the floor.

In later stages extensive wasting of the muscles occurs, and the limbs and spine may assume grotesque deformities. Respiratory infections become more difficult to control and frequently are the cause of death. A second cause of death is involvement of the heart muscle. In recent years the use of antibiotics has helped to prolong the life of the child with muscular dystrophy.

Facioscapulohumeral muscular dystrophy is a second type that involves both sexes. Symptoms of this type may appear during the early teens or sometimes later in life. It is not as incapacitating as pseudohypertrophic muscular dystrophy, and most of these patients may live a relatively long and useful life.

Limb-girdle, a third type of muscular dystrophy, has its onset usually in the second or third decade of life. It develops more rapidly and may incapacitate the individual within a few years.

Cause. The cause of pseudohypertrophic muscular dystrophy is unknown. There is a definite hereditary factor, and it is transmitted frequently in the same manner as hemophilia—through an unaffected mother to the male children. At the present time no cure is known, and the prognosis is poor. Much research has been and is being done, however, in an attempt to find the cause and thus a method of treatment.

Care. Even though the prognosis is poor, much can be done to help these children live useful and happy lives. Education for the muscular dystrophy child should not be neglected. Attendance at a regular school is desirable as long as his physical condition permits. When this is no longer possible, his education should be continued in a school for handicapped children. As the disease progresses and the physical activities that he can participate in lessen, reading may become his chief means of entertainment.

Muscular dystrophy children should be encouraged and taught to help themselves as much as possible and for as long as possible. They may be slow and clumsy, but active use of their muscles helps maintain strength, which, when lost, is never regained. Parents need help in understanding this, and because muscular dystrophy is a slow progressive disease the parents or family must assume most of the responsibility for the child's care. Preventing joint contractures is of the utmost importance. It is necessary that the family be taught the value of a foot support to prevent drop foot and proper bed positions to prevent knee and hip flexion contractures or other deformities.

Overweight frequently becomes a problem as the child grows older and is less active. Overeating is to be guarded against.

The nurse should remember that the

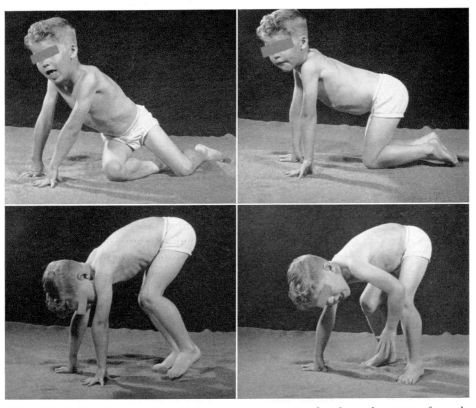

Fig. 354. Child with pseudohypertrophic progressive muscular dystrophy arising from the floor in a typical fashion. After getting on his hands and knees he braces his hands against his thighs and pushes himself to an upright position (Gowers' sign).

Continued.

family of the muscular dystrophy child needs guidance and assistance in securing equipment that facilitates care and at the same time lessens the demands on the mother's physical strength. Rehabilitation aids, such as a trapeze for the bed or a lift for moving the patient from bed to wheelchair, should be made available.

Many muscular dystrophy patients have received assistance through the Muscular Dystrophy Association of America. This organization was founded in 1950 by the parents and families of muscular dystrophy victims, and through local and state agencies it assists the needy muscular dystrophy patient by providing school facilities, physical therapy, braces, wheelchairs, and other items needed for his care. It also has made provision for grants to finance research pertaining to this disease.

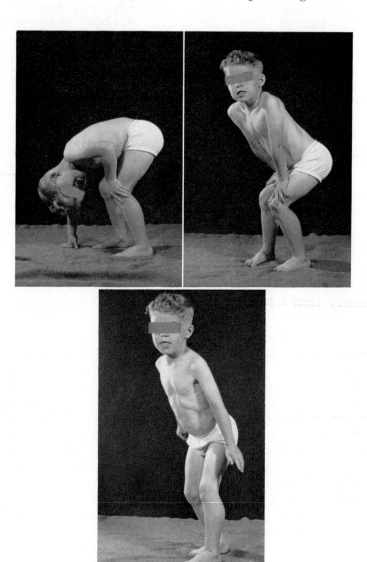

Fig. 354—cont'd. For legend see preceding page.

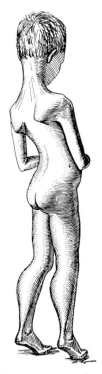

Fig. 355. Moderately advanced case of infantile pseudohypertrophic progressive muscular dystrophy. Note enlarged calves, contracted heel cords, sway-back, and winged shoulders.

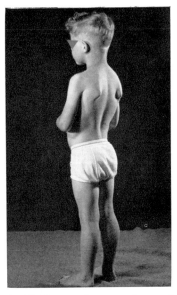

Fig. 356. Child in early stage of muscular dystrophy. Note winging of scapulae, lumbar lordosis, and enlarged calf muscles.

Birth palsy (Erb's paralysis)

Cause. Birth palsy consists in a paralysis of the arm caused by damage to the brachial plexus during the process of birth. It may occur spontaneously during a relatively difficult labor, or it may result from the use of instruments or traction on the arm in abnormal labor.

Types. There are two common types (both are becoming less frequent with improved obstetric methods): the milder type in which only the muscles about the shoulder are paralyzed (Erb's paralysis) and the severe type in which the whole arm is paralyzed (Aaron-Duchenne type). In both types the arm is rotated inward by the unparalyzed pectoral and scapular muscles. These become contracted if the condition remains untreated for any great length of time, and the deformity becomes fixed.

The prognosis in the Erb's type of paralysis is good. It is poor in that of the whole arm or the lower arm (Klumpke).

Treatment. In the milder type of birth palsy the nerves are injured and the paralysis is usually caused by the pressure of hemorrhage on the brachial nerve trunks. Recovery usually takes place, but the arm must be maintained

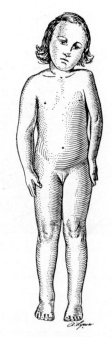

Fig. 357. Birth palsy (Erb's) of the left arm in a child 6 years of age. There is inward rotation, adduction, and atrophy.

in a position of abduction and external rotation to protect the paralyzed muscles and to prevent contracture of the unparalyzed internal rotators and adductors. The treatment should be started very soon after birth, and immobilization may be accomplished either by means of an abduction splint that extends from the pelvis to the tip of the fingers or by means of a plaster of paris cast. If the splint is used, daily applications of heat and massage and the use of active and passive exercises speed up recovery.

When the cast is used, the upper portion over the arm should be removed at the end of 2 or 3 weeks so that treatments can be carried out. Recovery usually takes place in from 6 to 10 weeks.

In the severe whole arm paralysis, there is usually formidable damage or complete severance of some of the roots of the brachial plexus. Inspection by operation and suturing of these nerve roots will sometimes lead to partial recovery. The arm should be splinted also, but recovery, if it occurs, is at a very slow rate.

Nursing care. Early recognition of birth paralysis is not difficult. It is frequently suspected by the obstetrician as he delivers the child. The causative factor is a forcible separation of head and shoulder during delivery. This produces a tearing injury of the nerves of the brachial plexus. The nurse giving the initial bath will note the characteristic position of the arm hanging flaccidly with the elbow in extension, the shoulder adducted and rotated inwardly (often accompanied by a cupping appearance of the shoulder), and the hand pronated, palm facing the back. The infant does not use the arm and will object to its being moved for him during the first days of life. This gradually subsides, and the arm can be moved without pain to the child.

Difficult, prolonged labor seems to play a definite part in the etiology of this condition, since anesthesia is employed in these cases, and considerable muscular relaxation is present during birth. In cases with extreme tearing, Sever says unequal pupils (Horner's signs) can frequently be observed.

Treatment is ordered immediately, although it may be only a tying of the child's wrist to the crib head. The purpose of treatment is to prevent stretching of the paralyzed muscle and contracture of the unaffected groups. The arm is therefore secured in a position in which strong muscles cannot become shortened and contracted. This is done by casts or splints, and the position is the so-called "Statue of Liberty" attitude in which the arm is abducted and elevated, the shoulder is rotated externally, and the hand is in a position of supination.

Physicians' orders as to care and handling of these patients may vary in

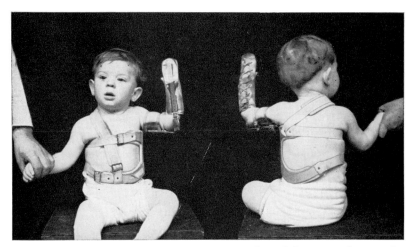

Fig. 358. Abduction arm brace. The arm is maintained in abduction and external rotation. The thoracic and iliac portions ensure stability of the brace, and a part of the weight of the apparatus is distributed to the normal shoulder. (Courtesy University Hospitals, Iowa City, Iowa.)

some degree. Constant protection of the affected muscles to prevent them from being stretched by the opposing group is the usual order. Therefore the nurse must be able to improvise methods of support for the arm when the brace or splints are removed during the bath and exercise. In an infant or young child this is not a very easy assignment. The nurse should not remove the brace until she has everything in readiness to bathe the part. Securing the wrist to the head of the crib with a clove hitch of muslin bandage is frequently done. A linen splint, devised originally at Michael Reese Hospital for protection of the deltoid in patients with infantile paralysis, would provide an excellent means of maintaining good position at

such times, because sometimes the brace must remain off for hours—for repair, cleaning, or the like.

Other surgeons will alternate protection with periods of supervised activity or manipulation, during which the joints of the upper extremity are passively put through their full range of motion.

The type of physical therapy is ordered by the surgeon and is carried out by a physical therapist if one is available. If it is necessary for the nurse to perform this function, she should ask the doctor to demonstrate the treatment to her before she assumes the responsibility. It will usually consist of light massage and manipulation of the affected extremity.

Charcot joints and other neuromuscular affections (neuropathies)

Charcot joints are not truly neuromuscular affections but are allied enough to be included in this chapter.

It has been established clinically and roentgenographically that the bone, cartilage, and ligaments can at times literally melt away, leaving a very misshapen, unstable, unserviceable, and yet quite painless joint. This is known as a neuropathy and occurs particularly in association with certain nervous tissue disorders such as neurosyphilis, diabetic neuritis, syringomyelia, and occasionally paraplegia. The name Charcot has been applied to these joints.

There is no specific treatment except to treat the underlying cause: penicillin for neurosyphilis, diet and insulin to control the diabetes, and radiation therapy for syringomyelia. The unstable joint does not heal, but occasionally the progression of the process can be checked. Attempts at fusion or application of braces will benefit the affected joints.

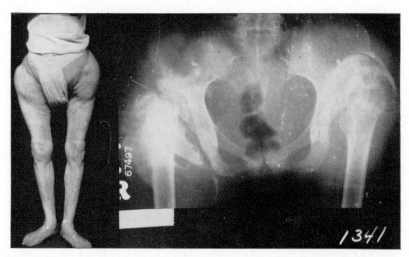

Fig. 359. Charcot joints. Roentgenogram illustrates extensive destruction of bone. The patient experiences little or no pain, but such joints are quite unstable and weight bearing is difficult.

STUDY QUESTIONS

1. Be prepared to discuss the three types of brachial palsy concerning nerve roots and muscles involved and loss of motion. Describe the typical position of the arm.

2. What is the treatment of brachial palsy and what are the nursing responsibilities related to early diagnosis; to nursing care; and to provision for adequate follow-up care?

REFERENCES

Deaver, G. G.: Rehabilitation program in muscular dystrophy, Crippled Child **34**:6-7, 29, 1956.

Fischer, K. A.: Erb's palsy, Physiotherapy Rev. **20**:328-332, 1940.

Gucker, T.: The orthopedic management of progressive muscular dystrophy, J. Am. Phys. Ther. A. **44**:243-246, 1964.

MacGinniss, O.: Muscular dystrophy, Nursing Outlook **10**:588-591, 1962.

Milhorat, A. T.: Therapy in muscular dystrophy, M. Ann. District of Columbia **23**: 15-21, 70, 1954.

The Muscular Dystrophies, J.A.M.A. **159**:21-23, 1955.

Morris, A. G., and Vignos, P. J.: A self-care program for the child with progressive muscular dystrophy, Am. J. Occup. Ther. **14**: 301-305, 1960.

Steindler, A.: Orthopedic operations, Springfield, Ill., 1950, Charles C Thomas, Publisher.

Chapter 15

Medicolegal aspects of nursing

The purpose of this chapter is to convey a basic general background of the legal liability of the nurse. It is necessarily limited to a survey of the most general points, and attention is directed to the list of references at the end of this chapter for the reader who desires a more detailed knowledge of the subject. If any trend is ascertainable in this field, it is the growing awareness that nursing is being recognized as a true profession with a corresponding increase of responsibilities and accompanying legal obligations. However, a great variety of treatment of this subject and many areas of inconsistency in court decisions of the various states still exist.

Any discussion of the legal aspects of nursing is necessarily interwoven with the relationship of the nurse to the physician and hospital and the complex series of legal obligations and duties of each to the other and of all to the patient. The basic approach will be to ascertain the standards applied to determine if the nurse has been negligent in the performance of her functions and then to determine who else may also be liable for the same act.

DEFINITION

There is no agreed definition of nursing, and each state has attempted to establish the meaning through statute. Using a composite of the various statutes, the following is submitted as a definition of nursing: A nurse is one who engages and holds herself out as qualified in the application of biologic, physical, or social sciences for the observation of symptoms and reactions of patients, the accurate recordation of fact, and the carrying out of treatments and medications or other lawful orders under the direction of or supervision of a physician. In addition the average statute provides for the required educational and training requirements, distinguishes between the various subclasses of nurses—for example, registered, practical, and student—and provides an exception for those performing similar services in the home without claim of nursing qualifications.

To establish a common basis for a discussion of the various legal consequences of nursing acts it is necessary to deal with the various functions of a nurse, which seem to be historically classified as follows:

1. Independent nursing functions are the functions and duties a nurse can properly perform without direction, supervision, and control of the physician and can be further subdivided as follows:
   (a) The accurate observation of and recognition of symptoms and reactions of the patient
   (b) The accurate recordation of fact and maintenance of various required hospital records
   (c) The application of general nursing procedures concerned with hygiene of the patient, such as bathing the patient,

making beds, answering requests of the patient, etc.

(d) Supervision of the safety and security of the patient, for example, properly situating the patient in bed or chair or locking windows

2. Dependent nursing functions are the functions that can be performed by a nurse only under the direction and supervision of the physician, since they include acts normally included within the definition of the practice of medicine.

LIABILITY OF NURSE FOR NEGLIGENCE

One of the basic concepts of our legal system is that every person must govern his conduct so as to minimize the possibility of injury to others to the extent that a reasonably prudent man would do under the circumstances. This is known as the standard of due care, the violation of which results in a negligent act. This standard is accurately defined in the case of *Heaven* vs. *Pender* as follows:

"Whenever one person is by circumstances placed in such a position with regard to another that everyone of ordinary sense, who did think, would at once recognize that if he did not use ordinary skill and care in his own conduct with regard to those circumstances he would cause danger of injury to the person or property of another, a duty to use ordinary care and skill to avoid such danger exists."

This same standard applies to the nurse, who offers herself to the public as a person trained and skilled in her profession. The nurse, therefore, must conduct herself as a reasonable, prudent nurse, possessing the skill and training of the nurses in her community. If she fails to meet this test in a particular situation and if this failure is the cause of injury to the patient she will be subject to civil liability for damages caused thereby.

It is not possible to provide the nurse with a list of various situations with the corresponding acts necessary to avoid

liability. There is a tremendous amount of litigation regarding this question in specific situations; however, it is not the purpose of this article to analyze it but to provide a broad pattern based on these decisions with a few illustrations drawn from them.

It is important to note that the law does not require the nurse or physician to be an absolute ensurer of the patient's welfare through the course of care and treatment. If the nurse conducts herself with due care in accordance with established nursing practices in her community and injury to the patient results, she will not be liable for the damages. By analogy to the field of medical malpractice, which uses the same standard to determine the presence or absence of negligence, a recent case of *Thompson* vs. *Lillehei*, et al., 273 Federal 2d 376 (1959), will serve to illustrate this point. In this situation an attempted surgical repair of a ventricular septal defect in an 8-year-old girl by using the mother as a donor under the technique of cross control circulation resulted in an air embolism in the donor, which in turn resulted in permanent brain damage and corresponding mental deficiency. After carefully reviewing the evidence and expressing sympathy for the plight of the donor-plaintiff, the court ruled that the doctors had taken every precaution then known to medical science and the injury occurred nevertheless, but without negligence on the part of the doctors.

Using the classic definition of nursing functions as set forth, the following are some of the most litigated areas of nursing liability and will serve to illustrate the application of the standard of due care to the typical nursing duties.

1. A nurse is required to recognize and record symptoms in patients. Although she is not required to perform this function to the extent and with the skill of a physician, failure of the

nurse to recognize abnormal reactions to prescribed treatment or drugs or the improper administration of treatments or drugs have resulted in liability for the nurse.

2. An error in the recordation of fact can obviously have serious consequences for the patient.

3. In applying the more menial nursing skills such as bathing the patient or assisting him into a wheelchair, administering ice or hot packs, frequent injuries have occurred. For example, placing the patient in bath water that results in a burn or failing to properly support a patient during his transfer to a wheelchair have incurred liability for the nurse.

4. One of the most difficult areas is in the so-called dependent nursing functions that require the direction and supervision of the physician. If one of these functions were performed without the direction or supervision required, the act itself would be negligent and an improper nursing activity. Even though proper supervision and direction exist, the act can be improperly performed and result in negligence by the nurse.

A major cause of the difficulty in this area is that the nurse normally has some independent diagnostic and remedial functions that require no physician's directions or supervision. For example, the nurse in checking the pulse of a patient, in administering a simple medication and noting the patient's reaction, is making a diagnosis that is in the realm of her legitimate functions. Just where the line must be drawn between this type of diagnosis and treatment and more extensive ones is a matter of confusion and disagreement among the court decisions. Acts such as suturing, changing dressings, and administration of anesthetics have usually been held to require the direction and supervision of the physician.

Another problem in this field is that as a practical matter physicians cannot and do not exercise direct physical control and supervision over some dependent nursing functions. The only guide available to the nurse is the advice that, if it has been generally accepted in the immediate medical community, a certain act can be performed by an experienced nurse without direct supervision of the physician. Such an act will probably not incur liability for negligence by mere performance of the act. For example, in many areas it is a common practice for the nurse to administer intravenous and hypodermic injections upon the request of the physician but without any supervision by him.

5. The nurse has the unpleasant legal duty to question the order of a physician that is obviously incorrect and that will result in injury to the patient if she carries out the instructions. At the risk of becoming unpopular the only safe course of conduct for the nurse is to inquire when in doubt.

6. A nurse's normal functions can be extended in the emergency situation, which is defined as one in which there is immediate danger of death or serious injury to the patient if prompt remedial action is not taken and in which a physician is not available to perform the same. In this situation the nurse may properly perform functions normally beyond the scope of authorized nursing activities with this important limitation—she may never perform an act for which she was not trained, such as surgery. She could, for example, clean a wound and suture the same if immediately necessary. One consolation for the nurse is that under the pressure of the moment the law does not expect cool detached reflection that will produce 100% accuracy in diagnosing the actual existence of an emergency condition as defined but only requires that under the circumstances reasonably prudent persons would have reached the same conclusion.

In the final analysis the application of the aforementioned standard of due care to the alleged negligent act of the nurse will turn upon the particular communities feelings, as expressed through the jury members, of what is just, sensible, and proper under the circumstances. Inability to predict the results of this process makes any positive guide for the nurse inadequate.

LIABILITY OF OTHERS FOR NURSE'S NEGLIGENT ACTS

Once the liability of the nurse for her negligent acts has been established, the next step is to determine if the hospital, physician, or both are also liable. This depends upon the classification of the nurse as either an employee or an independent contractor within the basic concepts of agency law. Subject to the limitations of oversimplification, these concepts state that, if the nurse was the employee of the physician or hospital and the injury to the patient occurred within the course of her employment, the employer (physician or hospital) will also be liable. If the nurse is not hired by either hospital or doctor, however, but directly by the patient, the nurse only will be liable for her negligence. Perhaps the only example of the independent contractor nurse is the private duty nurse who is usually furnished by a listing service and is hired and paid directly by the patient.

The usual problem is to determine whose employee the nurse was at the time of injury, that of the physician or hospital. Obviously, an injury by the physician's own office nurse incurs the former's liability. The nurse who is employed by the hospital as a member of the regular nursing force will incur liability upon the hospital for injury caused by the performance of her independent nursing functions as defined previously.

The real problem exists in the area of the dependent nursing functions that must be performed under direction and supervision of the physician. The majority and historic rule is that, if the physician has this control and supervision as he is theoretically required to do, he should be held liable for acts of the nurse performed under this control and supervision. Several additional theories are advanced in support of this view. One is based upon the borrowed servant theory in the field of agency law. Applied here, the argument would be that although the nurse is primarily the hospital's employee she temporarily becomes the physician's employee at the time he takes over the direction and control of her actions in performing a certain act. Another theory is that the physician cannot delegate his responsibility for the performance of these dependent nursing functions and therefore remains liable. The most impressive theory and the real basis for the majority

view in my opinion is that our society desires to place the responsibility on the physician because this is the person who is selected by and relied upon by the patient and who usually has the financial ability to pay for the damages.

As a result of the majority view the surgeon is held responsible for all of the actions of the nurses in the operating room because he is deemed to be in complete control of all personnel during the operation. Therefore, if the nurse fails to count the sponges correctly and one is inadvertently left in the patient, the surgeon as well as the nurse is liable for the injuries caused.

There is a growing minority that maintains that the physician is not liable in such situations unless he has actual physical supervision or was negligent in permitting the nurse to attempt the act causing injury. The theory in support of this view is that the physician does not in fact have the opportunity to exercise such supervision and he should be free to concentrate upon his major functions rather than these secondary duties. In addition, it is argued that the physician should be able to rely upon the hospital providing qualified and competent nurses. In final analysis the confusion arises because of the elasticity of the distinction between medical and nursing duties, caused in part by the medical profession's willingness to admit the increasingly professional characteristic of nursing only as a means of reducing the physician's legal responsibilities and at the same time refusing to allow the nurse to encroach upon the functions historically labeled as the practice of medicine.

NURSE'S LIABILITY FOR INTENTIONAL ACTS

The nurse will usually encounter the area of personal liability for intentional acts in only two situations; namely, assault and battery and false imprisonment. It should be noted that acts subject the nurse to civil liability for both compensable or actual damages and punitive damages.

Assault is the act of putting another in immediate fear of personal injury, whereas battery is the act of harmful or offensive contact against another. Both acts must be intentional as contrasted to accidental and must be without legal justification. The nurse may have occasion to restrain a patient from an act that is harmful to the latter's condition even though the patient may think otherwise. Certainly, when the patient is mentally ill, restraint is required; and when no more force than necessary is applied, there can be no action for assault and battery. The same result occurs when restraint is necessary to prevent the pain-racked patient from injuring himself. If the physical contact with the patient is not justifiable as necessary medical treatment to which the patient has expressedly or impliedly consented, the nurse will be liable for damages of the type set forth previously. It is essential that the patient consent to the treatment involved, since the mentally competent patient can refuse to accept any treatment offered. When such a refusal occurs, the remedy is to require the patient to either consent to the treatment or leave the hospital. The patient must comply with hospital rules and must limit himself to areas of the hospital in which the rules permit his presence. If the patient violates these rules, physical restraint to enforce them should be no more violent than necessary (which does not include an act that would produce great bodily injury) and be followed by a request for his departure from the hospital. The nurse has the right to prevent the patient from injuring other patients, hospital personnel, and guests so long as only a reasonable amount of force is used; and of course, she has the right of self-defense in the event of a physical attack by a patient.

False imprisonment is total restraint against a person's will by violence or a threat of violence from an actor who intends to restrain and upon a victim who is aware of the restraint. If a nurse refuses to permit a patient to leave the hospital and uses violence or the threat of violence to enforce the restraint, she will be subject to civil liability for false imprisonment. Again, restraint based upon justifiable medical treatment that the patient has expressedly or impliedly consented to will not create liability. If a patient is told under threat of violence that he cannot leave the hospital until his bill is paid, false imprisonment occurs, and if the nurse has so advised the patient she will be subject to civil action.

REFERENCES

Code of Iowa, 1958, Chaps. 148 and 152.

The doctor and the law, Vols. 2 and 3, Fort Wayne, Ind., 1959. By the Law Department of The Medical Protective Co.

Harrison, G.: Nurse and the law, Philadelphia, 1945, F. A. Davis Co.

Hayt, E., and Hayt, L.: Legal guide for American hospitals, New York, 1950, Hospital Textbook Co.

Hershey, N.: The law and the nurse—nurse, hospital, and emergency care, Am. J. Nursing 63:105-106, 1963; 63:121-122, 1963.

Restrictions and safety, Am. J. Nursing 63: 124-125, 1963.

Who may authorize an autopsy, Am. J. Nursing 63:103-105, 1963.

Obtaining consent for the use of body tissues, Am. J. Nursing 63:105-106, 1963.

Court role of legal counsel, Am. J. Nursing 63:127-128, 1963.

The immunity doctrines, Am. J. Nursing
63:108-109, 1963.

Res ipsa loquitur, Am. J. Nursing **63:**101-
102, 1963.

A sharp remark provoketh wrath—and a
law suit, Am. J. Nursing **63:**105-106,
1963.

The apparently erroneous order, Am. J.
Nursing **64:**111-112, 1964.

When in doubt about admitting a patient,
Am. J. Nursing **64:**125-126, 1964.

The private duty nurse, Am. J. Nursing
64:121-122, 1964.

Layman's law is like layman's medicine,
Am. J. Nursing **64:**135-136, 1964.

Lesnik, M. J., and Anderson, B. E.: Nursing
practice and the law, Philadelphia, 1955,
J. B. Lippincott Co.

Lott, J., and Gray, R.: Law in medical and
dental practice, Chicago, 1942, Foundation
Press.

Scheffel, C.: Jurisprudence for nurses. New
York, 1945, Lakeside Publishing Co.

Glossary

achondroplasia a form of dwarfism in which the trunk and head are of almost normal size but the limbs are short and sometimes distorted; caused by a disturbance in epiphyseal growth that originates in intrauterine life; definitely congenital and frequently inherited.

acromegaly (gigantism) overgrowth of stature, enlargement of the jaw, shoulder girdle, pelvis, hands, and feet; usually develops during periods of rapid growth in adolescents but may occur in adult life.

actinomycosis (blastomycosis lumpy jaw) infection usually first manifested in the bones of the jaw; in small proportion of patients spine is affected; destructive areas, of interest to orthopedists, found in spine, and usually some abscess formation; diagnosis made by the ray-fungus obtained by aspiration of abscess; treatment by drainage, evacuation of abscessed area, or radiation therapy that usually leads to cure within 6 months or a year.

adactylism absence of the fingers or the toes.

amputation neuroma enlargement at the end of a cut nerve usually composed of jumbled scar and regenerating nerve tissue and often painful.

amyotonia congenita inherited weakness of the muscles; may persist through adult life or may respond to antirachitic therapy in earlier life.

ankylosis stiffening of a joint; caused by scar tissue or bone growth between the two surfaces of a joint; occurs as result of infection or irritation.

arthrodesis surgical fusion of a joint.

arthrogryposis flexion contractures of the limbs (congenital).

arthroplasty operative creation of a new joint to replace a stiff or ankylosed joint.

arthrotomy operative exploration of a joint.

brachydactylism congenital shortening of the fingers or toes.

Brodie's abscess localized circumscribed osteomyelitic abscess, usually of the long bones; virulence of organism low; treatment by drainage and curettage and infiltration with powdered sulfanilamide; prolonged sulfonamide therapy may be required.

calcaneovalgus sometimes called congenital flatfoot; consists in a deformity in which the tibialis anticus is contracted and the gastrocnemius (heel cord group) is weak; a deformity in which, at birth, toes and top of foot may lie against anterior surface of leg.

cartilaginous exostoses (multiple) see dyschondroplasia.

cavus hollowfoot (contracture of the plantar fascia).

cervical rib a congenital anomaly; consists of a supernumerary rib attached to one of the cervical vertebrae; because of pressure rib may produce sensory, motor, and vasomotor symptoms in upper extremity.

Charcot joint degenerative proliferative joint lesion of tertiary syphilis causing instability and enlargement but lacking in pain.

Charcot-Marie-Tooth disease characterized by atrophy and paralysis of muscles as a result of degenerative changes in the peripheral nerves; peroneal muscles usually affected first; progresses slowly, has familial tendency, and occurs more frequently in males than in females.

chondritis inflammation of a cartilage.

chondrodystrophy (hypertrophic) see dyschondroplasia.

cineplasty a type of operation in which a skin tunnel is constructed through muscle belly in an arm amputation; by a pulley arrangement the tunneled muscle is made to activate the artificial hand.

Clutton's joints bilateral synovitis of the knees and elbows as a result of congenital syphilis.

congenital absence of the clavicle (cleidocranialdyscrasy, sternocleidodysostosis) ab-

467

sence of the clavicles associated with delay in closure of frontal sutures of skull; causes box-head deformity of skull and groove down center of forehead.

coxa hip.

coxa plana flattened head of the femur.

coxa valga increase of the angle between the neck and shaft of femur.

coxa vara decrease of the angle between the neck and shaft of femur.

cretinism representing type of dwarfism caused by insufficient function of thyroid gland; persons affected have large tongues, thick lips, flattened noses, and puffy eyelids, and should be treated by the administration of thyroid extract.

cubitus elbow.

Dupuytren's contracture scar formation in superficial skin tissues of palm as a result of trauma and focal infection; one, two, or more fingers flexed toward palm; treatment by elimination of foci and complete operative removal of scar.

dyschondroplasia (Ollier's disease) more common in males than females; an overgrowth of bone or bony prominences (exostoses) near epiphysis caused by congenital misplacement or abnormal distribution of growth cells; characterized by multiple overgrowth of bones near joints; if bony projections interfere with joint function or are subject to local irritation, they should be removed.

echinococcus cyst destructive bone lesions infected by the *Taenia echinococcus* when the parasite lodges within bone tissue.

epiphysitis (acute) disease of epiphyseal region near joints; characterized by pain and tenderness near joint; motion usually normal; treatment by immobilization in plaster cast for mild cases and incision and drainage for more active ones.

equinus (like the foot of a horse) consists in contracture of Achilles tendon to extent that ball of foot in walking makes contact with ground but heel cannot touch.

fibrositis rheumatoid involvement of superficial tissues of bony surfaces and of intramuscular and periarticular tissues of bony surfaces; "muscular rheumatism, periarthritis"; pain usually referred to joint but motions not much limited; fibrous nodules found in hands, back, and hips; patient feels stiff and has many spots of tenderness; treatment by removal of focal infection with physical

therapy treatments and probably use of vaccines.

flat feet (rigid) in certain young persons, pain and stiffness of ankles without apparent cause; characterized by progressive knock-ankle deformity and limitation of motion in joints of foot; result of an inherent congenital weakness or to inflammatory changes resulting from focal infection; treated by manipulation (under anesthesia) with correction of deformity and application of plaster cast; corrective procedure combined with removal of any detectable focal infection; for fixed deformity reconstructive operation to restore arch may be required.

Friedreich's ataxia characterized by weakness of leg muscles and caused by degenerative changes in nerve fibers in dorsal and lateral tracts of spinal cord; a progressive condition; familial; treatment by bracing and muscle reeducation; stabilization operations may be helpful.

Gaucher's disease generalized bone disease associated with pathology of spleen; bone lesions similar to hyperparathyroidism.

genu knee.

genu valgum knock-knees.

genu varum bowlegs.

genu recurvatum hyperextended position of the knee (back-knee position).

gigantism disease of youth as a result of overactivity of anterior portion of pituitary gland; bony growth usually symmetric, and person may attain height of 7 to 9 feet.

"glass" arm athlete's arm weakened by presence of subdeltoid bursitis or epicondylar bursitis.

glioma malignant tumor of brain or nerve cells.

goniometer special protractor used to measure joint motion.

gout caused by overindulgence in beers and wines and meats; disease usually seen in acute attacks that may involve various joints but most commonly the first metatarsophalangeal joint; acute attacks accompanied by extreme pain, redness, and swelling, and usually caused by some dietary indiscretion; when the result of excessive intake of purine foods, treatment usually immobilization in splints combined with elimination of purines and administration of neocinchophen.

Gowers' sign "climbing up the legs" to attain an erect position in progressive muscular dystrophy.

Guillian-Barré syndrome (polyneuritis) symmetric paralysis that develops slowly; frequently follows some mild infection; often confused with poliomyelitis; respiratory embarrassment may develop and necessitate a tracheotomy and use of respirator; prognosis good for return of normal muscle power.

hallux great toe.

hallux valgus bunion position.

Heberden's nodes enlargements about finger joints accompanying chronic arthritis; enlargements partly bony and partly composed of gelatinous material.

hemophiliac joints occur frequently when disease is present; joints assume a fusiform swelling; areas of subcutaneous hemorrhage; tend to subside with administration of cold packs and vitamin K; immobilization and blood transfusions important factors in preventing further bleeding; joints, after repeated attacks become ankylosed; any surgery distinctly contraindicated.

involucrum new bone that grows around the sequestrated shaft of an old bone, such as in osteomyelitis.

intermittent hydrarthrosis usually occurs between 30 and 40 years of age; occurs most frequently in knee or both knees and is transient; swelling characteristically painless, lasts a few days, and then disappears only to recur in a month or two; absence of pain or tenderness or of any abnormality in roentgenographic findings in joints; thought that disturbance of allergic or endocrine nature responsible; spontaneous disappearance of disease may occur in pregnancy, but as a rule synovectomy offers best prospect of cure.

Kümmel's disease delayed collapse of an injured vertebra in which a minor fracture or no fracture was demonstrated roentgenographically immediately following injury; collapse may occur as late as 5 or 6 months after injury.

kyphosis increase in posterior curve of thoracic vertebrae (hunchback).

Little's disease congenital cerebral palsy or spastic paralysis.

lordosis anterior flexion of lower part of back causing hollow back deformity.

macrodactylia congenital enlargement of one or several digits of hand or foot; may be hereditary.

Madelung's deformity deformity of wrist in which distal end of radius displaced anteriorly; causes dorsal prominence of distal end

of ulna and limitations in dorsiflexion of wrist.

Marfan syndrome (arachnodactyly) characterized by weakness of muscles, hypermobility of joints, marked scoliosis long thin extremities, including bones of hands and feet (spider fingers and toes).

Marquio's disease syndrome of mild dwarfism that is hereditary and involves body asymmetrically as compared to achondroplasia.

melorheostosis (flowing bones) extremely rare condition in which cortical portion of bone is overgrown and gives a flowing appearance; usually confined to a single extremity.

meningococcus arthritis joint infection following meningitis; surrounding tissues more involved than joints; prognosis good when immobilization and sulfonamide injection used; ankylosis not infrequent.

mongolianism accidental nonhereditary body type having characteristic features of Mongol race combined with idiocy.

myelomas, multiple cancerlike type of generalized bone destruction; always fatal.

myositis inflammation of a muscle.

myositis ossificans (progressiva) rare disease of unknown origin in which the muscles and fascia are converted into bone; childhood disease involving first the spinal muscles and gradually spreading to other parts of the body.

Nelton's line extends from the anterosuperior iliac spine to ischial tuberosity.

osteitis deformans (Paget's disease) disease of unknown origin that affects persons of middle age and manifests itself by gradual thickening and bowing of shafts of long bones and thickening of skull; cystic areas in bone that are filled with gelatinous and fibrous material with great increase in vascularity; trunk may gradually become shortened and chest barrel-shaped; legs and arms may become bowed; roentgenograms show characteristic bone changes; patient usually complains of aching pains in spine and extremities; treatment directed toward support or correction of deformities.

osteitis fibrosa cystica (von Recklinghausen's disease) decalcification of bone caused by hypersecretion of parathormone from parathyroid glands; excretion of calcium and phosphorus markedly increased; formation of renal calculi is not uncommon; bone fractures may result from decalcification process.

osteitis of Gerry (chronic diffuse sclerosing)

usually occurs in shafts of long bones in late childhood; thickening of bone and cortex; may be redness, tenderness, and a dull ache; treatment by excision of thickened bone cortex or drilling of holes through it.

osteochondromatosis formation of multiple loose cartilaginous bodies within joints.

osteoclasis fracturing a bone surgically by means of an osteoclast.

osteogenesis imperfecta (fragilitas osseum, brittle bones) congenital or inherited disease in which calcium content and size of bones is far below normal; numerous fractures usually result from even mildest types of trauma; represent a difficult nursing problem on this account; healing of fractures normal; dwarfism common; eyes have peculiar bluish discoloration of sclera; condition has a tendency to disappear after puberty but is distinctly hereditary in character; prevention of deformities and later correction of deformities are orthopedic problems.

osteomalacia deficiency disease of bone in which decalcification takes place and bones may collapse; characterized by heart-shaped pelvic ring.

osteopetrosis (marble bones) thickening of bone cortex throughout bones of body including the pelvis, vertebrae, and skull; blindness frequently associated with the disease.

osteopoikilosis (spotted bones) a rare condition in which there is scattered spotting in ends of long bones usually discovered accidentally by roentgenography; usually no symptoms.

osteoporosis decalcification of the bone.

osteosclerosis group of diseases characterized by abnormal increase in calcium content of bone as shown in roentgenograms; thickening of cortex and narrowing of medullary canal; cause unknown.

osteotomy cutting of bone.

plantar wart ordinary wart that occurs on weight-bearing surface of foot and is usually extremely painful on pressure.

pneumococcus arthritis usually follows pneumonia in about 2 weeks with an active and painful joint infection; pus formation; poor prognosis held for joint; treatment by drainage, splinting, and the administration of sulfonamides.

polydactylism excessive number of fingers or toes.

podagra gouty inflammation of great toe.

Raynaud's disease vasomotor constrictor disturbance that may affect upper or lower extremities or both.

renal rickets dwarfism; rare disease of childhood in which there is replacement of red bone marrow by fat; seen in combination with chronic interstitial nephritis.

Schüller-Christian disease (xanthomatosis) childhood disease characterized by deposit of fat in bone as result of disturbed fat metabolism; roentgenographic findings of multiple cystic areas characteristic.

scorbutus scurvy.

scurvy caused by dietary deficiency of vitamin C (antiscorbutic vitamin); characterized by subperiosteal and submucous hemorrhages.

sequestrum usually refers to dead bone that acts as medius for continuing drainage, as in osteomyelitis.

spasmodic wryneck characterized by jerking motions of head and neck as a result of chronic nerve irritation; treatment by long immobilization in plaster cast that includes head, shoulders, and chest.

spondylitis inflammation of vertebra.

Still's disease generalized rheumatoid arthritis in children.

subluxation incomplete dislocation.

synostosis when two contiguous bones become united as variant from normal; congenital synostosis of the radius and ulna is example; trauma can be productive of synostosis.

synovitis inflammation of the synovial membrane lining joint capsule.

talipes refers to ankle.

tenodesis securing tendon to bone.

tenotomy cutting of tendon.

tuberculous dactylitis tuberculous infection of bones of fingers and toes; develops in early childhood; areas of destruction in phalanges and metacarpals, usually accompanied by pus formation and bone sequestration; responds to conservative treatment with rest and sunshine.

typhoid spine typhoid bacillus infection of vertebra coincidental with typhoid fever; characterized by extreme pain in back and extremities and elevation of temperature; roentgenograms show localized destruction and proliferation of bone in low dorsal or lumbar region; treatment usually by immobilization in plaster casts; recovery usually takes place, but there may be permanent but localized stiffness.

Index

X